AF333503

Molecular Neurosurgery With Targeted Toxins

MOLECULAR NEUROSURGERY WITH TARGETED TOXINS

Edited by

RONALD G. WILEY, MD, PhD

*Departments of Neurology and Pharmacology,
Vanderbilt University School of Medicine*
and
*Neurology Service, Veterans Affairs Tennessee Valley Healthcare System,
Nashville, TN*

and

DOUGLAS A. LAPPI, PhD

Advanced Targeting Systems, San Diego, CA

HUMANA PRESS ✳ TOTOWA, NEW JERSEY

PREFACE

The use of targeted cytotoxins in experimental neurobiology is a new field. This strategy involves producing highly selective neural lesions by targeting a cytotoxin into specific neurons based on their binding to surface membrane targets, such as neurotransmitter or growth factor receptors, and so on. The goal is to produce lesions of unprecedented selectivity to match the staggering complexity of the organization of the nervous system. Indeed, a considerable body of evidence exists that the expression of surface membrane molecules correlates with the function of specific types of neurons.

Molecular Neurosurgery With Targeted Toxins seeks to provide a selected collection of examples of this approach that have been implemented with great success. Included are introductory considerations and background on the toxins, followed by five chapters reviewing the use of the immunotoxin 192 IgG-saporin to lesion the cholinergic basal forebrain. This approach has been highly successful, and as pointed out by the authors, has provided a valuable animal model of Alzheimer's disease. However, it is hardly the only application of targeted toxins in neuroscience. Subsequent chapters include reviews of some of the varied uses of another immunotoxin, anti-DBH-saporin, which is used to make remarkably selective lesions of catecholaminergic neurons, and a chapter on hypocretin–saporin that can be used to produce narcoleptic animals. A variety of other saporin conjugates, such as neuropeptide–saporin conjugates, are proving valuable in pain research; these are reviewed in two chapters, followed by a chapter on the novel application of cholera toxin B chain-saporin to produce a model of CNS demyelination.

The chapter authors were asked to provide both overview perspectives and, in some cases, more practical details to enable the reader to appreciate exactly what is involved in using these agents. We, the editors, have been intimately involved in the development of the agents discussed in this volume and present this body of information as an introduction to those who would use this approach in their own experiments.

Ronald G. Wiley, MD, PhD
Douglas A. Lappi, PhD

CONTENTS

CONTRIBUTORS

HARRY F. BAKER • *Department of Experimental Psychology, School of Veterinary Medicine, Cambridge, UK*

THOMAS G. BEACH • *Civin Laboratory for Neuropathology, Sun Health Research Institute, Sun City, AZ*

CARLOS BLANCO-CENTURION • *Department of Neurology, Harvard Medical School and Veterans Administration Medical Center, West Roxbury, MA*

JOHN P. BRUNO • *Department of Psychology, Ohio State University, Columbus, OH*

KISHOR BUGARITH • *Programs in Neuroscience, Washington State University, Pullman, WA*

FRANK DESARNAUD • *Department of Neurology, Harvard Medical School and Veterans Administration Medical Center, West Roxbury, MA*

THU T. DINH • *Programs in Neuroscience, Washington State University, Pullman, WA*

R. A. DURHAM • *Pfizer Pharmaceuticals, Ann Arbor, MI*

M. R. EMMERLING • *Pfizer Pharmaceuticals, Ann Arbor, MI*

A. FISHER • *Israel Institute for Biological Research, New Ziona, Israel*

DMITRY GERASHCHENKO • *Department of Neurology, Harvard Medical School and Veterans Administration Medical Center, West Roxbury, MA*

PATRICE G. GUYENET • *Department of Pharmacology, University of Virginia, Charlottesville, VA*

CHRISTOPHER N. HONDA • *Department of Neuroscience, University of Minnesota, Minneapolis, MN*

W. G. HONER • *Department of Psychiatry, University of British Columbia, Vancouver, Canada*

LUC JASMIN • *Departments of Anatomy and the W. M. Keck Foundation Centre for Integrative Neuroscience and Neurological Surgery, University of California, San Francisco, CA*

KANWARJIT KELLEY • *Departments of Anatomy and the W. M. Keck Foundation Centre for Integrative Neuroscience and Neurological Surgery, University of California, San Francisco, CA*

DOUGLAS A. LAPPI • *President and Chief Scientific Officer, Advanced Targeting Systems, San Diego, CA*

K. J. LAYNE • *Civin Laboratory for Neuropathology, Sun Health Research Institute, Sun City, AZ*

ERIC MURILLO-RODRIGUEZ • *Department of Neurology, Harvard Medical School and Veterans Administration Medical Center, West Roxbury, MA*

A. J. Newell • *Civin Laboratory for Neuropathology, Sun Health Research Institute, Sun City, AZ*

Peter T. Ohara • *Departments of Anatomy and the W. M. Keck Foundation Centre for Integrative Neuroscience and Neurological Surgery, University of California, San Francisco, CA*

M. E. Poston • *Civin Laboratory for Neuropathology, Sun Health Research Institute, Sun City, AZ*

P. E. Potter • *Department of Pharmacology, Midwestern University, Glendale, AZ*

P. K. Rauschkolb • *Department of Pharmacology, Midwestern University, Glendale, AZ*

Rosalind M. Ridley • *Department of Experimental Psychology, School of Veterinary Medicine, Cambridge, UK*

Sue Ritter • *Programs in Neuroscience, Washington State University, Pullman, WA*

A. E. Roher • *Longtine Center for Molecular Biology, Sun Health Research Institute, Sun City, AZ*

Dawna M. Salter • *Programs in Neuroscience, University of Southern California, Los Angeles, CA*

Martin Sarter • *Department of Psychology, University of Michigan, Ann Arbor, MI*

K. Sawada • *Department of Psychiatry, University of British Columbia, Vancouver, Canada*

Reinhard Schliebs • *Deparment of Neurochemistry, University of Leipzig, Paul Flechsig Institute for Brain Research, Leipzig, Germany*

Ann M. Schreihofer, PhD • *Department of Physiology, Medical College of Georgia, Augusta, GA*

S. Scott • *Civin Laboratory for Neuropathology, Sun Health Research Institute, Sun City, AZ*

Priyattam J. Shiromani, PhD • *Department of Neurology, Harvard Medical School and Veterans Administration Medical Center, West Roxbury, MA*

Fiorenzo Stirpe, MD • *Dipartimento di Patologia Sperimentale, Universita di Bologna, Bologna, Italy*

Ruth L. Stornetta, PhD • *Department of Pharmacology, University of Virginia, Charlottesville, VA*

L. I. Sue • *Sun Health Research Institute, Sun City, AZ*

Lucy Vulchanova • *Deparment of Veterinary PathoBiology, University of Minnesota, St. Paul, MN*

Jerene J. Waite • *University of California, San Diego, CA, Veteran's Medical Research Foundation, San Diego, CA*

D. G. Walker • *Laboratory for Neuroinflammation, Sun Health Research Institute, Sun City, AZ*
S. D. Webster • *Department of Molecular Biology and Biochemistry, University of California, Irvine, CA*
Ronald G. Wiley • *Departments of Neurology and Pharmacology, Vanderbilt University School of Medicine and Neurology Service, Veterans Affairs Tennessee Valley Healthcare System, Nashville, TN*

1

Introduction to Molecular Neurosurgery

Ronald G. Wiley and Douglas A. Lappi

The term *molecular neurosurgery* has been applied to several different experimental strategies, including a variety of genetic manipulations. For the purposes of this book, the term is used to refer to the use of targeted cytotoxins to produce highly selective neural lesions. Used in this sense, the term is relevant to both experimental and potential clinical applications. The body of work addressed in this volume grew out of initial experiments in the laboratory of Donald J. Reis in 1980–1981. The initial experimental challenge was how to selectively destroy baroreceptor afferents that make up a small portion of the vagus and glossopharyngeal nerves. The strategy chosen was to develop a technique using toxin retrogradely transported from an application site on the peripheral baroreceptor nerves in the neck. First attempts used low-molecular-weight cytotoxic drugs, such as doxorubicin, and were unsuccessful. Reasoning that the initial lack of success reflected inadequate delivery of toxin to the cell bodies, a plan was developed to attach these drugs to a well-transported agent, such as wheat germ agglutinin, which at the time was introduced as a highly effective anatomical tracer *(1)*. However, a simpler option seemed attractive. If a lectin such as wheat germ agglutinin was well transported, then perhaps a toxic lectin such as ricin or abrin would work. In retrospect, Harper and colleagues *(2)* had previously shown evidence for retrograde axonal transport of ricin, but this publication was discovered only after the initial suicide transport experiments applied ricin to the vagus nerve *(3)*.

This suicide transport technique had obvious limitations, but drawing on work done in the cancer field, the toxic lectins eventually led to immunotoxins and most recently neuropeptide-toxin conjugates. Success in this transition to highly selective lesioning agents rests heavily on the work

From: *Molecular Neurosurgery With Targeted Toxins*
Edited by: R. G. Wiley and D. A. Lappi © Humana Press Inc., Totowa, NJ

of Fiorenzo Stirpe. Stirpe did extensive work on ribosome-inactivating proteins, including saporin, the agent of choice for making antineuronal immunotoxins and neuropeptide-toxin conjugates. In Chapter 2, he reviews some of this extensive body of work.

Chapters 3–5 present three reviews of work using the immunotoxin 192 immunoglobulin G (IgG)-saporin (192 IgG-sap). This agent was the second antineuronal immunotoxin developed. The first, OX-7-saporin (OX-7-sap), was made by Stirpe and colleagues for studies in cancer research, and subsequently shown to be an effective suicide transport agent *(4)*. Based on success using OX-7-sap as a suicide transport agent, an antineuronal immunotoxin using a monoclonal antibody (192 IgG) to the low-affinity neurotrophin receptor (p75^{NTR}) was made next *(5)*. Widespread use has been made of 192 IgG-sap for selective lesions of the cholinergic basal forebrain (CBF) neurons in rats.

Chapters 3–5 present the accumulated experience of three of the most active groups using 192 IgG-sap to lesion the CBF, each for different experimental purposes. Chapter 3 covers the behavioral and neurochemical experiments of Waite and colleagues in rats with selective lesions of the CBF. Their experience illustrates some of the practical and theoretical challenges inherent in attempts to analyze behavior using selective neural lesions. Chapter 4 is a comprehensive review of the prolific contributions of Schliebs and colleagues that have focused on neurochemical issues in rats treated with intracerebroventricular (icv) 192 IgG-sap. Chapter 5 presents the use of 192 IgG-sap as a selective suicide transport agent to make anatomically restricted cortical cholinergic denervations rather than the typical strategy of destroying the entire CBF. In this application, 192 IgG-sap is used to retrogradely kill CBF neurons.

A limiting feature of 192 IgG-sap has been that it only works in rats. This drawback reflects the specificity of the 192 IgG monoclonal antibody for rat p75^{NTR} *(6)*. Chapter 6 shows that substituting the ME20.4 monoclonal antibody made against human p75^{NTR} results in an effective agent that has made possible a particularly revealing series of behavioral studies in primates. Chapter 7 describes use of ME20.4-saporin in rabbits, in which a provocative series of experiments suggests a relationship between cholinergic denervation and β-amyloid deposition in the cortex. Together, Chapters 3–7 provide an overview of past and present experiments using saporin-containing immunotoxins to lesion the CBF selectively. This line of investigation remains of interest in understanding Alzheimer's disease as well as the behavioral functions of the CBF.

Chapter 8 describes a series of neuroendocrine studies by Ritter and colleagues using the immunotoxin antidopamine β-hydroxylase-saporin (anti-DβH-sap). This chapter illustrates the usefulness of this approach for producing selective lesions of central noradrenergic neurons. Chapter 9 provides a critical description of the use of anti-DβH-sap in brainstem autonomic circuits including interesting comparison of lesions made by retrogradely transported anti-DβH-sap vs local application of anti-DβH-sap to target cell bodies.

Chapters 10 and 11 shift focus to the relatively new group of targeted toxins made of neuropeptides conjugated to saporin. Chapter 10 provides a review of the various agents developed so far and some applications of these agents to specific experimental questions, particularly pain. Chapter 11 goes into detail about the use of hypocretin-2/orexin B-saporin conjugate in studies on narcolepsy.

Chapters 12 and 13 involve studies with two new suicide transport agents. In Chapter 12, a conjugate of saporin to the lectin IB4 (isolectin B4 from *Griffonia simplicfolia*), which selectively destroys nonpeptidergic primary nociceptive sensory neurons that respond to glial cell line-derived neurotrophic factor (GDNF). The tracer toxin cholera toxin B subunit-saporin (CTB-sap) is the subject of Chapter 13, which describes the unusual use of this toxin to produce demyelination in the spinal cord. Although CTB-sap also is highly effective as a suicide transport agent *(7)*, Chapter 13 describes creative use of this toxin to destroy central nervous system oligodendroglia.

Within a reasonable size volume, it is not possible to cover all of the antineuronal cytotoxins that have been reported or the creative use of these agents in a variety of experimental settings. Table 1 provides a listing of agents currently in use. Among immunotoxins not included in the present volume are the recently reported antidopamine transporter (anti-DAT-sap) *(8)* and antiserotonin transporter (anti-SERT-sap) *(9)* immunotoxins with saporin. The development of neuropeptide-toxin conjugates is moving rapidly, including dermorphin–saporin (derm–sap) *(10)* and corticotrophin-releasing factor-saporin (CRF-sap) *(11)*. Undoubtedly, new antineuronal immunotoxins and neuropeptide-toxin conjugates will be forthcoming for experimental and possibly therapeutic use.

The present volume offers examples of some of the most-used agents that are hoped to prove valuable to current investigators and to those who would adopt this strategy as part of their experimental armamentarium. A previous volume covered more details of the early development of suicide transport and immunolesioning agents *(12)*.

Table 1
Currently Available Molecular Neurosurgery Agents

	Molecular targets	Neural targets
Suicide transport agent		
Ricin/abrin	–N-Acetyl-D-galactosamine	Peripheral sensory and motor
Modeccin/volkensin	–Gal or –GalNAc (?)	Central and peripheral
Cholera B-saporin	GM1 ganglioside	Central and peripheral
IB4-saporin	–α-D-galactose	Ret+ peripheral sensory
OX7-saporin	Thy 1	All neurons
Immunolesioning agent		
192 IgG-sap/ME20.4-sap	p75[NTR]	CBF, primary sensory, sympathetic postganglionic
Anti-DβH-saporin	Dopamine β-hydroxylase	Adrenergic and noradrenergic
Anti-DAT-saporin	Dopamine transporter	Midbrain dopaminergic
Anti-SERT-saporin	Serotonin transporter	Serotonergic (brainstem)
Neuropeptide–toxin conjugate		
Substance P-saporin	Substance P receptor (NK-1R)	NK-1R expressing (central nervous system)
Dermorphin-saporin	Mu opiate receptor (MOR)	MOR expressing
Hypocretin-2/orexin-B-sap	Orexin-2 receptor (OX2R)	OX2R expressing
Corticotrophin-releasing factor-saporin	CRF1 receptor	CRF1 expressing
Acetylated LDL-saporin	LDL receptor	Microglia/macrophages

NK-1R, neurokinin-1 receptor; LDL, low-density lipoprotein; Gal, galictose; Qa1 NAc, *N*-acetylgalactosamine.

A number of caveats about the practical use of antineuronal targeted toxins have arisen as experience has increased. The first is the requirement for pilot experiments to determine optimal dose and effectiveness in any given experimental application. This concern is particularly important when considering that the selective agents (immunotoxins, neuropeptide–toxin conjugates) are relatively, but not absolutely, selective. The ideal dose should be just enough to make the desired lesion, but no more. At high local concentrations, nonspecific uptake (bulk fluid-phase endocytosis) can result in cells internalizing toxic amounts of saporin. Intraparenchymal injections seem more demanding in this regard than injecting toxin into the cerebrospinal fluid. One approach to deliver sufficient toxin to a large structure deep within the brain is to use the slow, low-concentration/high-volume infusion techniques developed by Oldfield and coworkers *(13–15)*; these prevent high local toxin concentrations and distribute toxin by bulk fluid flow through the tissue rather than by diffusion.

A second caveat is the importance of postmortem anatomic evaluation of the lesions whenever possible. There are at least two reasons for doing this. First, the lesions obtained can vary among animals even using the most consistent toxin dose and injection techniques. Second, correlations between extent of toxin-induced cell loss and changes in behavior (or neurochemical parameters) are a powerful addition to the analysis of such data. Although often overlooked, such correlations can be used to test hypotheses and to enhance power of statistical analyses.

Similarly, time course studies are often revealing. As might be expected, selective removal of one particular type of neuron may promote compensatory changes in remaining neurons of the same type (*see* Chapter 3) or plastic adaptation of other types of neurons *(16)*. In some instances, the primary effect of the lesion completely disappears within a few weeks (ref. *17* and Wiley, Kline, and Vierck, 2004, unpublished). A particularly striking example is rewiring that occurs in the oculomotor system after selective destruction of medial rectus motor neurons by retrogradely transported ricin *(18–20)*. Time course studies permit assessment of the primary effect of destroying the target neurons and of the secondary remodeling/adaptations. Without time course studies, erroneous conclusions may be drawn about the function of the targeted neurons.

Last, there is the challenging issue of what constitutes the appropriate control conditions/treatments. Several approaches have been used:

1. Inject control animals with vehicle, usually saline.
2. Inject control animals with unconjugated saporin in comparable doses to the targeted toxin.

3. Inject targeted toxin pretreated with dithiothreitol to reduce the disulfide bond holding saporin to the targeting vector.
4. Inject an irrelevant saporin conjugate that does not target any neurons *per se*.
5. Inject a second saporin conjugate that targets different neurons.
6. Pretreat animals with antagonist of the targeted receptor to prevent binding of targeting vector.

Each approach has some relevance, but no one control condition/injection is likely to be fully adequate. The last alternative is particularly attractive, but not available for all of the current targeted toxins.

The experiments described in the present volume all involve the introduction of biologically active protein into specific cells. Proof of internalization of the protein responsible for the biological activity (saporin) is demonstrated by a simple readout, cell death. Introduction of therapeutic and biologically active molecules into nervous system cells will probably have important clinical application. This volume clearly shows that a foreign substance can be delivered into specific cell types based on a common property, markers on the cell surface.

As the present volume attests, the use of cell surface markers to define populations of neurons has already found many applications. This likely represents an evolutionary trend in the identification/description of nervous system organization fostered by molecular neurosurgery, which makes possible new ways to demonstrate neuronal function and systems neurobiology. In this capacity, molecular neurosurgery provides a bridge from the intensely focused molecular biology of individual neurons to the macroscopic functions of neural systems such as behavior. The development of molecular neurosurgery has been dependent on the availability of methods and reagents for identifying or "seeing" cell surface markers. At present, there are limited targeting reagents in use (i.e., lectins, antibodies, receptor ligands, etc.). There are many potential reagents waiting to be used to make targeted toxins, and with time, many new ones will emerge. The future is bright and filled with opportunity for expanded use of targeted toxins, molecular neurosurgery, to characterize the complexities of nervous system organization and potentially treat neurological disorders.

As experience accumulates and additional antineuronal toxins become available, new strategies and approaches will undoubtedly develop. The present volume is offered to help those who would use these approaches as well as those wishing to assess the validity of data collected using these agents. It is hoped these examples will facilitate and encourage others to consider the usefulness of these powerful techniques in their own research.

REFERENCES

1. Mesulam M-M, ed. *Tracing Neural Connections With Horseradish Peroxidase.* New York: Wiley; 1982.
2. Harper CG, Gonatas JO, Mizutani T, Gonatas NK. Retrograde transport and effects of toxic ricin in the autonomic nervous system. Lab Invest 1980;42:396–404.
3. Wiley RG, Blessing WW, Reis DJ. Suicide transport: destruction of neurons by retrograde transport of ricin, abrin, and modeccin. Science 1982;216:889–890.
4. Wiley RG, Stirpe F, Thorpe P, Oeltmann TN. Neuronotoxic effects of monoclonal anti-Thy 1 antibody (OX7) coupled to the ribosome inactivating protein, saporin, as studied by suicide transport experiments in the rat. Brain Res 1989;505:44–54.
5. Wiley RG, Oeltmann TN, Lappi DA. Immunolesioning: selective destruction of neurons using immunotoxin to rat NGF receptor. Brain Res 1991;562:149–153.
6. Chandler CE, Parsons LM, Hosang M, Shooter EM. A monoclonal antibody modulates the interaction of nerve growth factor with PC12 cells. J Biol Chem 1984;259:6882–6889.
7. Llewellyn-Smith IJ, Martin CL, Arnolda LF, Minson JB. Retrogradely transported CTB-saporin kills sympathetic preganglionic neurons. NeuroReport 1999;10:307–312.
8. Wiley RG, Harrison MB, Levey AI, Lappi DA. Destruction of midbrain dopaminergic neurons by using immunotoxin to dopamine transporter. Cell Mol Neurobiol 2003;23:839–850.
9. Nattie EE, Li A, Richerson GB, Lappi DA. Medullary serotonergic neurons and adjacent neurons that express neurokinin-1 receptors are both involved in chemoreception in vivo. J Physiol 2004; 556:235–253.
10. Porreca F, Burgess SE, Gardell LR, et al. Inhibition of neuropathic pain by selective ablation of brainstem medullary cells expressing the μ-opioid receptor. J Neurosci 2001;21:5281–5288.
11. Maciejewski-Lenoir D, Heinrichs SC, Liu XJ, et al. Selective impairment of corticotropin-releasing factor1 (CRF1) receptor-mediated function using CRF coupled to saporin. Endocrinology 2000;141:498–504.
12. Wiley RG, Lappi DA. *Suicide Transport and Immunolesioning.* Austin, TX: Landes Co. Molecular Biology Intelligence Unit; 1994.
13. Wood JD, Lonser RR, Gogate N, Morrison PF, Oldfield EH. Convective delivery of macromolecules into the naive and traumatized spinal cords of rats. J Neurosurg 1999;90(Suppl 1):115–120.
14. Lieberman DM, Laske DW, Morrison PF, Bankiewicz KS, Oldfield EH. Convection-enhanced distribution of large molecules in gray matter during interstitial drug infusion. J Neurosurg 1995;826:1021–1029.
15. Morrison PF, Laske DW, Bobo H, Oldfield EH, Dedrick RL. High-flow microinfusion: tissue penetration and pharmacodynamics. Am J Physiol 1994;266(1 pt 2):R292–R305.

16. Harrison MB, Roberts RC, Wiley RG. A selective lesion of striatonigral neurons decreases presynaptic binding of [3H]hemicholinium-3 to striatal interneurons. Brain Res 1993;630:169–177.
17. Vulchanova L, Olson TH, Stone LS, Riedl MS, Elde R, Honda CN. Cytotoxic targeting of isolectin IB4-binding sensory neurons. Neuroscience 2001;108:143–155.
18. de la Cruz RR, Pastor AM, Delgado-Garcia JM. Influence of the postsynaptic target on the functional properties of neurons in the adult mammalian central nervous system. Rev Neurosci 1996;7:115–149.
19. de la Cruz RR, Pastor AM, Delgado-Garcia JM. Long-term effects of selective target removal on brainstem premotor neurons in the adult cat. Eur J Neurosci 1993;5:232–239.
20. de la Cruz RR, Baker R, Delgado-Garcia JM. Response of adult cat abducens internuclear interneurons to selective removal of their target motoneurons. Exp Brain Res 1991;84:167–172.

2

Ribosome-Inactivating Proteins

Fiorenzo Stirpe

INTRODUCTION

The designation of *ribosome-inactivating proteins* (RIPs; reviews in refs. *1–4*) has been applied to plant proteins that enzymatically damage ribosomes in a catalytic manner, thus inhibiting protein synthesis (Table 1). The first identified RIPs were two potent toxins, known for more than a century: ricin, from the seeds of *Ricinus communis*, and abrin, from the seeds of *Abrus precatorius*.

Subsequently, many more RIPs were identified; they can be divided into type 1 RIPs, single-chain proteins of approx 30 kDa, and type 2 RIPs, consisting of two peptide chains, an A chain of about 30 kDa with enzymatic activity, linked to a B chain of about 35 kDa with lectin activity, capable of binding to oligosaccharides containing galactose. A category of type 3 RIPs has been proposed for a maize b-32 RIP, which is synthesized as a proenzyme and is activated after the removal of a short internal peptide segment leaves two segments of 16.5 and 8.5 kDa *(5)*, and for JIP60, an RIP from barley in which a segment similar to type 1 RIP is combined with another segment of similar size but no known function *(6)*. It seems unjustified to define a new class of proteins on the basis of two disparate cases, and for the time being, it seems preferable to consider these two proteins as peculiar type 1 RIPs. A schematic representation of RIP structure is shown in Fig. 1.

Type 2 RIPs can bind to galactose residues on cell membranes, thus agglutinating the cells. Furthermore, this binding leads to entry of the molecule into the cells. Ricin, which contains mannose, also is taken up by Kupffer cells and other macrophages via mannose receptors *(7–9)*. The entry into cells and the intracellular fate of type 2 RIPs and of ricin A chain has been well studied. It has been found that they are transported to the Golgi

From: *Molecular Neurosurgery With Targeted Toxins*
Edited by: R. G. Wiley and D. A. Lappi © Humana Press Inc., Totowa, NJ

Table 1
Purified Ribosome-Inactivating Proteins

Family, genus, species, and plant tissues	Name
Type 1 ribosome-inactivating proteins	
Angiospermae	
Aizoaceae	
Mesembryanthemum crystallinum	
cDNA	
Amarantaceae	
Amaranthus viridis	
Leaves	Amaranthin
Asparagaceae	
Asparagus officinalis	
Seeds	Asparins
Basellaceae	
Basella rubra	
Seeds	
Caprifoliaceae	
Sambucus ebulus	
Leaves	Ebulitins
Sambucus nigra	
Bark	Nigritin
Caryophyllaceae	
Agrostemma githago	
Seeds	Agrostins
Dianthus barbatus	
Leaves	Dianthin 29
Dianthus caryophyllus	
Leaves	Dianthins
Dianthus sinensis	
Leaves	
Gypsophila elegans	
Leaves	Gypsophilin
Lychnis chalcedonica	
Seeds	Lychnin
Petrocoptis glaucifolia	
Whole plant	Petroglaucin
Petrocoptis grandiflora	
Whole plant	Petrograndin
Saponaria ocymoides	
Seeds	Ocymoidin

(continued on next page)

Saponaria officinalis
Leaves, roots, seeds — Saporins
Stellaria aquatica
Leaves — Stellarin
Vaccaria pyramidata
Seeds
Chenopodiaceae
β *vulgaris*
Seedling cDNA — Betavulgin
Spinacia oleracea — *Spinacia oleracea* protein
leaves — (SOP)
Cucurbitaceae
Bryonia dioica
Leaves, roots — Bryodins
Citrullus colocynthis
Seeds — Colocins
Cucurbita moschata
Sarcocarp — Cucurmosin
Cucurbita pepo
Sarcocoarp — Pepopcin
Luffa acutangola
Seeds — Luffaculin
Luffa cylindrica
Seeds — Luffins
Marah oreganus
Seeds — MOR
Momordica balsamina
Seeds — Momordin II
Momordica charantia
Seeds — Momordins
Momordica cochinchinensis
Seeds — Momorcochin
Sechium edule
Seeds — Sechiumin
Trichosanthes sp. Bac Kan 8-98 — Trichobakin
Trichosanthes anguina
Seeds — Trichoanguin
Trichosanthes cucumeroides
Tubers — β-Trichosanthin
Trichosanthes kirilowii
Roots, seeds — Trichosanthins, trichokirin,
Trichosanthins antiviral proteins
(TAP 29)

(continued on next page)

Tubers

Euphorbiaceae
Gelonium multiflorum
Seeds — Gelonin
Hura crepitans
Latex — *H. crepitans* RIP
Manihot palmata
Seeds — Mapalmin
Manihot utilissima
Seeds — Manutins
Iridaceae
Iris hollandica
Bulbs — Iris RIPs (IRIPs)
Lamiaceae
Clerodendron aculeatum
Leaves cDNA
Lauraceae
Cinnamomum camphora
Seeds — Camphorin
Liliaceae
Asparagus officinalis
Seeds — Asparins
Muscari armeniacum
Bulbs — Musarmins
Yucca recurvifolia — YLP
leaves
Nyctaginaceae
Bougainvillea spectabilis — Bouganin
Leaves
Mirabilis expansa
Roots, cell cultures — ME_1
Mirabilis jalapa
Seeds, roots, tissue culture — Mirabilis antiviral protein (MAP)
Phytolaccaceae
Phytolacca americana
Leaves, seeds, tissue culture, roots — Pokeweed antiviral protein (PAP)
Phytolacca dioica
Seeds, leaves — *Phytolacca dioica* RIPs
Phytolacca dodecandra
Leaves, tissue culture — Dodecandrins
Phytolacca insularis
Leaves, cDNA — Insularin (Phytolacca insularis protein [PIP])

Poaceae

Trichomaglin

(continued on next page)

Hordeum vulgare
Seeds   Barley RIP
Secale cereale
Seeds   *Secale cereale* RIP
Triticum aestivum
Germ, seeds   Tritins
Zea mays
Seeds   Maize RIP
Sambucaceae
Sambucus ebulus
Leaves   Ebulitin
Cryptogamia
Laminaria japonica
Leaves   Lamjapin
Mushrooms*a*
Volvariella volvacea   *V. volvacea* RIP
Fruiting bodies

Type 2 ribosome-inactivating proteins
Toxic ribosome-inactivating proteins
Euphorbiaceae
Ricinus communis
Seeds   Ricins, *Ricinus* agglutinin
Fabaceae
Abrus precatorius
Seeds   Abrins
Passifloraceae
Adenia digitata
Roots   Modeccins
Adenia volkensii
Roots   Volkensin
Viscaceae
Phoradendron californicum
Leaves   *P. californicum* lectin
Viscum album
Leaves   Mistletoe lectin I, viscumin
Nontoxic ribosome-inactivating proteins
Cucurbitaceae
Momordica charantia
Seeds   *M. charantia* lectin
Euphorbiaceae
Ricinus communis   *R. communis* agglutinin
Iridaceae
Iris hollandica
Bulbs   IRA

(continued on next page)

Lauraceae	
Cinnamomum camphora	
Seeds	Cinnamomin
Cinnamomum porrectum	
Seeds	Porrectin
Liliaceae	
Polygonatum multiflorum	
Leaves	PM RIP
Ranunculaceae	
Eranthis hyemalis	
Bulbs	EHL
Sambucaceae	
Sambucus ebulus	
Leaves	Ebulin 1

[a]The isolation of RIPs from other mushrooms (*Boletus affinis*, *Flammulina velutipes*, *Hypsizigus marmoreus*, *Lentinus edodes*, *Lyophyllum shimeji*, and *Pleurotus tuber-regium*) has been reported. However, these proteins do not appear to meet the stringent criteria required to identify RIPs.

and endoplasmic reticulum and subsequently translocate to the cytoplasm. The matter has been exhaustively reviewed *(10–12)* and is not dealt with here. Once inside the cytoplasm, the A chains, through their enzymatic activity, cause irreversible damage to ribosomes and possibly other structures, eventually killing the cell (*see* Fig. 2). However, some type 2 RIPs have been identified with a structure very similar to that of the toxins, but with much less toxicity.

Type 1 RIPs, devoid of a binding chain, are internalized much less efficiently by cells, mainly by fluid phase pinocytosis *(13)* or through the α2-macroglobulin receptor *(14)*, and consequently have relatively low toxicity. However, they can be rendered as toxic as type 2 RIPs if they can enter, or are forced into, cells. This occurs when they are included in liposomes *(15)*; in erythrocyte ghosts that can be fused with cells *(16)*; in viral envelopes *(17)*; when cells are infected by viruses *(18)*; when RIPs are linked to proteins capable of binding to cells, such as lectins, antibodies, growth factors, and cytokines; and when cells are permeabilized with complement *(19)*. Entry of RIPs into cells can be facilitated also by electrical pulses *(20)*, shock waves *(21,22)*, or photochemical internalization *(23)*. A summary of the properties of types 1 and 2 RIPs is given in Table 2.

DISTRIBUTION IN NATURE

Ribosome-inactivating proteins are widely present in the plant kingdom, with type 1 found more frequently. Most RIPs were isolated from plants

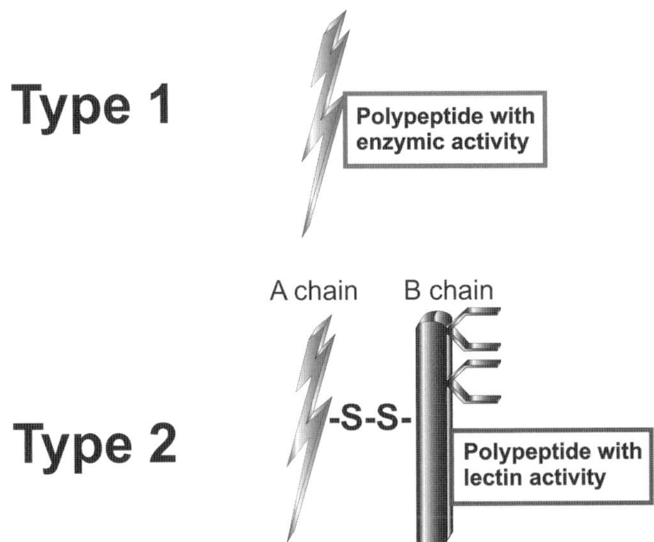

Fig. 1. Schematic representation of the structure of type 1 and 2 ribosome-inactivating proteins (RIPs). The prototypical type 1 RIP is saporin that consists only of the enzymatic polypeptide without any binding capacity. The prototype for type 2 RIPs is ricin, which consists of a binding polypeptide (B chain) disulfide connected to the enzymatically active A chain. Both saporin and ricin A chain have been artificially attached to binding moieties to produce toxins with specific targeting properties determined by the binding moiety. Examples include substance P-saporin, which targets cells expressing the neurokinin-1 receptor, and OX7-ricin A chain, which targets cells expressing Thy 1.

belonging to the Angiospermae, but at least one was found also in a mushroom (*Volvariella volvacea*; *24*) and one in an alga (*Laminaria japonica*; *25*). They can be detected in virtually all tissues examined (roots, stems, leaves, flowers, fruits, seeds, latex, cultured cells), sometimes in different forms in the same tissue. Others are more restricted in distribution; for instance, ricin is present in the seeds but not in other tissues of *Ricinus communis*, compared to the several forms of saporin, which are found in seeds, leaves, and roots of *Saponaria officinalis (26)*. A higher level of RIP has been found in stressed, senescent, or virally infected plant tissues *(27–29)*.

Many plant materials (more than 300 in our laboratory) were examined for the presence of RIPs, and type 1 RIPs appeared to be more frequent than type 2 and preferentially distributed among plants belonging to some families (e.g., *Caryophyllaceae, Cucurbitaceae, Euphorbiaceae*). It should be noted, however, that most screening studies were performed not to study the distribution of RIPs, but to find materials containing a high level of them.

ENZYMATIC MECHANISM OF ACTION OF RIPs ON 80 S RIBOSOMES

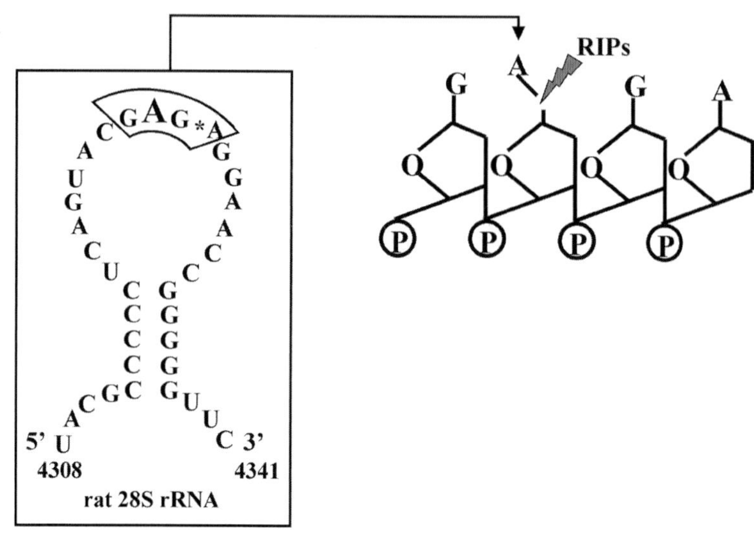

*α-Sarcin target

Fig. 2. Schematic representation of the biochemical action of ribosome-inactivating proteins (RIPs) such as ricin and saporin. The enzymatic activity is directed at removing an adenine within the α-sarcin site on the large (28S) ribosomal subunit, which results in failure of binding of elongation factor-2 and cessation of protein synthesis by the altered ribosome.

Consequently, plants belonging to families in which RIPs had been found were tested more frequently, and materials showing activity below a set threshold were excluded.

RIP activity was detected in some plants, but even when the presence of a RIP was excluded not all tissues were examined, an RIP could have been present at a very low concentration below detection level, and the search for these proteins was based on the effect of crude extracts on protein synthesis, generally using a rabbit reticulocyte lysate. RIPs acting on different ribosomes could have been missed. Thus, RIPs could be more widespread, even ubiquitous, in the plant kingdom. Furthermore, the bacterial Shiga and shigalike toxins are RIPs *(30)*, and an enzymatic activity similar to that of RIPs has been detected in animal cells and tissues *(31)*. Consequently, the issue of the distribution of RIPs in nature remains open.

Table 2
General Properties of Ribosome-Inactivating Proteins

	Type 1	Type 2	
Structure	One chain	Two chains	
		Toxic	Nontoxic
Molecular weight	26 kDa	60–65 kDa	56–58 kDa
Inhibition of protein synthesis		(IC_{50}, nM)	
Cell free	0.002–4.0	45–48	ND
		A chain 0–3.5	A chain 0.1–0.3
HeLa cells	140–33,000	0.0003–0.008	>200
Toxicity to mice (LD50, µg/kg)	950–40,000	0.7–80	>1600

MECHANISM OF ACTION

The first clue to the mechanism of action of RIPs came from studies on ricin. It was found that this toxin inhibits protein synthesis in cells and in cell-free extracts. This was because of irreversible damage to ribosomes, produced in a catalytic manner, suggestive of an enzymatic activity. This was studied in detail by Endo and colleagues, who found that ricin cleaves the glycosidic bond of a single adenine residue (A_{4324} in rat liver ribosomal ribonucleic acid [rRNA]) from 28S rRNA, thus removing the base from RNA *(32)*. This key residue is adjacent to the site of cleavage of rRNA by α-sarcin in a tetranucleotide $GA_{4324}GA$ of a highly conserved loop at the top of a stem, now termed the α-sarcin/ricin loop. This observation was extended to other RIPs, which were officially classified as rRNA *N*-glycosidases (rRNA *N*-glycohydrolases, EC 3.2.2.22).

It was found that some RIPs remove more than one adenine from ribosomes, and subsequently that all RIPs remove adenine from deoxyribonucleic acid (DNA) and some from other polynucleotides *(33,34)*. Consequently, the denomination of polynucleotide adenine glycosylase was proposed for these proteins *(31)*. This activity is variable from RIP to RIP and from one substrate to another. These new findings shed a different light on the mechanism of cytotoxicity and antiviral activity of RIPs, as is discussed in the section on antiviral activity. Hudak et al. *(35)* found that pokeweed antiviral protein (PAP) removes adenine from capped but not from uncapped BMV RNA and concluded that these proteins could inhibit protein synthesis by depurinating capped messenger RNA (mRNA). Presumably, whenever RIPs reach nucleic acids inside a cell, they would create unstable abasic sites liable to be cleaved.

A controversial matter is the lyase activity of RIPs reported by several investigators (reviewed in ref. *4*). In at least two laboratories, it was clearly shown that the nuclease activity of RIPs was caused by contamination by nucleases *(36,37)* and that the glycosylase is the only enzymatic activity of RIPs *(38)*.

TOXICITY AND CYTOTOXICITY

Toxicity to Animals

The first RIPs identified, ricin and abrin, are potent toxins, and when their structure became known, it was ascertained that their B chain with lectinic properties binds to galactosyl residues on the cell membrane. This allows and actually facilitates the entry of the toxin into cells, in which the A chain exerts its enzymatic activity, damaging ribosomes and inhibiting protein synthesis. These findings were extended and confirmed for other type 2 RIPs subsequently identified and led to the conclusions that:

1. Type 2 RIPs were toxins.
2. This was the mechanism through which type 2 RIPs exerted their toxic action.

These two concepts were accepted for several years, until new information was obtained both on the properties of RIPs and on the mechanism of their enzymatic activity.

The toxic RIPs include (besides ricin and abrin, known for more than a century) the more recently identified modeccin, volkensin, viscumin, and a *Phoradendron californicum* lectin. These toxic RIPs have a very similar structure, and still their median lethal doses (LD$_{50}$'s) are different, sometimes by two orders of magnitude, as in the case of RIPs from taxonomically related plants, such as modeccin and volkensin (both from Passifloraceae). Also, the LD$_{50}$ for different animal species may vary. The LD$_{50}$ of volkensin for rats is 20-fold lower than that for mice, and its value of 50–60 ng/kg makes volkensin the most potent known toxin from a plant *(39)*.

Different lesions result from the various toxins. Thus, only ricin affects primarily Kupffer cells *(7)*; modeccin *(40)* and volkensin (unpublished results from our laboratory) cause very severe necrotic changes in the liver of rats. Ricin poisoning also causes severe inflammation of intestinal and lymphoid organs and consistently stimulates the production of inflammatory cytokines by blood mononuclear cells *(41)*. In contrast, abrin did not affect liver and brought about necrosis of acinar pancreatic cells *(42)* and apoptotic changes in the intestine and lymphoid tissues of the rat *(43)*. No lesions that could account for death were observed in rats poisoned with viscumin or with doses of volkensin high enough to cause death within 6–8 h (unpublished observations from our laboratory). This, together with seizures observed just before death, suggests the possible involvement of damage to the nervous system. This is consistent with the following observations:

1. All toxic type 2 RIPs tested are retrogradely transported along peripheral nerves, although only modeccin and volkensin undergo a similar "suicide transport" if injected in the central nervous system (reviewed in refs. *44* and *45*).
2. Ricin injected outside the nerves into several tissues reaches the relevant autonomic ganglia (reviewed in ref. *1*).

Some lectins identified from *Sambucus* species, camphor tree and iris, have a structure very similar to that of ricin and related toxins in that they consist of an A chain with enzymatic activity and of a B chain with similar lectin properties, but they still have much lower cytotoxicity. The reasons for this difference are not known yet, although in a comparative study of ricin and nigrin, a nontoxic lectin, it was found that the two lectins enter equally well into cells, but nigrin undergoes more rapid degradation and excretion than ricin *(46)*.

The less-toxic type 1 RIPs were discovered more recently, and very few studies of their toxicity to animals are reported. The pathology of mice given lethal doses of various type 1 RIPs consisted of cell necrosis in the liver, kidney, and spleen *(47)*. Liver lesions induced by saporin were histologically very similar to those induced by ricin, although a difference was observed in the effects on liver xanthine oxidoreductase, which was converted from the dehydrogenase into the oxidase form in ricin-poisoned but not in saporin-poisoned rats and leaked from the liver into blood only in the latter animals *(48)*.

Cytotoxicity

At the cellular level, it was found that RIPs, either type 2 *(43,49)* or type 1 *(50,51)*, induce apoptosis and subsequently, or at higher doses, necrosis both in organs of poisoned animals *(43)* and in a variety of cultured cells *(52–56)*.

The mechanism through which ricin induces apoptosis has been studied. The involvement of various caspases, caspase-like and serine proteases *(54–56)*, and poly(ADP-ribose) [poly(adenosine 5'-diphosphate-ribose)] cleavage *(57)* was reported. It was suggested also *(56)* that protein synthesis inhibition was not the sole cause of ricin-induced apoptosis. Very early nuclear changes observed in cells poisoned by ricin or Shiga toxin appear to be independent of the inhibition of protein synthesis because they were not seen when a comparable inhibition of protein synthesis was induced by cycloheximide *(57)*. Changes in genomic DNA also were observed in cells exposed to saporin, and it was ascertained that both rRNA *N*-glycosidase and internucleosomal DNA fragmentation contribute to cytotoxicity *(58)*. This suggests that the effect of RIPs on both RNA and DNA may contribute to the pathogenesis of cell damage.

It is noteworthy that the toxicity of each RIP to different cells varies, with IC_{50}'s ranging over two orders of magnitude *(1)*, at least partly related to pinocytotic activity of the cells. Those with normally high pinocytotic/phagocytic activity (e.g., macrophages) are more highly sensitive to ricin *(8,9)*.

All RIPs are immunogenic. Ricin is a potent allergen and brings about formation of immunoglobulin E (IgE) against ricin itself and other antigens (reviewed in ref. *1*), and many type 1 RIPs were found to cause allergy (unpublished observations from our laboratory).

ANTIPARASITIC ACTIVITY

Antiviral Activity

It has been known since 1925 that a pokeweed leaf extract has antiviral activity against plant viruses *(59)*. After 50 yr, the antiviral factor was purified as PAP, and it was found that it inhibited protein synthesis *(60)* by inactivating ribosomes *(61)* and thus was the first purified RIP. Subsequently, it was found that all RIPs, either type 1 or 2, had antiviral activity against plant viruses *(62)*. Investigations were extended to animal viruses, and it was found that several type 1 RIPs inhibited replication of poliovirus, influenza virus, herpes simplex virus, and human immunodeficiency virus (HIV) (reviewed in refs. *63* and *64*).

These findings led to the investigation of possible practical applications. Attempts to treat patients infected with HIV were unsuccessful and actually caused mental *(65)* or neurological adverse reactions *(66,67)*.

More promising were the attempts to use RIPs to protect plants against viruses; several plants transfected with RIPs genes actually showed resistance to viral infections. However, transfected plants had an altered phenotype when PAP *(68)* or barley jasmonate-induced protein (JIP60) *(69)* was expressed at a high level, indicating that these RIPs also damaged plants.

The mechanism of the antiviral activity of RIPs is still not completely clear. It was thought for some years that the subcellular segregation of RIPs was broken as a consequence of cell damage caused by viral infection, and then the proteins could reach and inactivate ribosomes, thus killing the infected cells and preventing viral replication. This notion is supported by the sensitivity of plant ribosomes to conspecific RIPs *(70)*, but is not consistent with some observations:

1. Trichosanthin inhibited HIV replication at concentrations lower than that inhibiting protein synthesis *(71)*.
2. A mutant of PAP that did not damage pokeweed ribosomes still was able to prevent viral replication *(72)*.

Together, these results indicate that ribosomal damage cannot account entirely for the antiviral activity of RIPs. The observations about the depurination of nucleic acids other than rRNA suggest possible damage to viral RNA or to the virus-induced DNA as an alternative or at least parallel mechanism.

Antifungal Activity

It was reported that barley RIPs, in association with glucanase and chitinase, have antifungal activity *(73)* and confer resistance against fungal attack to transfected plants *(74)*. Presumably, the other enzymes are necessary to disrupt the tegument of fungi, thus allowing the entry of RIPs into cells. Increased resistance to *Rhizoctonia solani* was found in plants transfected with maize b-32 RIP *(75)* or PAP (reviewed in ref. *76*). It was reported that three RIPs (ricin A chain, saporin-S6, and an RIP from *Mirabilis expansa*) have antifungal activity and inactivate fungal ribosomes *(77)*.

CELL TARGETING

Experimental Studies

Ribosome-inactivating proteins have been used in attempts to eliminate unwanted cells in a selective manner for both experimental and therapeutic purposes. The subject has been exhaustively reviewed and is discussed here in general terms only.

The general principle was to link the proteins to appropriate molecules capable of entering, or at least binding to, the cells to be killed. Antibodies were used in most of experiments as the carriers with the highest specificity, but growth factors, lectins, hormones, neuropeptides, and cytokines were also employed. Both type 1 and type 2 RIPs have been used; the latter are highly toxic, but have the disadvantage of binding to virtually any cell through their B chains. Thus, conjugates were prepared as follows:

1. With ricin with blocked B chain binding site.
2. With isolated A chains of type 2 RIPs (mostly ricin A chain).
3. With type 1 RIPs.

Conjugates were prepared either chemically, introducing a link, most often a disulfide bond, between the RIP and the carrier or as fusion recombinant proteins.

For experimental purposes, the most widely used conjugates are those made with saporin and monoclonal antibodies against components of the central nervous system, as described elsewhere in this book. Few conjugates were prepared for other experimental purposes, which is surprising because these should be very useful experimental tools to remove any kind of cells selectively, as shown by the removal of fibroblasts from pancreatic cells in culture *(78)*.

The great majority of conjugates prepared for clinical use were against tumor cells (reviewed in ref. *79*) or against immunoreactive cells for the treatment of autoimmune diseases (reviewed in ref. *80*), graft-vs-host reaction (reviewed in ref. *81*), or to prevent graft rejection (reviewed in ref. *82*). In other more limited studies, immunotoxins were prepared against various cells, such as corneal endothelial cells, to prevent corneal vascularization *(83)*; retinal pigment epithelial cells *(84)*; or muscle cells for the experimental therapy of muscular spasms *(85)*.

Clinical Trials

Several clinical trials were performed with immunotoxins, most of them prepared with modified ricin or ricin A chain (reviews in refs. *86–89*) or with type 1 RIPs momordin *(90)*, PAP, and saporin (reviewed in ref. *79*). The great majority concerned the experimental therapy not only of tumors, graft-vs-host disease, and autoimmune diseases, but also of other ailments, such as diabetes *(91)* and opacification of the posterior capsule of the eye *(92)*. Immunotoxins either were administered to patients or were used for ex vivo purging of cell suspensions (e.g., bone marrow) to be infused in patients.

The results were often encouraging, possibly more than those obtained with the early trials of chemotherapeutic agents, particularly in the case of hematological malignancies *(87)*. The main limitations resulting from these studies were:

1. The poor penetration of the conjugates inside solid tumors.
2. Adverse side effects, such as myalgias, fatigue, fever, capillary leak syndrome.
3. The immune response against both the antibody and the toxin, which prevented repeated administrations.

The poor penetration into solid tumors could be overcome using smaller conjugates (e.g., with scFv fragments or with immunotoxins against endothelial cells of tumour vasculature), which would cause thrombosis with consequent ischemia of the tumor *(93)*. The peculiar capillary leak syndrome, the most important side effect *(94)*, might be reduced in various ways (reviewed in ref. *95*) and controlled with careful dosage of the immunotoxins.

The immune response is currently the major obstacle to the use of immunotoxins in the clinic because their administration cannot be repeated except in severely immunodeficient patients. It is hoped that this difficulty may be overcome in the future using conjugates of human antibodies linked to the human enzymes, perhaps eventually including the equivalent of RIPs *(31)*.

For the time being, immunotoxins constructed with RIPs or other toxic moieties, in addition to usefulness as experimental tools, could be employed in the clinic for ex vivo purging and therapy of topical tumors (i.e., of bladder cancer), as suggested by in vitro studies *(96,97)* and clinical trials *(90,98)*. Finally, it is common opinion among many scientists working in the field (e.g., *99*) that, because the decrease of tumor masses was observed after a short-term treatment in some clinical trials, one or two administrations of an immunotoxin could eliminate completely small groups of cells and even now might be useful in the treatment of the minimal residual disease.

SUMMARY

The RIPs from plants were described. The known RIPs are divided into type 1, consisting of a single chain with enzymatic properties, and type 2, consisting of an enzymatic A chain linked to B chain with the properties of a lectin specific for sugar with the galactose structure. Some type 2 RIPs are potent toxins, ricin being the best known, whereas others are much less toxic. All RIPs damage irreversibly ribosomes, by removing an adenine residue from rRNA, and depurinate also other nucleic acids. The distribution in nature, the mechanism of action, the toxicity and the main biological properties of RIPs were described, as well and their use as components of conjugates with antibodies (immunotoxins) and other carriers were mentioned.

NOTE ADDED IN PROOF

Reviews coverings several aspects of ribosome-inactivating protein appeared in ref *100*.

REFERENCES

1. Barbieri L, Battelli MG, Stirpe F. Ribosome-inactivating proteins from plants. Biochim Biophys Acta 1993;1154:237–282.
2. Nielsen K, Boston RS. Ribosome-inactivating proteins: a plant perspective. Annu Rev Physiol Plant Mol Biol 2001;52:785–816.

3. Peumans WJ, Hao Q, Van Damme EJM. Ribosome-inactivating proteins from plants: more than RNA *N*-glycosidases? FASEB J 2001;15:1493–1506.

4. Van Damme EJM, Hao Q, Barre A, et al. Ribosome-inactivating proteins: a family of plant proteins that do more than inactivate ribosomes. Crit Rev Plant Sci 2001;20:395–465.

5. Walsh TA, Morgan AE, Hey TD. Characterization and molecular cloning of a proenzyme form of a ribosome-inactivating protein from maize—novel mechanism of proenzyme activation by proteolytic removal of a 2.8-kilodalton internal peptide segment. J Biol Chem 1991;266:23,422–23,427.

6. Reinbothe S, Reinbothe C, Lehmann J, Becker W, Apel K, Parthier B. JIP60, a methyl jasmonate-induced ribosome-inactivating protein involved in plant stress reactions. Proc Natl Acad Sci USA 1994;91:7012–7016.

7. Derenzini M, Bonetti E, Marinozzi V, Stirpe F. Toxic effects of ricin. Studies on the pathogenesis of liver lesions. Virchows Arch B Cell Pathol 1976;20:15–28.

8. Skilleter DN, Paine AJ, Stirpe F. A comparison of the accumulation of ricin by hepatic parenchymal and non-parenchymal cells and its inhibition of protein synthesis. Biochim Biophys Acta 1981;677:495–500.

9. Simmons BM, Stahl PD, Russell JH. Mannose receptor-mediated uptake of ricin toxin and ricin A chain by macrophages. Multiple intracellular pathways for A chain translocation. J Biol Chem 1986;261:7912–7920.

10. Sandvig K, van Deurs B. Entry of ricin and Shiga toxin into cells: molecular mechanisms and medical perspectives. EMBO J 2000;19:5943–5950.

11. Sandvig K, van Deurs B. Transport of protein toxins into cells: pathways used by ricin, cholera toxin and Shiga toxin. FEBS Lett 2002;529:49–53.

12. Sandvig K, Grimmer S, Lauvrak U, et al. Pathways followed by ricin and Shiga toxin into cells. Histochem Cell Biol 2002;117:131–141.

13. Madan S, Ghosh PC. Interaction of gelonin with macrophages. Effect of lysosomotropic amines. Exp Cell Res 1991;198:52–58.

14. Cavallaro U, Nykjaer A, Nielsen M, Soria M. α2-Macroglobulin receptor mediates binding and cytotoxicity of plant ribosome-inactivating proteins. Eur J Biochem 1995;232:165–171.

15. McIntosh DP, Heath TD. Liposome-mediated delivery of ribosome inactivating proteins to cells in vitro. Biochim Biophys Acta 1982;690:224–230.

16. Foxwell B, Long J, Stirpe F. Cytotoxicity of erythrocyte ghosts loaded with ribosome-inactivating proteins following fusion with CHO cells. Biochem Int 1984;8:811–819.

17. Sargiacomo M, Barbieri L, Stirpe F, Tomasi M. Cytotoxicity acquired by ribosome-inactivating proteins carried by reconstituted Sendai virus envelopes. FEBS Lett 1983;157:150–154.

18. Fernández-Puentes C, Carrasco L. Viral infection permeabilizes mammalian cells to protein toxins. Cell 1980;20:769–775.

19. Goldmacher VS, Anderson J, Blättler WA, Lambert JM, Senter PD. Antibody complement-mediated cytotoxicity is enhanced by ribosome-inactivating proteins. J Immunol 1985;135:3648–3651.

20. Mir LM, Banoun H, Paoletti C. Introduction of definite amounts of nonpermeant molecules into living cells after electropermeabilization: direct access to cytosol. Exp Cell Res 1988;175:15–25.
21. Delius M, Adams G. Shock wave permeabilization with ribosome inactivating proteins: a new approach to tumor therapy. Cancer Res 1999;59:5227–5232.
22. Kodama T, Doukas AG, Hamblin MR. Delivery of ribosome-inactivating protein toxin into cancer cells with shock waves. Cancer Lett 2003;189:69–75.
23. Selbo PK, Hogset A, Prasmickaite L, Berg K. Photochemical internalisation: a novel drug delivery system. Tumour Biol 2002;23:103–112.
24. Yao Q-Z, Yu MM, Ooi LSM, et al. Isolation and characterization of a type 1 ribosome-inactivating protein from fruiting bodies of the edible mushroom (*Volvariella volvacea*). J Agric Food Chem 1998;46:788–792.
25. Liu RS, Yang JH, Liu WY. Isolation and enzymatic characterization of lamjapin, the first ribosome-inactivating protein from cryptogamic algal plant (*Laminaria japonica* A). Eur J Biochem 2002;269:4746–4752.
26. Ferreras JM, Barbieri L, Girbés T, et al. Distribution and properties of major ribosome-inactivating proteins (28 S rRNA *N*-glycosidases) of the plant *Saponaria officinalis* L. (Caryophyllaceae). Biochim Biophys Acta 1993;1216:31–42.
27. Reinbothe S, Mollenhauer B, Reinbothe C. JIPs and RIPs: the regulation of plant gene expression by jasmonate in response to environmental cues and pathogens. Plant Cell 1994;6:1197–1209.
28. Stirpe F, Barbieri L, Gorini P, Valbonesi P, Bolognesi A, Polito L. Activities associated with the presence of ribosome-inactivating proteins increase in senescent and stressed leaves. FEBS Lett 1996;382:309–312.
29. Girbés T, de Torre C, Iglesias R, Ferreras JM, Méndez E. RIP for viruses. Nature 1996;379:777–778.
30. Reisbig R, Olsnes S, Eiklid K. The cytotoxic activity of *Shigella* toxin. Evidence for catalytic inactivation of the 60S ribosomal subunit. J Biol Chem 1981;256:8739–8744.
31. Barbieri L, Valbonesi P, Bondioli M, et al. Adenine glycosylase activity in mammalian tissues: an equivalent of ribosome-inactivating proteins. FEBS Lett 2001;505:196–197.
32. Endo Y, Mitsui K, Motizuki K, Tsurugi K. The mechanism of action of ricin and related toxic lectins on eukaryotic ribosomes. The site and characteristics of the modification in 28S ribosomal RNA caused by the toxins. J Biol Chem 1987;262:5908–5912.
33. Nicolas E, Goodyer ID, Taraschi TF. An additional mechanism of ribosome-inactivating protein cytotoxicity: degradation of extrachromosomal DNA. Biochem J 1997;327:413–417.
34. Barbieri L, Valbonesi P, Bonora E, Gorini P, Bolognesi A, Stirpe F. Polynucleotide:adenosine glycosidase activity of ribosome-inactivating proteins: effect on DNA, RNA and poly(A). Nucleic Acids Res 1997;25:518–522.
35. Hudak KA, Bauman JD, Tumer NE. Pokeweed antiviral protein binds to the cap structure of eukaryotic mRNA and depurinates the mRNA downstream of the cap. RNA 2002;8:1148–1159.

36. Day PJ, Lord JM, Roberts LM. The deoxyribonuclease activity attributed to ribosome-inactivating proteins is due to contamination. Eur J Biochem 1998;258:540–545.
37. Valbonesi P, Barbieri L, Bolognesi A, Bonora E, Polito L, Stirpe F. Preparation of highly purified momordin II without ribonuclease activity. Life Sci 1999;65:1485–1491.
38. Barbieri L, Valbonesi P, Righi F, et al. Polynucleotide:adenosine glycosidase is the sole activity of ribosome-inactivating proteins on DNA. J Biochem 2000;128:883–889.
39. Stirpe F, Barbieri L, Abbondanza A, et al. Properties of volkensin, a toxic lectin from *Adenia volkensii*. J Biol Chem 1985;260:14,589–14,595.
40. Sperti S, Montanaro L, Derenzini M, Gasperi-Campani A, Stirpe F. Effect of modeccin on rat liver ribosomes in vivo. Biochim Biophys Acta 1979;562:495–503.
41. Licastro F, Morini MC, Bolognesi A, Stirpe F. Ricin induces the production of tumour necrosis factor-α and interleukin-1β by human peripheral blood mononuclear cells. Biochem J 1993;294:517–520.
42. Barbieri L, Gasperi-Campani A., Derenzini M., Betts CM, Stirpe F. Selective lesions of acinar pancreatic cells in rats poisoned with abrin. A morphological and biochemical study. Virchows Arch B Cell Pathol 1979;30:15–24.
43. Griffiths GD, Leek MD, Gee DJ. The toxic plant proteins ricin and abrin induce apoptotic changes in mammalian lymphoid tissues and intestine. J Pathol 1987;151:221–229.
44. Wiley RG, Lappi DA. *Suicide Transport and Immunolesioning*. Austin, TX: RG Landes; 1995.
45. Wiley RG, Kline RH IV. Neuronal lesioning with axonally transported toxins. J Neurosci Methods 2000;103:73–82.
46. Battelli MG, Citores L, Buonamici L, et al. Toxicity and cytotoxicity of nigrin b, a two-chain ribosome-inactivating protein from *Sambucus nigra*: a comparison with ricin. Arch Toxicol 1997;71:360–364.
47. Battelli MG, Barbieri L, Stirpe F. Toxicity of, and histological lesions caused by, ribosome-inactivating proteins, their IgG-conjugates, and their homopolymers. Acta Pathol Microbiol Immunol Scand 1990;98:585–593.
48. Battelli MG, Buonamici L, Polito L, Bolognesi A, Stirpe F. Hepatotoxicity of ricin, saporin or a saporin immunotoxin: xanthine oxidase activity in rat liver and blood serum. Virchows Arch 1996;427:529–535.
49. Büssing A. Induction of apoptosis by the mistletoe lectins: a review on the mechanisms of cytotoxicity mediated by *Viscum album* L. Apoptosis 1996;1:25–32.
50. Bergamaschi G, Perfetti V, Tonon L, et al. Saporin, a ribosome-inactivating protein used to prepare immunotoxins, induces cell death via apoptosis. Brit J Haematol 1996;93:789–794.
51. Bolognesi A, Tazzari PL, Olivieri F, Polito L, Falini B, Stirpe F. Induction of apoptosis by ribosome-inactivating proteins and related immunotoxins. Int J Cancer 1996;68:349–355.

52. Hughes JN, Lindsay CD, Griffiths GD. Morphology of ricin and abrin exposed endothelial cells is consistent with apoptotic cell death. Human Exp Toxicol 1996;15:443–451.
53. Williams JM, Lea N, Lord JM, Roberts LM, Milford DV, Taylor CM. Comparison of ribosome-inactivating proteins in the induction of apoptosis. Toxicol Lett 1997;91:121–127.
54. Komatsu N, Oda T, Muramatsu T. Involvement of both caspase-like proteases and serine proteases in apoptotic cell death induced by ricin, modeccin, diphtheria toxin, and *Pseudomonas* toxin. J Biochem 1998;124:1038–1044.
55. Gan YH, Peng SQ, Liu HY. Molecular mechanisms of apoptosis induced by ricin in HeLa cells. Acta Pharmacol Sin 2000;21:243–253.
56. Hu R-G, Zhai, Q-W, Liu, W-Y, Liu, X-Y. An insight into the mechanism of cytotoxicity of ricin to hepatoma cell: roles of Bcl-2 family proteins, caspases, Ca(2+)-dependent proteases and protein kinase C. J Cell Biochem 2001;81:583–593.
57. Brigotti M, Alfieri R, Sestili P, et al. Damage to nuclear DNA induced by Shiga toxin 1 and by ricin in human endothelial cells. FASEB J 2002;16:365–372.
58. Bagga S, Seth D, Batra JK. The cytotoxic activity of ribosome-inactivating protein saporin-6 is attributed to rRNA *N*-glycosidase and internucleosomal DNA fragmentation. J Biol Chem 2003;278:4813–4820.
59. Duggar BM, Armstrong JK. The effect of treating the virus of tobacco mosaic with the juices of various plants. Ann Mo Bot Gard 1925;12:359–366.
60. Irvin JD. Purification and partial characterization of the antiviral protein from *Phytolacca americana* which inhibits eukaryotic protein synthesis. Arch Biochem Biophys 1975;169:522–528.
61. Dallal JA, Irvin JD. Enzymatic inactivation of eukaryotic ribosomes by the pokeweed antiviral protein. FEBS Lett 1978;89:257–259.
62. Stevens WA Spurdon C, Onyon LJ, Stirpe F. Effect of inhibitors of protein synthesis from plants on tobacco mosaic virus infection. Experientia 1981;37:257–259.
63. Battelli MG, Stirpe F. Ribosome-inactivating proteins from plants. In: Chessin M, DeBorde D, Zipf A, eds. *Antiviral Proteins in Higher Plants*. Boca Raton, FL: CRC Press; 1995:39–64.
64. Wang P, Tumer NE. Virus resistance mediated by ribosome inactivating proteins. Adv Virus Res 2000;55:325–355.
65. Byers VS, Levin AS, Waites LA, et al. A phase I/II study of trichosanthin treatment of HIV disease. AIDS 1990;4:1189–1196.
66. Kahn JO, Gorelick KJ, Arri CJ, et al. Safety and pharmacokinetics of GLQ223 in subjects with AIDS and AIDS-related complex. Antimicrob Agents Chemother 1994;38:260–267.
67. Garcia PA, Bredesen DE, Vinters HV, et al. Neurological reactions in HIV-infected patients treated with trichosanthin. Neuropathol Appl Neurobiol 1993;19:402–405.

68. Lodge JK., Kaniewski K, Tumer NE. Broad-spectrum virus resistance in transgenic plants expressing pokeweed antiviral protein. Proc Natl Acad Sci USA 1993;90:7089–7093.

69. Görschen E, Dunaeva M, Hause B, Reeh I., Wasternack C, Parthier B. Expression of the ribosome-inactivating protein JIP60 from barley in transgenic tobacco leads to an abnormal phenotype and alterations on the level of translation. Planta 1997;202:470–478.

70. Prestle J, Schönfelder M, Adam G, Mundry K-W. Type 1 ribosome-inactivating protein depurinate plant 25S rRNA without species specificity. Nucleic Acids Res 1992;20:3179–3182.

71. Lee-Huang S, Huang PL, Kung H-F, et al. TAP 29: An anti-human immunodeficiency virus protein from *Trichosanthes kirilowii* that is nontoxic to intact cells. Proc Natl Acad Sci USA 1991;88:6570–6574.

72. Tumer NE, Hwang D-J, Bonness M. C-terminal deletion mutant of pokeweed antiviral protein inhibits viral infection but does not depurinate host ribosomes. Proc Natl Acad Sci USA 1997;94:3866–3871.

73. Leah R, Tommerup H, Svendsen I, Mundy J. Biochemical and molecular characterization of three barley seed proteins with antifungal properties. J Biol Chem 1991;266:1564–1573.

74. Jach G, Gornhardt B, Mundy J, et al. Enhanced quantitative resistance against fungal disease by combinatorial expression of different barley antifungal proteins in transgenic tobacco. Plant J 1995;8:97–109.

75. Maddaloni M, Forlani F, Balmas V, et al. Tolerance to the fungal pathogen *Rhizoctonia solani* AG4 of transgenic tobacco expressing the maize ribosome-inactivating protein b-32. Transgenic Res 1997;6:393–401.

76. Tumer NE, Hudak K, Di R, Coetzer C, Wang P, Zoubenko O. Pokeweed antiviral protein and its applications. Curr Top Microbiol Immunol 1999;240:139–158.

77. Park SW, Stevens NM, Vivanco JM. Enzymatic specificity of three ribosome-inactivating proteins against fungal ribosomes, and correlation with antifungal activity. Planta 2002;216:227–234.

78. Beattie GM, Lappi DA, Baird A, Hayek A. Selective elimination of fibroblasts from pancreatic islets monolayers by basic fibroblast growth factor-saporin mitotoxin. Diabetes 1990;39:1002–1005.

79. Frankel AE, Kreitman RJ, Sausville EA. Targeted toxins. Clin Cancer Res 2000;6:326–334.

80. Wu M. Are immunoconjugates useful for therapy with autoimmune diseases? Int J Immunopharmacol 1997;19:83–93.

81. Vallera DA. Targeting T cells for GVHD therapy. Semin Cancer Biol 1996;7:57-64.

82. Knechtle SJ. Treatment with immunotoxin. Phil Trans R Soc Lond B 2001;356:681–689.

83. Fulcher S, Lui G, Houston LL, et al. Use of immunotoxin to inhibit proliferating human corneal endothelium. Invest Ophthalmol Visual Sci 1988;29:755–759.

84. Jaffe GJ, Earnest K, Fulcher S, Durham NC, Lui GM, Houston LL. Antitransferrin receptor immunotoxin inhibits proliferating human retinal pigment epithelial cells. Arch Ophthalmol 1990;108:1163–1168.

85. Hott JS, Dalakas MC, Sung C, Hallett M, Youle RJ. Skeletal muscle-specific immunotoxin for the treatment of focal muscle spasm. Neurology 1998;50:485–491.

86. Frankel AE, Tagge EP, Willingham MC. Clinical trials of targeted toxins. Semin Cancer Biol 1995;6:307–317.

87. Engert A, Sausville EA, Vitetta E. The emerging role of ricin A-chain immunotoxins in leukemia and lymphoma. Curr Top Microbiol Immunol 1998;234:13–33.

88. Ghetie MA, Ghetie V, Vitetta ES. Immunotoxins for the treatment of B-cell lymphomas. Mol Med 1997;3:420–427.

89. O'Toole JE, Esseltine D, Lynch TJ, Lambert JM, Grossbard ML. Clinical trials with blocked ricin immunotoxins. Curr Top Microbiol Immunol 1998;234:35–56.

90. Yu L, Gu F, Zhang C, Xie S, Guo Y. Targeted diagnosis and treatment of superficial bladder cancer with monoclonal antibody BDI-1. Chin Med J 1998;111:404–407.

91. Skyler JS, Lorenz TJ, Schwartz S, et al. Effects of an anti-CD5 immunoconjugate (CD5-plus) in recent onset type I diabetes mellitus: a preliminary investigation. The CD5 Diabetes Project Team. J Diabetes Complications 1993;7:224–232.

92. Clark DS, Emery JM, Munsell MF. Inhibition of posterior capsule opacification with an immunotoxin specific for lens epithelial cells: 24 month clinical results. J Cataract Refract Surg 1998;24:1614–1620.

93. Veenendaal LM, Jin H, Ran S, et al. In vitro and in vivo studies of a VEGF121/rGelonin chimeric fusion toxin targeting the neovasculature of solid tumors. Proc Natl Acad Sci USA 2002;99:7866–7871.

94. Vitetta ES. Immunotoxins and vascular leak syndrome. Cancer J 2000;suppl 3:S218–S224.

95. Pennell CA, Erickson HA. Designing immunotoxins for cancer therapy. Immunol Res 2002;25:177–191.

96. Thiesen H-J, Juhl H, Arndt R. Selective killing of human bladder cancer cells by combined treatment with A and B chain ricin antibody conjugates. Cancer Res 1987;47:419–423.

97. Battelli MG, Polito L, Bolognesi A, Lafleur L, Fradet Y, Stirpe F. Toxicity of ribosome-inactivating proteins-containing immunotoxins to a human bladder carcinoma cell line. Int J Cancer 1996;65:485–490.

98. Zang Z, Xu H, Yu L, et al. Intravesical immunotoxin as adjuvant therapy to prevent the recurrence of bladder cancer. Chin Med J 2000;113:1002–1006.

99. Flavell DJ. Saporin immunotoxins. Curr Top Microbiol Immunol 1998;234:57–61.

100. Stirpe F. (ed.). Ribosome-inactivating proteins. Mini Rev Med Chem 2004;4:461–595.

3

Biochemical, Physiological, and Behavioral Characterizations of the Cholinergic Basal Forebrain Lesion Produced by 192 IgG-Saporin

Jerene J. Waite

BACKGROUND

The Cholinergic Hypothesis

Selective lesioning of the cholinergic neurons in the basal forebrain nuclei was a highly sought goal for use as an animal model of Alzheimer's disease. Autopsy studies of Alzheimer's-diseased brain tissue found that a substantial loss of the cholinergic innervation of the cerebral cortex and hippocampus was a prominent feature of this disease, and the degree of this neuron loss was highly correlated with the degree of dementia *(1,2)*. Subsequent research confirmed that cholinergic neurons originating in the nucleus basalis of Meynert, the diagonal band of Broca, and the medial septal nucleus, which terminate mainly in the cortex, olfactory bulb, and hippocampus *(3,4)*, are destroyed in the progression of Alzheimer's disease. This loss occurred earlier than the degeneration of other types of neurons, and the scale of this cholinergic cell death was massive. The similarity to dopaminergic depletion in Parkinson's disease was evident, and the cholinergic hypothesis for the dementia of Alzheimer's disease was proposed. The need for an animal model to test therapeutic strategies fueled basic research about the function of this cholinergic basal forebrain (CBF) system.

Unselective CBF Lesions

Lesioning methods already in use on rat brains included mechanical lesions such as fimbria/fornix transections to remove cholinergic (and other)

From: *Molecular Neurosurgery With Targeted Toxins*
Edited by: R. G. Wiley and D. A. Lappi © Humana Press Inc., Totowa, NJ

input to the hippocampus and radio-frequency or electrolytic lesioning of discrete regions. Excitotoxins, many of which are potent agonists at glutamate receptors that destroy cells bearing these receptors by excessive excitation or calcium ion overload, were a considerable improvement over mechanical lesions because perikarya, but not fibers en passage, are destroyed *(5,6)*. Unfortunately, many different kinds of cells (including glia) bear glutamate receptors and, although cholinergic neurons are susceptible to these toxins as demonstrated by depletion of cholinergic markers, histological examination has demonstrated that other cell types, especially GABA-ergic (γ-aminobutyric acid) neurons, are destroyed when excitotoxins are infused into the nucleus basalis magnocellularis of rats *(7–9)*.

The ethylcholine aziridinium ion AF64A was developed in a well-reasoned attempt to produce greater specificity for cholinergic neuron destruction. It targeted a specific membrane protein present on cholinergic neurons, the high-affinity choline transporter *(10)*. Unfortunately, the specificity of this toxin for cholinergic neurons in vivo was difficult to ensure because of the high alkylating reactivity of the aziridinium ion. When injected intracerebroventricularly (icv), it can destroy cholinergic innervation of the hippocampus, but its utility as a specific cholinotoxin is less than was originally hoped *(11,12)*.

Development of 192 Immunoglobulin G-Saporin

Ultimately, the goal of producing a selective lesion of CBF neurons was achieved by the collaboration between groups led by Dr. Douglas Lappi and Dr. Ronald Wiley and the coupling of two compounds, saporin and an antibody against the rat low-affinity (p75) nerve growth factor receptor (NGF-R). This immunotoxin, 192 immunoglobulin G-saporin (IgG-sap), built on the idea of coupling a compound selective for cholinergic neurons with a toxin. Saporin is cytotoxic only when it gains access to the interior of cells and inhibits protein synthesis. The immunotoxic compound relies on internalization of the antibody for the desired selectivity. Such chimeric suicide transport agents were under investigation for targeting malignant cells, as well as other uses for selective cell destruction in a living organism. Of the toxins tested, saporin proved to have the greatest efficacy in cell destruction when coupled to a molecule that conferred specificity and applied to neurons in the central nervous system *(13–17)*.

A monoclonal antibody to the rat p75 nerve growth factor-receptor (NGF-R), 192 IgG is endocytosed on binding to the receptor and is retrogradely transported from axon terminals to cell bodies *(18)*. When radioiodinated and injected icv, it was found to accumulate preferentially in the basal forebrain cholinergic neurons *(19,20)*. Thus, although in vitro immunohistochemistry using [125]I-192 IgG detects low-affinity binding in other brain regions, intraventricular infusion produced more selective targeting to long-axon projection neurons bearing a high density of p75 NGF-R, namely, the cholinergic neurons of the basal forebrain nuclei.

Saporin is a single-chain (type 1), ribosome-inactivating protein obtained from seeds of the soapwort plant *Saponaria officinalis (16)*. It is a specific *N*-glycosidase at the 60S ribosomal subunit *(21)*. The enzymatic nature of this protein implies that a single molecule, once gaining access to the intracellular compartment, could eventually destroy the cell by inhibition of translation (protein synthesis). The antibody coupling of saporin renders an immunotoxin with at least a 10-fold greater cytotoxicity for the targeted cell type compared to the effects of saporin alone *(22)*.

Both groups of researchers were independently studying the effects of disulfide coupling of saporin to proteins that would yield a desired selectivity. Lappi was working on a project using basic fibroblast growth factor conjugated to saporin *(23,24)*. Wiley's group successfully used the Thy-1 antibody OX7 coupled to saporin to produce neuron loss in the striatum and cerebellum *(13,22)*. The Thy-1 antigen, a glycoprotein, is present on all neurons, although when OX7-sap is infused into the lateral ventricles, it destroys Purkinje cells in the cerebellum. When Schweitzer reported that ventricularly infused 192 IgG would bind to and be retrogradely transported into the particular NGF-R-bearing neurons of the CBF *(19,20)*, a convergence of effort led to the development of the first immunotoxin of high CBF neuronal selectivity combined with better efficacy than had been produced by any excitotoxin *(15)*.

DEVELOPMENT OF USE

Time Course of Cell Loss

The study of a new pharmacological agent always requires both a time course and a dose-dependence assessment. The question is, Which to do first? We knew from other investigators that low-microgram quantities of the toxin produced a great degree of cholinergic cell loss with intracerebroventricular administration. A short study of a small number of doses indicated that approx 4 mg of 192 IgG-sap was needed for reliable production of the maximal depletion of the enzyme for acetylcholine (ACh) synthesis, choline acetyltransferase (ChAT), as measured by its activity in cortical and hippocampal homogenates. We then proceeded to do a more careful assessment of the time course of onset of CBF destruction at this high dose *(25)*.

Although ChAT is not the rate-limiting enzyme in ACh production, it is a useful marker for loss of cholinergic axon terminals. The quantitative reliability of the assay of ChAT activity by incorporation of [^{14}C]acetyl coenzyme A (CoA) into ACh has made it a useful tool in the evaluation of cholinergic lesions *(26)*.

We expected that the circulation of the cerebrospinal fluid would ensure equivalent distribution of a high dose of the immunotoxin bilaterally even if only a single icv infusion was performed. This was generally true, although small differences between left and right hemisphere ChAT activity were detected from animals sacrificed nearest the time of infusion. By 7 d postlesion, there were no significant lateral differences in any brain region tested.

The immunotoxin 192 IgG-sap proved to be the most efficacious CBF toxin developed. Frontal and parietal cortex retained less than 20% ChAT activity a week after surgery. Hippocampal activity was less than 10%. The olfactory bulbs, innervated by cholinergic neurons of the diagonal band, were most depleted, yielding undetectable levels of ChAT activity. The destruction was complete by 7 d. For comparison, the ChAT activity measured subsequent to intraparenchymal infusions of the highly efficacious excitotoxin α-amino-3-hydroxy-5-methyl-4-isoxazole propionic acid (AMPA) was 34% and 16% in frontal and parietal cortex, respectively, and 44% in the hippocampus *(27)*. Other excitotoxins were less effective.

In corroboration of earlier studies, no changes at all in ChAT activity were found in the cerebellum, pons, or striatum, underscoring the remarkable selectivity of this lesioning agent *(28,29)*. Our high-performance liquid chromatographic assessment of tissue monoamine and monoamine metabolite levels also resembled results of other investigators in this sense: There were significant increases from control levels of certain monoamines in some tissues at some time-points. However, these differences were not sustained and not consistently detected in different studies *(28,30,31)*. The consensus was that the immunotoxin did not directly affect monoamine levels, but that responses to the dramatic cholinergic loss were most likely affecting other neurotransmitter systems, particularly at earlier time-points.

Investigations of Selectivity

Results from intracerebroventricular administration of 192 IgG-sap were particularly compelling because the immunotoxin was potentially accessible to the entire central nervous system with this type of lesion induction, underscoring its amazing selectivity for the CBF. The ability to lesion only cholinergic neurons in the CBF with a single unilateral or, at most, a pair of infusions into the lateral ventricles was highly appealing. Prior attempts to lesion this system using excitotoxins required as many as two bilateral infusions into the medial septum and two bilateral infusions into the nucleus basalis, producing much greater nonspecific mechanical damage and difficulty limiting the diffusion to relevant structures *(27)*.

Many laboratories were conducting histological studies around this time, all looking for nonselective (non-CBF) changes. GABA-ergic neurons were unaffected in the CBF and terminal fields *(32–35)*. Neuronal peptides, other cholinergic neurons, and monoamine-containing axons were unaffected by either icv or intraparenchymal infusions of the toxin *(34,36)*.

The study of the selectivity for the CBF was also included in our next experiment, in which we turned to the question of dose dependence *(30)*. This larger experiment tested different doses of 192 IgG-sap first on rat behaviors and then for biochemical and histological effects.

Perhaps the most interesting aspect of our histological analysis involved immunohistochemistry with the monoclonal antibody 192 IgG. If the immunotoxin destroyed every cell in the brain bearing the p75 NGF-R, we would have seen no antibody binding in brain sections from lesioned animals with this method. What we found was that, in areas (other than the CBF) where high densities of NGF-R are normally stained in control brain slices, there was no reduction in labeling—no loss of cells bearing NGF-R (also described in ref. *34*). These cells are not necessarily cholinergic and not necessarily neurons. We speculated that the immunotoxin did not have access to these cells, or that the NGF-R on these cells may not endocytose if the immunotoxin did have access *(30)*.

The only cell type discovered susceptible to 192 IgG-sap administered intracerebroventricularly—other than CBF neurons—is the cerebellar Purkinje cell *(37)*. (Changes in ChAT activity did not occur in the cerebellum because the Purkinje cells are GABA-ergic.) Cerebellar Purkinje cells do not have a high density of NGF-R, but the icv infusions of 192 IgG-sap present the immunotoxin to the extensive dendritic fields, destroying Purkinje cells closest to the dorsal cerebellar surface *(30,31,34)*. Our dose-dependence study found that the pattern of Purkinje loss diminished gradually from the outermost dorsal layer to no cell loss on the inner layers, even at the highest dose (4 µg) of 192 IgG-sap used *(30)*. A subsequent experiment quantitated the Purkinje loss per layer and compared it with that produced by OX7-sap, also injected intracerebroventricularly (Table 1) *(38)*.

This, unfortunately, was a spoiler for the icv administration of the immunotoxin, especially for its use in behavioral studies. Ultimately, intraparenchymal administration had to be developed to produce lesions restricted to the CBF and, for some studies, lesions restricted to parts of the CBF or its terminal fields.

Table 1
Cerebellar Purkinje Cell Number/20 mm (Means ± SEM)

Band no.	PBS-Control	1.6 µg 192-sap	2.6 µg 192-sap	3.3 µg 192-sap	2 µg OX7-sap
1	56 ± 3.7	50 ± 3.9	28 ± 5.1[a]	22 ± 4.4[a]	26 ± 5.4[a]
2	65 ± 3.9	58 ± 3.4	43 ± 4.6[a]	42 ± 3.0[a]	39 ± 5.5[a]
3	56 ± 6.7	66 ± 7.1	50 ± 3.7	48 ± 4.9	50 ± 4.4
4	57 ± 9.1	64 ± 5.2	54 ± 7.8	54 ± 4.2	50 ± 6.8

[a]Reduced number of Purkinje cells. Hematoxylin/eosin-stained Purkinje cells were counted from coronal sections 10 mm on both sides of midline, beginning with the most dorsal layer (band 1) and continuing ventral to band 4. Control and 1.6 mg 192 IgG-sap groups had a uniform number of cells in all four bands. The two higher doses of 192 IgG-sap and the OX7-sap group had reduced cell numbers in the two dorsal bands, but bands 3 and 4 were equivalent to controls. The Purkinje cell loss was the same for these three groups (38).

SEM, standard error of the mean; PBS, phosphate-buffered saline.

Development of Intraparenchymal Infusion Methods

Direct infusion of 192 IgG-sap required some experimentation to accomplish similar degrees of CBF destruction to the degree obtained using icv administration without concomitant nonspecific or nonselective damage at the infusion site. Placement of infusion needles or capillaries and limitation of diffusion to the area of interest was again a concern. Other investigators have worked on this with varied success.

Application of toxin to the cortex is feasible, and retrograde neuronal loss in the nucleus basalis was observed *(39)*. Broad lesioning of cortical innervation is still more easily accomplished, however, by toxin placement within the nucleus basalis using either one or two infusion sites per hemisphere. Although hippocampal infusions were also successful *(40,41)*, this structure is unusually sensitive to mechanical damage *(42)*. Thus, for hippocampal lesions, medial septal infusions are also preferable to application of the toxin into the terminal fields.

Early studies found that a high degree of lesioning was possible with direct infusions into the nucleus basalis or medial septum, but there was considerable nonselective loss of cholinergic (ChAT-positive) interneurons in the striatum after infusions into the nucleus basalis *(34,35)*. Other investigators obtained less unwanted damage, but the CBF cell loss was not as complete as that obtained from icv infusion *(36,43,44)*. Some found higher gliotic responses (compared with icv infusions) or necrotic damage at infusion sites *(33,45,46)*. Method development was hindered by the use of different preparations of the immunotoxin by different laboratories.

For our purposes, clean and near-complete lesions of the entire CBF were required, measured by cholinergic markers in the terminal fields—especially the cortex and hippocampus—as well as histological assessment of ChAT-positive neurons in the CBF nuclei. Doses much lower than those used originally coupled with very slow rates of infusion were ultimately successful at producing cholinergic neuron loss with minimal damage to other neurons *(32,33,46–48)*. We found that the medial septum was more sensitive to direct infusions than the nucleus basalis, and one infusion per hemisphere of 37 ng of immunotoxin in 0.5 μL, at a rate of 0.05 μL/min, yielded greater than 90% reduction of ChAT activity in the hippocampus with no remaining ChAT-positive neurons in the medial septum *(47)*. Using 75 ng per 0.5 μL in one infusion per hemisphere into the nucleus basalis, cortical ChAT activity was reduced 70–80%, approximately the extent of ChAT depletion attainable with icv administration. Thus, four total intraparenchymal infusions could reproduce, without extraneous damage, the cholinergic lesion obtained with icv administration *(47)*.

Gross Physiological Changes

Observations of the rats after icv administration of high doses (e.g., 4 µg) of 192 IgG-sap indicated that there were some apparent difficulties at about 7 d postsurgery, when control animals had already recovered from the surgical aftermath. It is at this time that weight loss and hypophagy are most apparent. Difficulty with locomotor activity and reduced olfactory-driven responses to novel odors, if observable at all, occur at this time. All of these difficulties, however, disappeared within a few days. The reduction of ChAT activity we found nearly maximal by 7 d postlesion correlates with this impairment stage, but it does not correlate with subsequent physiological recovery. Mere observation of rat behavior on handling or behavior in the home cage gives no indication of the extent of CBF cell loss. The small but detectable behavioral changes around the 7-d time-point may be caused by tissue responses to the neuronal destruction or to initial lack of compensation. Death of animals from administration of this toxin was rare and most likely caused by surgical complications rather than effects of the toxin.

BEHAVIORAL STUDIES

For the intended purpose of developing a more valid model of the cholinergic degeneration in Alzheimer's disease, the assessment and characterization of lesions produced by 192 IgG-sap must demonstrate not only selective CBF neuron loss, but also the presence of cognitive deficits in learning and memory relevant to dementia in humans. Many investigators have contributed to the large assembly of studies in this endeavor.

Spatial Learning and Memory: The Morris Water Maze

When 192 IgG-sap first became available to us, the current state of understanding of the cognitive effects of CBF lesions produced by excitotoxins was that much of the behavioral impairment observed in the Morris water maze task was caused by nonspecific, perhaps GABA-ergic, cell destruction in the nucleus basalis, produced particularly by ibotenic acid infusion *(49,50)*. The extent to which any of the learning or memory deficits was related to the cholinergic lesion was unclear. Thus, there was an immediate need to use this new immunotoxin for such studies.

Our initial studies resembled those of Nilsson et al. *(28)* and Berger-Sweeney et al. *(35)* in using the spatial learning paradigm of the Morris water maze as a primary means of cognitive assessment. The water maze results obtained by Nilsson et al. were encouraging, although a single high dose was used for the intracerebroventricular lesion induction (4.7 µg), and their rats seemed to have more physiological problems at about a week postlesion in terms of weight loss and lethal hypophagy. When we began our first water maze study, we were unaware of the results obtained by Berger-Sweeney et al. *(35)*.

We conducted three studies testing 192 IgG-sap-treated animals in the water maze. Two of these studies used comparable procedures *(30,38)*; the third required a different paradigm because of time restrictions in testing *(51)*. All three studies used animals given the toxin by icv infusion.

Dose-Dependent Differences in Water Maze Behavior

Having established that lesions produced by icv administration were complete by 2 wk after surgery, we initiated our first behavioral study, examining the effects of four doses of the immunotoxin *(30)*. We found, in the water maze, that animals receiving what we considered a moderate dose of toxin (2 µg, yielding somewhat less than maximal ChAT depletion) exhibited very modest deficiencies in learning to locate the submerged, hidden platform in the water maze. The acquisition of the task for these animals was significantly slower than for controls, but animals receiving a slightly higher dose (2.7 µg), and having a maximal CBF ChAT depletion in this study, exhibited grossly impaired performance in the task. In fact, this group of animals could hardly be said to have learned the procedure. There was a major disparity in the performance of these two groups, with immunotoxin doses differing by only 0.7 µg.

There was an additional unanticipated difficulty with animals that had received the highest dose (4 µg) of 192 IgG-sap in this study. Initial attempts to test their ability to swim in the water maze found them unable to swim normally. Normal rat behavior when placed in deep water is to extend their heads above the water and paddle their feet until they find a place to stand, such as the platform. Occasional animals, on acclimating to the water maze over a period of several days, have been observed to float on the surface slowly and not attempt immediate escape to the platform. These high-dose animals showed neither of these behaviors.

When placed in the water, they tended to dip their heads and flex their torsos inward, leading to submersion and, in some cases, tumbling under the water. Although I tried allowing them to acclimate and learn a different response in the first two water maze trials, these animals had to be rescued from under the water before the 90-s swim time was over. Their behavior during and after the trials suggested a heightened stress response to the experience. We decided to give this group of animals additional experience in the water maze without the platform to see if they could acclimate and be capable of swimming and performing the task. Shorter periods of time in the water over the course of a week did result in five of the eight animals in this group habituating, and they were able to swim for the two 90-s trials per day on the surface of the water.

We then tested these animals in the usual water maze paradigm in the presence of the submerged platform. We found that, even after regaining their ability to swim, animals in this group did not learn the procedure of swimming to the platform and staying there. In fact, as I attempted to guide them to the platform at the end of their trials, they would turn and avoid my hand, appearing to avoid placement on the platform. At the end of this assessment, I attached two wooden dowels to the platform, both dowels extending above the water and easily visible to the rats. The visible markers for the platform did not exactly induce these rats to escape from the water by swimming to the platform, however. They swam to the dowels and attempted to escape the water by climbing the dowels. This served the point of demonstrating that their vision was adequate, but did not demonstrate that they could learn (or were motivated to learn) the typical water maze procedure. Rats given 2.7 µg of the toxin, although they also did not learn the task, had no trouble swimming initially in the usual water maze procedure, and they did not show any deficiency or unusual behavior when tested with the visible dowels on the platform.

Subsequent lesion assessment showed that animals in groups given either 2.7 or 4 µg of immunotoxin had equivalent ChAT depletion in the CBF projection fields. However, not only was there a major difference in motoric behavior between these two groups, but also there was a major difference between these groups and the animals that had been lesioned with 2 mg of toxin. The ChAT depletion did not correlate linearly with the behavior in the water maze.

As noted, other investigators had described Purkinje cell loss that accompanied the icv administration of 192 IgG-sap. We confirmed that this had occurred in these animals, but a qualitative assessment of the amount of cerebellar damage did not appear to correlate with the degree of behavioral impairments observed, especially in the water maze. We saw very little difference in the amount of Purkinje cell loss in the animals given 2 µg and those given 4 mg of toxin. The need for a more quantitative comparison between the effects of Purkinje cell loss and the effects of CBF cell loss was evident.

At this time, the exploration of intraparenchymal infusions of 192 IgG-sap was producing mixed results in other laboratories. To improve on the excitotoxin model, the intraparenchymal infusions had to be both more selective and at least as effective in destroying the CBF neurons as had been found with excitotoxic lesioning, preferably equivalent to that obtained with icv immunotoxic lesions. If the cognitive deficit is small and difficult to detect with a loss of ChAT activity less than about 80–90%, then either the water maze is not a good behavioral test for changes subsequent to CBF lesion or the CBF lesion does not produce the expected behavioral deficits predicted by the cholinergic hypothesis.

Also about this time, two groups reported small or no spatial impairment in the water maze using 192 IgG-sap administered intraparenchymally into both the medial septum and the nucleus basalis *(52,53)*. The lesion assessments indicated that these were moderate lesions (both about 60% depletion in cortex; 78 and 60% in the hippocampus, respectively) compared to what seemed to be needed to observe behavioral deficits in the water maze. [More recently, my colleagues have reported results of a similar study comparing lesions produced by intraparenchymal infusions of both CBF nuclei with those produced by icv administration. Water maze behavioral deficits were small or absent despite about 75% ChAT depletion in the cortex and 92% in the hippocampus in the rats given intraparenchymal toxin *(54)*.] Perhaps the water maze task is not appropriate for testing behavioral consequences of selective CBF destruction.

Assessment of Attention in the Multiple-Choice Serial Reaction Time Task

Attention is tested in humans using a five-choice version of the serial reaction time (SRT) as part of the Cambridge Neuropsychological Test Automated Battery *(55)*. This test has been adapted to assess attention in rats *(56)*. Attentional impairments were discovered with excitotoxic lesions of specific CBF nuclei, especially the nucleus basalis, using this testing paradigm *(57,58)*. Studies testing the attention of rats lesioned with 192 IgG-sap also found attentional deficits using other paradigms *(45,46,59–61)*.

Another immunotoxin, OX7-sap, has been shown to destroy Purkinje cells when it is infused intracerebroventricularly, similar to the Purkinje cell destruction by 192 IgG-sap *(22,62)*. How would the immunotoxic destruction of Purkinje cells alone affect behavior, and could this be compared with the intracerebroventricularly induced lesion of 192 IgG-sap? We decided to compare the lesions produced by 192 IgG-sap with the pure Purkinje cell lesion produced by OX7-sap in the SRT paradigm used by Muir and Robbins for excitotoxin-lesioned rats. We chose this method because it retained the high degree of CBF lesion and minimal mechanical damage resulting from icv administration. We expected that the OX7-sap lesion would permit us to distinguish between CBF and cerebellar effects.

In the attentional task, all animals are trained to criterion performance and then lesioned. The baseline task in the five-choice SRT requires the animal to respond to the illumination of one of five rectangular ports arrayed on one wall of an operant chamber. The illumination typically lasts from 0.5 to 1 s. A food reward is delivered from the opposite wall after a correct response (nose poke) in the illuminated port, detected by interruption of an infrared beam. Reacquisition of this baseline task is the first test after recovery from surgery. Once all animals have regained criterion performance, variables are altered, challenging the animals to adjust to different conditions.

This study was done using a new batch of 192 IgG-sap with slightly less potency than the previous batch, necessitating a higher dose (3.3 µg) to obtain the same level of ChAT depletion in the hippocampus and cortex *(38)*. The pattern and amount of Purkinje cell loss were equivalent to that obtained with 2 µg of OX7-sap. We also conducted four other tests on these animals to characterize further the behavioral differences produced by the two immunotoxins *(63)*.

The assessment of attentional behavior in the SRT was successful in that the animals with the pure cerebellar lesion rarely showed the same type of behavior compared to the 192 IgG-sap-lesioned rats. Although we expected that the behavioral changes would be quantitatively different, with the CBF plus cerebellar lesion producing greater deficits, in fact the behavior profiles were qualitatively different in many respects. For example, under certain conditions, the 192 IgG-sap group perseverated less than controls, although under related conditions, the OX7-sap group perseverated more than controls. With a noise distraction, the OX7-sap rats performed better than controls, and the 192 IgG-sap rats performed worse.

Behaviors in the other tests (water maze, acoustic startle response, passive avoidance retention, and open field activity) also differed highly between the two lesion groups, but with these tests, the 192 IgG-sap group was unimpaired and the OX7-sap group demonstrated significant impairment with respect to controls. Notably, in this study, the 192 IgG-sap-lesioned rats performed very well in the water maze, learning as quickly and as well as controls. This was unexpected because ChAT depletion was nearly identical to that obtained using 2 µg in the prior water maze study, which had measured significant but unimpressive impairment in water maze acquisition and working memory. The OX7-sap group learned very poorly in the water maze, but did not exhibit the extreme severity of impairment observed with the two high-dose groups in the prior study of 192 IgG-sap *(30)*. (The water maze study of OX7-sap lesions was repeated and confirmed by another group; *64.*)

Clear differences were found between the 192 IgG-sap-lesioned rats and those lesioned with OX7-sap. Impaired inhibitory control with hyperkinetic behavior and decreased sensitivity to a visual stimulus and to auditory startle were found in rats given the Purkinje lesion alone. The behavioral profile of the 192 IgG-sap group showed impairment in particular conditions in the SRT in which the other group was not impaired. We concluded that the attentional task was a better test of the CBF lesion than the water maze. Spatial learning and memory, at least after a few weeks of recovery from the lesion induction, are not highly affected by loss of the cholinergic input to cortex and hippocampus.

Learning an Attentional Task: Intraparenchymal CBF Lesions

The prior experiment demonstrated that rats given extensive CBF lesions after learning the baseline SRT task had no difficulty reacquiring the task after surgery, and the rate of this reacquisition was the same as that of control animals. Yet, certain changes in the baseline procedure impaired their performance. We hypothesized that the spatial learning requirement of the water maze task is not challenging enough to uncover cognitive weakness in these animals, but that learning the baseline SRT task not only would challenge the rats more, but also would require different cognitive skills than the water maze task. The next experiment was designed to test the ability of CBF-lesioned rats to learn the attentional task of the SRT.

We used intraparenchymal infusions of 192 IgG-sap into both the medial septum and the nucleus basalis *(47)*, a sham-lesioned group to control for mechanical damage in the CBF (phosphate-buffered saline [PBS] vehicle), and a nonoperated "naïve" group to assess any impairment produced by the mechanical damage caused by fluid infusions. Acquisition was measured by counting the number of sessions required for an animal to meet predetermined criteria of performance.

The CBF lesion produced 70–78% reduction of ChAT activity in the cortex and 91% reduction in the hippocampus, determined at the end of the experiment, 10 mo postlesion (Table 2). The sham lesion produced a small decrement (0–14%) in ChAT activity, presumably reflecting the amount of nonspecific damage to noncholinergic cells as well.

Acquisition of the SRT task was accomplished in seven progressive stages after habituation to the operant chamber, reward pellets, and reward retrieval from the food magazine. When an animal retrieved pellets from the food tray, indicating adequate habituation, it was started on the training sessions. Each rat advanced through the stages of acquisition at its own rate, so the pattern of advancement was different for each rat. However, each training session was considered equivalent in counting the number of sessions to reach criterion performance in the final ("baseline") testing sequence. Sessions were daily, five per week, lasting 30 min or 100 trials, whichever came

Table 2
Lesion Assessment by ChAT Activity in SRT Acquisition Study

	Naïve $n = 15$	Sham $n = 15$	192-IgG Saporin $n = 14$
Cortex Frontal	52.7 ± 0.7	50.8 ± 0.5 (96%)	14.3 ± 2.2 (27%)[a]
Parietal	43.2 ± 0.7	40.0 ± 0.6 (92%)[b]	12.7 ± 1.9 (30%)[a]
Occipital	52.0 ± 0.7	45.1 ± 0.9 (87%)[b]	11.4 ± 1.3 (22%)[a]
Hippocampus	52.5 ± 1.2	45.1 ± 0.9 (86%)[b]	4.9 ± 1.8 (9%)[a]
Olfactory bulbs	31.3 ± 0.5	31.6 ± 0.5 (101%)	3.9 ± 1.8 (12%)[a]

[a]Significantly different from both naïve and sham.
[b]Significantly different from naïve (Fischer's Protected Least Significant Difference).

Intraparenchymal infusions into the medial septum and nucleus basalis with 192 IgG-sap or PBS (sham) or no infusion (naïve) constituted the three groups. One lesioned animal was removed from the study because of an excessively enlarged lateral ventricle. ChAT activity was measured in homogenates from bilateral tissue dissections by incorporation of [^{14}C]acetyl CoA into [^{14}C]acetylcholine and corrected for protein content. Means of the combined bilateral dissections in nanomoles ACh/h/mg protein plus or minus the standard error of the mean are shown. Percentages of the naïve control values are shown in parentheses after the raw data. n indicates number of rats per group.

first. Initial stages had longer times of port illumination (stimulus duration) and longer times in which a response (nose poke) would be counted (limited hold). In the first sequence, only the center port (port 5) was used. All subsequent sequences used the five odd-numbered ports (of the nine total ports), each spatially separated by an unused, covered port in the chamber. The parameters for progressive acquisition are shown in Table 3.

Despite the fact that the intracerebroventricularly infused, CBF-lesioned rats in the prior experiment had no problem performing the baseline five-choice SRT procedure after surgery, we found that the acquisition of this task by CBF-lesioned rats was highly impaired relative to either the sham-lesioned or the naïve groups (Table 4). It was necessary to institute a ceiling on the number of sessions allowed (75 sessions) because 10 of the 14 CBF-lesioned animals, 2 of 15 in the naïve group, and 3 of 15 in the sham group were not advancing.

The pattern of acquisition (or lack of it) is revealing. In the first sequence, animals must learn to respond to illumination of the single port to gain a reward (and advance to the next stage). The association of light, nose poke, and food is not always an easy step, even for unlesioned animals. In this experiment, without any extra shaping, all animals achieved this step. In the second sequence, the timing parameters were the same, but the number of ports was increased from one to five. Rats typically generalize to the five

Table 3
Parameter Settings for Acquisition Sequences
in the Five-Choice SRT Task

Sequence	Number of Ports	Stimulus duration (s)	Limited hold (s)	Intertrial interval (s)	Criterion for acquisition (% correct)
1	1	30	60	5	70
2	5	30	60	5	70
3	5	10	10	5	70
4	5	2.5	5	5	70
5	5	1.5	5	5	70
6	5	1.25	5	5	70
Baseline	5	1	5	5	85

Percentage correct is the percentage of correct responses of all trials in a single session. Each rat advanced through the sequences at its own rate. A single session of criterion performance moved the individual to the next sequence to avoid overtraining. Unused ports in a session were covered to reduce the probability of incorrect responses. The final criterion for baseline task acquisition was chosen from prior experience of the ability of unlesioned rats to achieve this level of performance.

ports quickly, in one or two sessions. In this experiment, most animals also generalized quickly, although two did not; one of the naïve and one of the sham group did not generalize and never did learn the task within the maximum number of sessions.

In the remaining sequences (third sequence through baseline), the animals must learn to perform the task with increasing speed and efficiency in response to progressively shorter stimulus durations; 1 naïve rat and 2 sham-lesioned rats were unable to succeed in this. However, 10 of the 14 CBF rats did not succeed. Half of the CBF group passed the sixth sequence, but only four of these were able to perform to criterion in the baseline sequence. The largest source of the difference in response among these groups was that the CBF-lesioned animals had a much greater number of omissions (no response to stimulus) compared with the other groups, although their accuracy in responding correctly *when they responded* was as good (for 11 of the 14) as that of animals in the other groups (Table 5). (Performance was determined by percentage correct, which included all trials within a session.) The sham group also showed significantly more omissions than the naïve group, although it was not nearly as severe as that shown by CBF-lesioned animals.

It must be concluded that the CBF-lesioned rats were able to learn the initial associations, generalize from one to five ports, but were not able to perform this procedure quickly and correctly. Motor impairment, lack of motivation, or inadequate attentional focus could account for this result.

Table 4
Acquisition of the Five-Choice SRT Task (Number of Sessions to Criterion)

Group	*n*	Mean ± SEM	Range	Mean rank	Number failing criterion
Naïve	15	42.3 ± 3.9	26–75	15.7	2
Sham-lesion	15	47.1 ± 4.1	31–75	19.2	3
192 IgG-sap	14	68.4 ± 3.2	38–75	33.3	10

Criterion was set at 85% correct responses in the baseline SRT sequence. The maximum number of sessions allowed was 75. Animals that did not make this criterion were assigned the ceiling value of 75. The 192 IgG-sap group was significantly impaired in learning the task compared with each of the other groups ($p < 0.0167$). (Overall comparisons were made using a nonparametric Kruskal–Wallis one-way ANOVA; $p = 0.0004$, H = 15.567, corrected for ties. Between-group comparisons were made with the Mann–Whitney U test with the α significance level adjusted to $p < 0.0167$.)

SEM, standard error of the mean.

Further testing in this study included a session in which the duration of intertrial interval (ITI) was variably lengthened (4.5–9 s). This challenged the animals' timing expectations, reduced the frequency of trials and thereby lessened the degree of vigilance required. We found that, in this session, the CBF-lesioned group had a higher number of premature responses (during the ITI). This was not unexpected because they have more time to make premature responses. The length of the ITI duration correlated positively with the amount of premature responding for all three groups, but the CBF-lesioned rats made significantly more premature nose pokes than either sham or naïve rats. If the lesioned rats were not motivated or if they were motor-impaired, we would not have seen this increased responding during the ITI. The amount of perseverative responding (repeated nose-poking after a correct response) was unchanged. This evidence supports our conclusion that motor or motivational impairments were not significant contributors to the lesion effect and that attentional impairement was a major behavioral aspect of the CBF lesion produced by intraparenchymally infused 192 lgG-sap.

PHYSIOLOGICAL STUDIES

Methods of Lesion Assessment

Throughout the experiments in which rats were lesioned with 192 IgG-sap and in past studies using excitotoxins, we have assessed the lesions by histology and/or postmortem, homogenate ChAT activity from relevant brain regions. As stated previously, the latter assay is performed to quantify the loss

Table 5
Performance of Five-Choice SRT Baseline Sequence

	Naïve ($n = 15$)	Sham ($n = 15$)	192 IgG-sap ($n = 11$)
Percentage accuracy	93.2 ± 0.6	94.0 ± 0.6	90.1 ± 1.2
Percentage omissions	15.5 ± 1.1	21.2 ± 1.5[a]	38.9 ± 2.7[b]

[a]Significantly different from naïve.
[b]Significantly different from both naïve and sham.
Four daily sessions of the baseline sequence were conducted subsequent to a rat attaining 90% accuracy within a single session on the baseline sequence. (Three lesioned animals were unable to achieve this.) Shown are the means for all four sessions combined plus or minus the standard error of the mean. Accuracy is the percentage correct of all trials in a session excluding omissions. Omissions are the percentage of trials with no response of all trials in a session.

of cholinergic terminals relative to controls. However, there are some indications from work done by others that cholinergic lesions may induce greater in vivo ChAT activity in cholinergic terminals that survive a lesion without affecting the expression of ChAT. That is, the in vivo production of ACh may increase under the circumstances of a cholinergic lesion, although the amount of ChAT present in the terminals does not change *(65,66)*. The effect of this would be an overestimate of the degree of lesion by homogenate ChAT activity compared to what actually occurs at cholinergic synapses.

To test this possibility, we used in vivo microdialysis, homogenate ChAT activity, and the in vivo synthetic rate of ACh production as independent measures of the extent of a cholinergic lesion produced by icv administration of 192 IgG-sap *(67)*. Frontal cortex and hippocampus were chosen for lesion assessment measurements, representing terminal fields of the two extreme ends of the CBF system.

Dialysate samples were quantified by high-pressure liquid chromatography. The rate of ACh synthesis was determined by intravenous injection of deuterated choline into the rat and sacrifice 1 min later by focused-beam microwave irradiation of the head. Gas chromatography/mass spectrometry was then employed to quantify the amounts of labeled and unlabeled choline and ACh *(68)*. Postmortem ChAT activity was measured by incorporation of [^{14}C]acetyl Co-A into [^{14}C]acetylcholine *(26)*, normalized to homogenate protein concentration *(69)*.

At 1 and 15 wk postlesion, microdialysis was conducted on lesioned and sham-lesioned rats in the frontal cortex and lateral hippocampus. Assessment of the ACh synthesis rate was done at 16 wk. ChAT activity had to be determined from different animals given the same toxin and control treatments. ChAT activity was also assessed at 1 and 15 wk postlesion.

Table 6
Lesion Assessments (Percentage of Sham)

	ChAT activity	ACh synthesis rate	Microdialysis
Frontal cortex			
8 mg 192 IgG-sap	28.2 ± 1.9	33.9 ± 6.4[a]	8.4 ± 8
6 mg 192 IgG-sap	32.7 ± 3.5	35.3 ± 6.4	
Saporin (control)	103 ± 0.8	98 ± 14	
Hippocampus			
8 mg 192 IgG-sap	19.4 ± 6.1	38.5 ± 4.5[b]	33.7 ± 21
6 mg 192 IgG-sap	26.8 ± 7.2	75.8 ± 11[b]	
Saporin (control)	101 ± 2	98 ± 14	

[a]ACh synthesis rate was significantly higher than results from microdialysis ($p = 0.0087$, Scheffe post hoc test).

[b]ACh synthesis rate was significantly higher than ChAT activity. Two-way ANOVA: lesion group by method, significant effects of method [$F(1,28) = 13.85, p = 0.0009$] and lesion group [$F(2,28) = 30.3, p = 0.0001$] *(67)*.

ChAT activity and microdialysis were measured 15 wk postlesion in separate groups of animals. ACh synthesis rates were measured 16 wk postlesion in the animals subjected to microdialysis. Saporin (1.8 µg, equivalent to the saporin in 8 µg of immunotoxin), unconjugated to antibody, was given as a control for nonspecific effects of the toxin. Means plus or minus the standard error of the mean.

ChAT activity was compared to in vivo microdialysis of ACh in both the frontal cortex and the hippocampus of rats given the same surgical treatment (8 µg icv 192 IgG-sap, from a batch of toxin with much less potency, or PBS) at 1 wk postlesion. At this time-point the percentages relative to sham lesion were the same for both methods of measurement in both brain regions *(67)*.

At the longer postlesion time, all three measurements and two doses (6 and 8 µg) of 192 IgG-sap were compared (Table 6). At the high dose of immunotoxin, in frontal cortex the lesion assessment from microdialysis was significantly lower than that obtained from the rate of ACh synthesis. ChAT activity was not significantly different from either the rate of ACh synthesis ($p = 0.719$) or microdialysis ($p = 0.0674$). Results from the ChAT assay and the rate of ACh synthesis were also statistically indistinguishable both at the low dose of immunotoxin ($p = 0.755$) and with the nonselective toxin, saporin ($p = 0.564$). (The unconjugated saporin infusion had no effect on these measures of cholinergic activity compared to the sham-lesioned group in either frontal cortex or hippocampus.)

In hippocampus, however, for both doses of 192 IgG-sap, results from ChAT activity underestimated the available ACh as determined by the rate of ACh synthesis. Microdialysis results for the high dose of immunotoxin were not significantly different from either of the other two measures (one-way analysis of variance [ANOVA], $p = 0.9697$ vs ACh synthesis rate; $p = 0.7117$ vs ChAT activity). The high variability of the microdialysis measurements was at least partly because we did not use inhibitors of acetylcholinesterase in our dialysis medium to maintain realistic physiological conditions.

Thus, cholinergic terminals in the hippocampus that survived immunotoxic lesion by 192 IgG-sap compensated for the lesion by increased synthesis of ACh. Surviving terminals in the frontal cortex did not compensate in the same way. Hippocampal compensation was greatest in the group that received the low dose of immunotoxin and therefore had a greater residual level of cholinergic terminals. This study was in accord with others that suggested that cellular mechanisms for compensation after cholinergic neuron loss can differ depending on tissue type or brain region. Differences also are likely to depend on the method and degree of cholinergic terminal loss *(65,66,70–74)*. (Despite this finding, we—and others—continue to use ChAT activity, paired frequently with histology, to assess lesions because of its reliability and ease of use compared to the other two methods tested.)

Cholinergic Effects on Cerebral Blood Flow

The nucleus basalis, especially the cholinergic neurons originating in this region and projecting to the cerebral cortex, had been implicated by a number of studies *(75,76,77)* in the regulation of regional cerebral blood flow. Uncertainties remained, however, mainly because of the absence of effects from excitotoxic lesions of the nucleus basalis *(78–81)*. We hypothesized that lesions produced by the more selective 192 IgG-sap might give clearer results than excitotoxic lesions with their associated destruction of GABA-ergic neurons *(82)*. The experiment was designed to test not only changes in cortical blood flow subsequent to a bilateral CBF lesion, but also the effect of intravenous physostigmine on the resulting blood flow measurements *(83)*.

Rats were given bilateral icv infusions of 3.6 µg (total) of 192 IgG-sap, with PBS infusions as controls. At 6–8 wk postlesion, 4.2 µg/kg-min of physostigmine or saline were infused through a venous catheter for 50 min. Cerebral blood flow was determined by quantitative iodo-^{14}C-antipyrine autoradiography, with a 30-s infusion (100 µCi/kg in 0.6 mL) at the end of the 50-min period *(83,84)*. Cerebral blood flow in 154 cortical regions per brain was quantitated (eight coronal brain slices, 18–24 regions per slice). ChAT activity was determined from cortical tissue adjacent to areas assessed for cerebral blood flow.

ChAT activity in four neocortical areas was decreased 80–84% in lesioned animals. The highest regional cortical blood flow in controls was in the left medial temporal lobe, extending into the right posterior parietal lobe. The effect of the lesion was evident with a global decrease of cortical blood flow, the greatest decrease in regions where cerebral blood flow was highest in control animals, particularly the temporal cortex *(83)*.

The systemic physostigmine infusion significantly increased cortical blood flow as expected. The increase was greatest in those areas already having heightened blood flow. The overall cortical area of heightened blood flow induced by physostigmine infusion was larger in comparison to the unlesioned saline-infused control animals. Cortices from lesioned animals given physostigmine also had increased blood flow, also concentrated in the areas of the temporal and posterior parietal lobes and over a larger area. The increase caused by physostigmine in lesioned animals was generally not as great, however, as that in unlesioned brains treated with physostigmine. Overall, the effect of the physostigmine infusion on lesioned rats tended to bring blood flow up to levels observed in unlesioned rats without physostigmine treatment. Cortical regions that were least affected by the immunotoxic lesion, such as entorhinal cortex (about 40% ChAT decrease), produced no detectable reduction in blood flow and no elevation for either group treated with physostigmine *(83)*. These regions also had low cerebral blood flow levels in all groups. The elevation of cerebral blood flow observed in lesioned animals treated with physostigmine did not parallel the degree of lesion measured by ChAT activity, but the long infusion of the cholinesterase inhibitor might be expected to increase and build up synaptic ACh levels at residual terminals. The possibility of an underestimate of in vivo synaptic levels of ACh by assessments based on homogenate ChAT activity may also be relevant in this experiment.

These results confirmed conclusions based on other methods that the neurons of the CBF are involved in directing cerebral blood flow to focal cortical regions *(85–89)*. The spatial pattern of lesion-induced reduction in cortical blood flow resembled the observed cortical blood flow reduction found patients with Alzheimer's disease *(90–92)*. Thus, the immunotoxic lesion produced in rats convincingly models at least this aspect of the effects of cholinergic degeneration found in the human disease state.

SUMMARY

What have we learned from the use of 192 IgG-sap in rats? Spatial learning and memory as defined by the standard water maze paradigm were relatively unaffected by CBF degeneration. Although a number of studies detected significant cognitive impairment in this task subsequent to intracerebroventricularly induced lesions, further work by many investigators has convincingly demonstrated what was beginning to be suspected from the excitotoxin studies: Rats with massive, but selective, loss of CBF neurons can learn and perform the water maze task as well as controls.

This is not to say that there are no cognitive deficits resulting from this lesion. Other types of tests did find impairments in specific behaviors. Certain aspects of attentional behavior and other types of learning tasks were demonstrably impaired in rats given the selective immunotoxic lesion. Behavioral studies describing cognitive impairments continue to mount, begging for some generalizable, underlying principle to integrate the diverse findings (*see* ref. *93*).

How well does the CBF lesion in rats support the cholinergic hypothesis of Alzheimer's disease? One of the problems inherent in the cholinergic hypothesis is that it is too simple. Alzheimer's disease has never been a disease of only basal forebrain cholinergic neurons. This hypothesis was developed because it seemed that the cholinergic innervation of the cortex and hippocampus in Alzheimer's disease was perhaps the first system to deteriorate in the disease. The cholinergic hypothesis was always only one of a number of hypotheses proposed by researchers and clinicians seeking a clue to the etiology of this disease. Certainly, there are aspects of an extensive CBF lesion in rats that appear to reproduce some clinical symptoms of Alzheimer's disease accurately. One should never underestimate the possibility that one of these symptoms, expressed in an animal model, might be useful as an appropriate medium to develop therapeutic interventions.

For those focused on understanding how a part of the brain functions in behavior and physiology, the investigation of the cholinergic hypothesis has produced intriguing new knowledge, although we remain a long way from comprehensive understanding. The pathway toward understanding, however, is frequently dependent on the creative development of better tools, one of which is the immunotoxin 192 IgG-saporin.

REFERENCES

1. Whitehouse PJ, Price DL, Clark AW, Coyle JT, DeLong MR. Alzheimer disease: evidence for selective loss of cholinergic neurons in the nucleus basalis. Ann Neurol 1981;10:122–126.
2. Perry EK, Tomlinson BE, Blessed G, Bergmann K, Gibson PH, Perry RH. Correlation of cholinergic abnormalities with senile plaques and mental test scores in senile dementia. Br Med J 1978;25:1457–1459.
3. Bigl V, Woolf NJ, Butcher LL. Cholinergic projections from the basal forebrain to frontal, parietal, temporal, occipital, and cingulate cortices: a com-

bined fluorescent tracer and acetylcholinesterase analysis. Brain Res Bull 1982;8:727–749.

 4. Mesulam M-M, Mufson EJ, Wainer BH, Levey AI. Central cholinergic pathways in the rat: an overview based on an alternative nomenclature. Neuroscience 1983;10:1185–1201.

 5. Dekker AJAM, Connor DJ, Thal LJ. The role of cholinergic projections from the nucleus basalis in memory. Neurosci Biobehav Rev 1991;15:299–317.

 6. Choi DW. Excitotoxic cell death. J Neurobiol 1992;23:1261–1276.

 7. Dunnett SB, Whishaw IQ, Jones GH, Bunch ST. Behavioural, biochemical and histochemical effects of different neurotoxic amino acids injected into nucleus basalis magnocellularis of rats. Neuroscience 1987;20:653–669.

 8. Lindefors N, Boatell ML, Mahy N, Persson H. Widespread neuronal degeneration after ibotenic acid lesioning of cholinergic neurons in the nucleus basalis revealed by *in situ* hybridization. Neurosci Lett 1992;135:262–264.

 9. Page KJ, Sirinathsinghji DJS, Everitt BJ. AMPA-induced lesions of the basal forebrain differentially affect cholinergic and non-cholinergic neurons: lesion assessment using quantitative *in situ* hybridization histochemistry. Eur J Neurosci 1995;7:1012–1021.

10. Gaal G, Potter PE, Hanin I, Kakucska I, Vizi ES. Effects of intracerebroventricular AF64A administration on cholinergic, serotoninergic and catecholaminergic circuitry in rat dorsal hippocampus. Neuroscience 1986;19:1197–1205.

11. Nakamura S, Tani Y, Maezono Y, Ishihara T, Ohno T. Learning deficits after unilateral AF64A lesions in the rat basal forebrain: role of cholinergic and noncholinergic systems. Pharmacol Biochem Behav 1992;42:119–130.

12. Meana JJ, Johansson B, Herrera-Marschitz M, et al. Effect of the neurotoxin AF64A on intrinsic and extrinsic neuronal systems of rat neostriatum measured by in vivo microdialysis. Brain Res 1992;596:65–72.

13. Wiley RG, Stirpe F, Thorpe P, Oeltmann TN. Neuronotoxic effects of monoclonal anti-Thy 1 antibody (OX7) coupled to the ribosome inactivating protein, saporin, as studied by suicide transport experiments in the rat. Brain Res 1989;505:44–54.

14. Contestabile A, Stirpe F. Ribosome-inactivation proteins from plants as agents for suicide transport and immunolesioning in the nervous system. Eur J Neurosci 1993;5:1292–1301.

15. Wiley RG, Oeltmann TN, Lappi DA. Immunolesioning: selective destruction of neurons using immunotoxin to rat NGF receptor. Brain Res 1991;562:149–153.

16. Stirpe F, Gasperi-Campani A, Barbieri L, Falasca A, Abbondanza A, Stevens WA. Ribosome-inactivating proteins from the seeds of *Saponaria officinalis* L. (soapwort), of *Agrostemma githago* L. (corn cockle) and of *Asparagus officinalis* L. (asparagus), and from the latex of *Hura crepitans* L. (sandbox tree). Biochem J 1983;216:617–625.

17. Lappi DA, Esch FS, Barbieri L, Stirpe F, Soria M. Characterization of a *Saponaria officinalis* seed ribosome-inactivating protein: immunoreactivity and sequence homologies. Biochem Biophys Res Commun 1985;129:934–942.

18. Taniuchi M, Johnson EM Jr. Characterization of the binding properties and retrograde axonal transport of a monoclonal antibody directed against the rat nerve growth factor receptor. J Cell Biol 1985;101:1100–1106.
19. Schweitzer JB. Nerve growth factor receptor-mediated transport from CSF labels cholinergic neurons: direct demonstration by a double-labeling study. Brain Res 1989;490:390–396.
20. Schweitzer JB. Nerve growth factor receptor-mediated transport from cerebrospinal fluid to basal forebrain neurons. Brain Res 1987;423:309–317.
21. Stirpe F, Bailey S, Miller SP, Bodley JW. Modification of ribosomal RNA by ribosome-inactivating proteins from plants. Nucleic Acids Res 1988;16:1349–1357.
22. Davis TL, Wiley RG. Anti-Thy-1 immunotoxin, OX7-saporin, destroys cerebellar Purkinje cells after intraventricular injection in rats. Brain Res 1989;504:216–222.
23. Gonzalez AM, Lappi DA, Buscaglia ML, Carman LS, Gage FH, Baird A. Basic FGF-SAP mitotoxin in the hippocampus. Specific lethal effect on cells expressing the basic FGF receptor. Ann NY Acad Sci 1991;638:442–444.
24. Lappi DA, Martineau D, Baird A. Biological and chemical characterization of basic FGF-saporin mitotoxin. Biochem Biophys Res Commun 1989;160:917–923.
25. Waite JJ, Wardlow ML, Chen AC, Lappi DA, Wiley RG, Thal LJ. Time course of cholinergic and monoaminergic changes in rat brain after immunolesioning with 192 IgG-saporin. Neurosci Lett 1994;169:154–158.
26. Fonnum F. Radiochemical microassays for the determination of choline acetyltransferase and acetylcholinesterase activities. J Biochem 1969;115:465–479.
27. Waite JJ, Chen AD, Wardlow ML, Thal LJ. Behavioral and biochemical consequences of combined lesions of the medial septum/diagonal band and nucleus basalis in the rat when ibotenic acid, quisqualic acid, and AMPA are used. Exp Neurol 1994;130:214–229.
28. Nilsson OG, Leanza G, Rosenblad C, Lappi DA, Wiley RG, Björklund A. Spatial learning impairments in rats with selective immunolesion of the forebrain cholinergic system. NeuroReport 1992;3:1005–1008.
29. Book AA, Wiley RG, Schweitzer JB. Specificity of 192 IgG-saporin for NGF receptor-positive cholinergic basal forebrain neurons in the rat. Brain Res 1992;590:350–355.
30. Waite JJ, Chen AD, Wardlow ML, Wiley RG, Lappi DA, Thal LJ. 192 immunoglobulin G-saporin produces graded behavioral and biochemical changes accompanying the loss of cholinergic neurons of the basal forebrain and cerebellar Purkinje cells. Neuroscience 1995;65:463–476.
31. Walsh TJ, Kelly RM, Dougherty KD, Stackman RW, Wiley RG, Kutscher CL. Behavioral and neurobiological alterations induced by the immunotoxin 192-IgG-saporin: cholinergic and non-cholinergic effects following icv injection. Brain Res 1995;702:233–245.
32. Lee MG, Chrobak JJ, Sik A, Wiley RG, Buzsáki G. Hippocampal theta activity following selective lesion of the septal cholinergic system. Neuroscience 1994;62:1033–1047.

33. Torres EM, Perry TA, Blokland A, et al. Behavioural, histochemical, and biochemical consequences of selective immunolesions in discrete regions of the basal forebrain cholinergic system. Neuroscience 1994;63:95–122.

34. Heckers S, Ohtake T, Wiley FG, Lappi DA, Geula C, Mesulam MM. Complete and selective cholinergic denervation of rat neocortex and hippocampus but not amygdala by an immunotoxin against the p75 NGF receptor. J Neurosci 1994;14:1271–1289.

35. Berger-Sweeney J, Heckers S, Mesulam MM, Wiley RG, Lappi DA, Sharma M. Differential effects on spatial navigation of immunotoxin-induced cholinergic lesions of the medial septal area and nucleus basalis magnocellularis. J Neurosci 1994;14:4507–4519.

36. Wenk GL, Stoehr JD, Quintana G, Mobley S, Wiley RG. Behavioral, biochemical, histological, and electrophysiological effects of 192 IgG-saporin injections into the basal forebrain of rats. J Neurosci 1994;14:5986–5995.

37. Wiley RG. Neural lesioning with ribosome-inactivating proteins: suicide transport and immunolesioning. Trends Neurosci 1992;15:285–290.

38. Waite JJ, Wardlow ML, Power AE. Attention deficit associated with cholinergic basal forebrain immunotoxin lesion produced by 192-saporin; motoric/sensory deficit associated with Purkinje cell immunotoxic lesion produced by OX7-saporin. Neurobiol Learn Mem 1999;71:325–352.

39. Holley LA, Wiley RG, Lappi DA, Sarter M. Cortical cholinergic deafferentation following the intracortical infusion of 192 IgG-saporin: a quantitative histochemical study. Brain Res 1994;663:277–286.

40. Steckler T, Keith AB, Wiley RG, Sahgal A. Cholinergic lesions by 192 IgG-saporin and short-term recognition memory: role of the septohippocampal projection. Neuroscience 1995;66:101–114.

41. Ohtake T, Heckers S, Wiley RG, Lappi DA, Mesulam MM, Geula C. Retrograde degeneration and colchicine protection of basal forebrain cholinergic neurons following hippocampal injections of an immunotoxin against the P75 nerve growth factor receptor. Neuroscience 1997;78:123–133.

42. Winkler J, Connor DJ, Frautschy SA, et al. Lack of long-term effects after β-amyloid protein injections in rat brain. Neurobiol Aging 1994;15:601–607.

43. Dougherty KD, Salat D, Walsh TJ. Intraseptal injection of the cholinergic immunotoxin 192-IgG saporin fails to disrupt latent inhibition in a conditioned taste aversion paradigm. Brain Res 1996;736:260–269.

44. Bannon AW, Curzon P, Gunther KL, Decker MW. Effects of intraseptal injection of 192-IgG-saporin in mature and aged Long-Evans rats. Brain Res 1996;718:25–36.

45. McGaughy J, Kaiser T, Sarter M. Behavioral vigilance following infusions of 192 IgG-saporin into the basal forebrain: selectivity of the behavioral impairment and relation to cortical AChE-positive fiber density. Behav Neurosci 1996;110:247–265.

46. Chiba AA, Bucci DJ, Holland PC, Gallagher M. Basal forebrain cholinergic lesions disrupt increments but not decrements in conditioned stimulus processing. J Neurosci 1995;15:7315–7322.

47. Pizzo DP, Waite JJ, Thal LJ, Winkler J. Intraparenchymal infusions of 192 IgG-saporin: development of a method for selective and discrete lesioning of cholinergic basal forebrain nuclei. J Neurosci Methods 1999;91:9–19.
48. Baxter MG, Bucci DJ, Gorman LK, Wiley RG, Gallagher M. Selective immunotoxic lesions of basal forebrain cholinergic cells: effects on learning and memory in rats. Behav Neurosci 1995;109:714–722.
49. Bartus RT, Dean RL, Pontecorvo MJ, Flicker C. The cholinergic hypothesis: a historical overview, current perspective, and future directions. Ann NY Acad Sci 1985;444:332–358.
50. Dunnett SB, Everitt BJ, Robbins TW. The basal forebrain-cortical cholinergic system: interpreting the functional consequences of excitotoxic lesions. Trends Neurosci 1991;14:494–501.
51. Winkler J, Ramirez GA, Thal LJ, Waite JJ. Nerve growth factor (NGF) augments cortical and hippocampal cholinergic functioning after p 75 NGF receptor-mediated deafferentation but impairs inhibitory avoidance and induces fear-related behavior. J Neurosci 2000;20:834–844.
52. Baxter MG, Gallagher M. Intact spatial learning in both young and aged rats following selective removal of hippocampal cholinergic input. Behav Neurosci 1996;110:460–467.
53. Dornan WA, McCampbell AR, Tinkler GP, et al. Comparison of site-specific injections into the basal forebrain on water maze and radial arm maze performance in the male rat after immunolesioning with 192 IgG-saporin. Behav Brain Res 1996;82:247–265.
54. Pizzo DP, Thal LJ, Winkler J. Mnemonic deficits in animals depend upon the degree of cholinergic deficit and task complexity. Exp Neurol 2002;177:292–305.
55. Sahakian BJ, Owen AM, Morant NJ, et al. Further analysis of the cognitive effects of tetrahydroaminoacridine (THA) in Alzheimer's disease: assessment of attentional and mnemonic function using CANTAB. Psychopharmacology 1993;110:395–401.
56. Carli M, Robbins TW, Evenden JL, Everitt BJ. Effects of lesions to ascending noradrenergic neurones on performance of a 5-choice serial reaction task in rats; implications for theories of dorsal noradrenergic bundle function based on selective attention and arousal. Behav Brain Res 1983;9:361–380.
57. Robbins TW, Everitt BJ, Marston HM, Wilkinson J, Jones GH, Page KJ. Comparative effects of ibotenic acid- and quisqualic acid-induced lesions of the substantia innominata on attentional function in the rat: further implications for the role of the cholinergic neurons of the nucleus basalis in cognitive processes. Behav Brain Res 1989;35:221–240.
58. Muir JL, Everitt BJ, Robbins TW. Reversal of visual attentional dysfunction following lesions of the cholinergic basal forebrain by physostigmine and nicotine but not by the 5-HT3 receptor antagonist, ondansetron. Psychopharmacology 1995;118:82–92.
59. Turchi J, Sarter M. Cortical acetylcholine and processing capacity: effects of cortical cholinergic deafferentation on crossmodal divided attention in rats. Brain Res Cogn Brain Res 1997;6:147–158.

60. Baxter MG, Holland PC, Gallagher M. Disruption of decrements in conditioned stimulus processing by selective removal of hippocampal cholinergic input. J Neurosci 1997;17:5230–5236.
61. Baxter MG, Bucci DJ, Holland PC, Gallagher M. Impairments in conditioned stimulus processing and conditioned responding after combined selective removal of hippocampal and neocortical cholinergic input. Behav Neurosci 1999;113:486–495.
62. Zhang ZJ, Berbos TG, Wrenn CC, Wiley RG. Loss of nucleus basalis magnocellularis, but not septal, cholinergic neurons correlates with passive avoidance impairment in rats treated with 192-saporin. Neurosci Lett 1996;203:214–218.
63. Waite JJ, Wardlow ML, Power AE. Deficit in selective and divided attention associated with cholinergic basal forebrain immunotoxic lesion produced by 192-saporin; motoric/sensory deficit associated with Purkinje cell immunotoxic lesion produced by OX7-saporin. Neurobiol Learn Mem 1999;71:325–352.
64. Gandhi CC, Kelly RM, Wiley RG, Walsh TJ. Impaired acquisition of a Morris water maze task following selective destruction of cerebellar Purkinje cells with OX7-saporin. Behav Brain Res 2000;109:37–47.
65. Roßner S, Yu J, Pizzo D, et al. Effects of intraventricular transplantation of NGF-secreting cells on cholinergic basal forebrain neurons after partial immunolesion. J Neurosci Res 1996;45:40–56.
66. Lapchak PA, Jenden DJ, Hefti F. Compensatory elevation of acetylcholine synthesis in vivo by cholinergic neurons surviving partial lesions of the septohippocampal pathway. J Neurosci 1991;11:2821–2828.
67. Waite JJ, Chen AD. Differential changes in rat cholinergic parameters subsequent to immunotoxic lesion of the basal forebrain nuclei. Brain Res 2001;918:113–120.
68. Jenden DJ, Choi L, Silverman RW, Steinborn JA, Roch M, Booth RA. Acetylcholine turnover estimation in brain by gas chromatography/mass spectrometry. Life Sci 1974;14:55–63.
69. Lowry OH, Rosebrough NJ, Farr AL, Randall RJ. Protein measurement with the Folin phenol reagent. J Biol Chem 1951;193:265–275.
70. Leanza G, Nilsson OG, Bjorklund A. Compensatory changes of in vivo acetylcholine and noradrenaline release in the hippocampus after partial deafferentation, as monitored by microdialysis. Brain Res 1993;615:147–159.
71. Lapchak PA, Araujo DM, Pasinetti G, Hefti F. Differential alterations of cortical cholinergic and neurotensin markers following ibotenic acid lesions of the nucleus basalis magnocellularis. Brain Res 1993;613:239–246.
72. Wenk GL, Olton DS. Recovery of neocortical choline acetyltransferase activity following ibotenic acid injection into the nucleus basalis of Meynert in rats. Brain Res 1984;293:184–186.
73. Watson M, Vickroy TW, Fibiger HC, Roeske WR, Yamamura HI. Effects of bilateral ibotenate-induced lesions of the nucleus basalis magnocellularis upon selective cholinergic biochemical markers in the rat anterior cerebral cortex. Brain Res 1985;346:387–391.

74. Vickroy TW, Watson M, Leventer SM, Roeske WR, Hanin I, Yamamura HI. Regional differences in ethylcholine mustard aziridinium ion (AF64A)-induced deficits in presynaptic cholinergic markers for the rat central nervous system. J Pharmacol Exp Ther 1985;235:577–582.
75. Scremin OU, Rovere AA, Raynald AC, Giardini A. Cholinergic control of blood flow in the cerebral cortex of the rat. Stroke 1973;4:232–239.
76. Biesold D, Inannami O, Sato A, Sato Y. Stimulation of the nucleus basalis of Meynert increases cerebral cortical blood flow in rats. Neurosci Lett 1989;98:39–44.
77. Lacombe P, Sercombe R, Verrecchia C, Philipson V, MacKenzie ET, Seylaz J. Cortical blood flow increases induced by stimulation of the substantia innominata in the unanesthetized rat. Brain Res 1989;491:1–14.
78. Scremin OU, Torres C, Scremin AME, O'Neal M, Heuser D, Blisard KS. Role of nucleus basalis in cholinergic control of cortical blood flow. J Neurosci Res 1991;28:382–390.
79. Santos-Benito FF, Gonzalez JL, de la Torre F. Choline acetyltransferase activity in the rat brain cortex homogenate, synaptosomes, and capillaries after lesioning the nucleus basalis magnocellularis. J Neurochem 1988;50:395–399.
80. Namba H, Irie T, Fukushi K, Yamasaki T, Tateno Y, Hasegawa S. Lesion of the nucleus basalis magnocellularis does not affect cerebral cortical blood flow in rats. Neurosci Res 1991;12:463–467.
81. Peruzzi P, Lacombe P, Moro V, Vaucher E, Levy F, Seylaz J. The cerebrovascular effects of physostigmine are not mediated through the substantia innominata. Exp Neurol 1993;122:319–326.
82. Barbelivien A, Noel C, MacKenzie ET, Dauphin F. Cerebrovascular evidence for a GABAergic modulation of the cholinergic vasodilatatory basalocortical system in the rat. Brain Res 1999;834:223–227.
83. Waite JJ, Holschneider DP, Scremin OU. Selective immunotoxin-induced cholinergic deafferentiation alters blood flow distribution in the cerebral cortex. Brain Res 1999;818:1–11.
84. Sakurada O, Kennedy C, Jehle J, Brown JD, Carbin GL, Sokoloff L. Measurement of local cerebral blood flow with iodo[^{14}C]antipyrine. Am J Physiol Heart Circ Physiol 1978;3:H59–H66.
85. Nakai M, Ogata J, Fukui K, Nakai Y, Maeda M. Basal forebrain and cerebral cortical muscarinic receptors mediate increase in cortical blood flow provoked by periaqueductal gray matter. Neuroscience 1997;79:571–579.
86. Vaucher E, Borredon J, Seylaz J, Lacombe P. Autoradiographic distribution of cerebral blood flow increases elicited by stimulation of the nucleus basalis magnocellularis in the unanesthetized rat. Brain Res 1995;691:57–68.
87. Chedotal A, Umbriaco D, Descarries L, Hartman BK, Hamel E. Light and electron microscopic immunocytochemical analysis of the neurovascular relationships of choline acetyltransferase and vasoactive intestinal polypeptide nerve terminals in the rat cerebral cortex. J Comp Neurol 1994;343:57–71.
88. Elhusseiny A, Cohen Z, Olivier A, Stanimirovic D, Hamel E. Functional acetylcholine muscarinic receptor subtypes in human brain microcirculation: identification and cellular localization. J Cereb Blood Flow Metab 1999;19:794–802.

89. Sato A, Sato Y. Cholinergic neural regulation of regional cerebral blood flow. Alzheimer Dis Assoc Disord 1995;9:28–38.
90. Mielke R, Schroder R, Fink GR, Kessler J, Herholz K, Heiss W-D. Regional cerebral glucose metabolism and postmortem pathology in Alzheimer's disease. Acta Neuropathol 1996;91:174–179.
91. Hirsch C, Bartenstien P, Minoshima S, et al. Reduction of regional cerebral blood flow and cognitive impairment in patients with Alzheimer's disease: evaluation of an observer-independent analytic approach. Dementia Geriatr Cogn Disord 1997;8:98–104.
92. Herholz K, Bauer B, Wienhard K, et al. In-vivo measurements of regional acetylcholine esterase activity in degenerative dementia: comparison with blood flow and glucose metabolism. J Neural Transm 2000;107:1457–1468.
93. Butt AE, Bowman TD. Transverse patterning reveals a dissociation of simple and configural association learning abilities in rats with 192 IgG-saporin lesions of the nucleus basalis magnocellularis. Neurobiol Learn Mem 2002;77:211–233.

4

Basal Forebrain Cholinergic Lesion by 192 IgG-Saporin

A Tool to Assess the Consequences of Cortical Cholinergic Dysfunction in Alzheimer's Disease

Reinhard Schliebs

INTRODUCTION

Alzheimer's disease, the most common neurodegenerative disorder causing senile dementia, is characterized by two major morphopathological hallmarks. The deposition of extracellular neuritic, β-amyloid peptide-containing plaques (senile plaques) in hippocampal and cerebral cortical regions of patients with Alzheimer's disease is accompanied by the presence of intracellular neurofibrillary tangles that occupy much of the cytoplasm of particular pyramidal neurons.

Another hallmark of Alzheimer's disease is a progressive neuronal cell loss associated with region-specific brain atrophy. In particular, the cholinergic projection from the nucleus basalis of Meynert to areas of the cerebral cortex is the pathway that is very early and most severely affected in brains from those with Alzheimer's disease. A number of studies have demonstrated that the learning and memory deficits observed in patients with Alzheimer's disease are caused at least partly by the progressive loss of basal forebrain cholinergic neurons, which led to the cholinergic hypothesis of geriatric memory dysfunction *(1,2)*. For reviews, *see* refs. *3–5*.

Massive loss of basal forebrain cholinergic neurons was demonstrated by reductions in number of cholinergic markers such as choline acetyltransferase, muscarinic and nicotinic acetylcholine receptor binding, as well as levels of acetylcholine. In particular, the activity of choline acetyl transferase is highly

From: *Molecular Neurosurgery With Targeted Toxins*
Edited by: R. G. Wiley and D. A. Lappi © Humana Press Inc., Totowa, NJ

correlated with the clinical dementia ratings across the neocortex of patients with Alzheimer's disease *(6)*.

However, impaired cortical cholinergic neurotransmission may also contribute to β-amyloid plaque pathology in Alzheimer's disease. This has been evidenced by a number of studies in vitro and in vivo that demonstrated cholinergic control of expression and processing of the β-amyloid precursor protein (APP; *7–15*). The basal forebrain cholinergic system also plays a role in regulation of cerebral cortical blood flow mediated by activation of cholinergic receptors and nitric oxide (NO)-related mechanisms and affects cerebral cortical glucose utilization, which may contribute to the impaired cerebral glucose metabolism observed in Alzheimer's disease.

However, it is still unclear how cognitive deficits, basal forebrain cholinergic cell loss, energy dysfunction, and β-amyloid formation and deposition are interrelated in the pathogenesis of Alzheimer's disease. To address this question, adequate animal approaches are required to produce specific cholinergic deficits in vivo. These would allow detailed evaluation of the neurochemical, neuropathological, and behavioral sequela, as well as functional implications of plastic repair mechanisms following cholinergic hypofunction and provide information that cannot be or can only partially be obtained in humans.

Lesions of the cholinergic basal forebrain complex result in a cortical cholinergic denervation and have been exploited in a number of studies to produce an animal model to mimic dysfunctions of cortical cholinergic neurotransmission; for review, *see* the work of Härtig et al. *(16)*, for instance. Because of the unique topographical organization of the basal forebrain cholinergic system, cholinergic lesion studies face a number of difficulties to selectively and specifically destroy the cholinergic neurons giving rise to the cholinergic basalo-cortical pathway: First, cholinergic cells in the basal forebrain do not comprise a distinct nucleus with sharp boundaries (e.g., like the locus coeruleus for noradrenergic cells), but they are distributed within a number of distinct forebrain nuclei, forming an irregular shaped band of neurons with both a rostral–caudal and ventral–dorsal extension. Second, the basal forebrain nuclei that comprise the cholinergic cell population also contain a variety of noncholinergic cells like γ-aminobutyric acid-(GABA), neuropeptides-, or glutamate-containing neurons intermingled with cholinergic ones. In addition, there are also noncholinergic fiber bundles passing through the basal forebrain in the neighborhood of cholinergic nuclei.

A large number of different experimental paradigms have been introduced to produce cholinergic deficits (*see*, e.g., Schliebs et al. *[17]*), comprising invasive procedures, such as mechanical or chemical destruction of cholinergic areas in the basal forebrain, interruption of hippocampal afferents by fimbria fornix transection *(18)*, or specific targeting of cholinergic cells by selective immunotoxins (*see*, e.g., refs. *19–21*). To destroy cholinergic cell populations chemically, various cytotoxins have been applied, including excitotoxins *(22)* and cholinotoxins *(23)*, a procedure limited by the selectivity and specificity of the toxins available. However, the introduction of the immunotoxin strategy *(24)* to lesion basal forebrain cholinergic neurons in a number of species with greater specificity and selectivity compared to excitotoxins *(19,25–27)* has led to a reassessment of the importance of the corticopetal cholinergic afferents in mediating cognitive function *(28)*. Moreover, the spatial separation between site of injection (ventricle) and area of neuronal degeneration (basal forebrain) allows the study of neurodegenerative events at the lesion site in the absence of any mechanical damage *(29–31)*.

This chapter summarizes the usefulness of the cholinergic immunotoxin 192 immunoglobulin G-saporin (192 IgG-sap) to produce cortical cholinergic dysfunction in rats and to study the interrelationship of basal forebrain cholinergic system with a number of physiological events that also play a role in the pathogenesis of Alzheimer's disease, including processing of the β-APP, glucose metabolism, cerebral blood flow, and NO- and inflammation-related mechanisms (Fig. 1).

192 IGG-SAP AS A USEFUL TOOL TO PRODUCE SPECIFIC AND SELECTIVE BASAL FOREBRAIN CHOLINERGIC CELL LOSS

In 1991, Wiley et al. *(32)* introduced a novel approach for neuronal lesioning using immunotargeting of unspecific cytotoxins to specific cell types. Cholinergic neurons of the basal forebrain possess low-affinity p75 nerve growth factor (NGF) receptors (p75NTR), whereas other neurons in this region, including the cholinergic cells in the nearby striatum, do not express detectable levels of p75NTR *(33,34)*. It was demonstrated that a well-characterized monoclonal antibody to p75NTR , 192 IgG, accumulates bilaterally exclusively in cholinergic neurons of the basal forebrain following intracerebroventricular administration *(35)*. Employing these properties of 192 IgG, an immunotoxin was developed by chemical linking of 192 IgG to the ribosome-inactivating protein saporin (192 IgG-sap) *(24)*.

Intracerebroventricular administration of 192 IgG-sap conjugate resulted in substantial reductions in the activity of choline acetyltransferase and acetylcholinesterase in widespread areas of the cortex and hippocampus and in

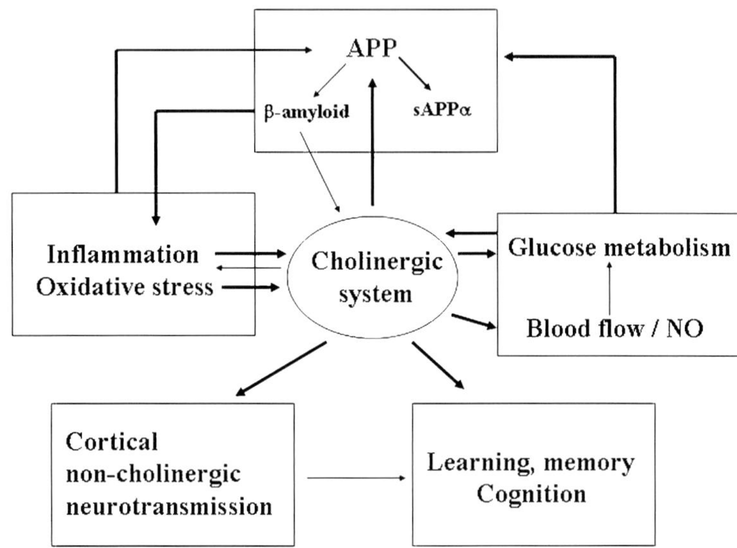

Fig. 1. Schematic depiction of interrelationships of the basal forebrain cholinergic system with expression and processing of the amyloid precursor protein (APP), glucose metabolism, blood flow, and NO-mediated processes, as well as cortical noncholinergic neurotransmission and degeneration-induced inflammation. As outlined in this chapter, dysfunction of basal forebrain cholinergic system produced by application of the cholinergic immunotoxin 192 IgG-sap results in impaired glucose metabolism and blood flow, increased processing of APP through the β-secretory, amyloidogenic pathway, in differentially altered noncholinergic cortical transmitter receptors, as well as in mild gliosis.

a nearly complete disappearance of choline acetyltransferase-positive, p75[NTR]-immunoreactive neurons in the medial septum, in both the vertical and horizontal limbs of the nucleus of the diagonal band of Broca, and in the nucleus basalis magnocellularis, whereas cholinergic interneurons in the striatum were not affected *(14,15,36–43)*. Moreover, a 40% decrease in m2 muscarinic receptor messenger ribonucleic acid (mRNA) in nuclei of the basal forebrain complex was observed after immunolesion, thus further emphasizing the loss of cholinergic cells *(40)*.

Noncholinergic septal neurons containing parvalbumin and noncholinergic substantia innominata neurons containing calbindin-D28k or nicotinamide adenine dinucleotide phosphate-diaphorase were not affected by 192 IgG-sap *(38)*. Similarly, the number of parvalbumin-containing GABA-ergic projection neurons in the septum-diagonal band of

Broca complex and nucleus basalis of Meynert was not reduced following intraventricular 192 IgG-sap application *(43–45)*. Moreover, 192 IgG-sap did not destroy neurotensin, galanin, somatostatin, or neuropeptide neurons within the basal forebrain *(46)*. Corresponding to the topographic location of cholinergic neurons in the basal forebrain, a dramatic increase in microglia has been demonstrated *(41,47)*, suggesting that the immunotoxin is lethal to cholinergic cells in the basal forebrain rather than suppressing the expression of cholinergic markers (e.g., choline acetyltransferase) in these cells *(48)*.

Selective lesions of septal hippocampal cholinergic neurons with 192 IgG-sap resulted in differential changes in cholinergic markers in cholinoceptive cortical target regions, including cholinergic receptors, choline uptake sites, vesicular acetylcholine transporter; acetylcholine release, muscarinic receptor coupling with G protein and phosphoinositide breakdown *(40,42,49,50)*.

The 192 IgG-sap affected two neuronal groups outside the basal forebrain that express p75[NTR]: NGF-reactive cerebellar Purkinje cells after intraventricular injection and cholinergic striatal interneurons after injections into the substantia innominata *(38)*. There are choline acetyltransferase-positive, but p75[NTR]-negative, neurons in the rat nucleus basalis-substantia innominata complex innervating the amygdala and parts of the rhinal paralimbic areas *(51,52)*, which are spared or only partially affected by the immunotoxin *(38)*. Similarly, cholinergic neurons in the ventral pallidum and sublenticular substantia innominata not expressing p75[NTR] are not affected by the immunotoxin.

Following selective cholinergic lesion by 192 IgG-sap, a number of studies failed to reveal impairments in behavioral paradigms seen after basal forebrain lesions produced with less-selective neurotoxins *(20)*. Apparently, many of the behavioral impairments observed following lesions with nonselective excitotoxins resulted from damage to noncholinergic cells or passing fibers in the basal forebrain, which led to reassessment of the importance of the corticopetal cholinergic afferents in mediating cognitive function. For overviews, *see* the work of Butt and Bowman *(53)*; McGaughy et al. *(28)*; Pizzo et al. *(54)*.

In conclusion, the detailed characterization of 192 IgG-sap suggested that cholinergic immunolesion by 192 IgG-sap is a valuable tool to produce specific cholinergic deficits in rats, which can be used as a model to study the impact of basal forebrain cholinergic system dysfunction on normal brain function.

CHOLINERGIC IMMUNOLESION AFFECTS CORTICAL NONCHOLINERGIC NEUROTRANSMISSION AT THE SYNAPTIC LEVEL

Alzheimer's disease is usually referred to as a multitransmitter disorder because a number of transmitter systems display dysfunctions. But, the basal forebrain cholinergic neuronal cell loss is a very early and consistent feature of Alzheimer's disease, and the question arose whether the changes in other neurotransmitter systems observed in brains from patients with Alzheimer's disease are consequences of cortical cholinergic deficits. To address this question, the effect of basal forebrain cholinergic cell loss on a number of transmitter receptors of various transmitter systems was studied by quantitative receptor autoradiography in brain sections from rats subjected to cholinergic immunolesion by intracerebroventricular 192 IgG-sap for various periods of survival time.

Neurotransmitter receptors are one of the decisive links in the chain of synaptic information processing. They can markedly respond to alterations in neuronal activity by adaptive mechanisms like sub- or supersensitivity or downregulation, which makes them an appropriate tool to monitor for interactive changes in the neuronal activity of a particular transmitter system. Quantitative receptor autoradiography and acetylcholinesterase histochemistry (indicating the extent of cholinergic lesion) were performed in adjacent brain sections, which allows simultaneous detection of the consequences of lesions on various parameters in a distinct cortical area and thus provides an appropriate tool to reveal correlations between cortical cholinergic hypoactivity and lesion-induced adaptive response in distinct cholinoceptive target regions.

N-Methyl-D-aspartate (NMDA) receptor binding was markedly reduced in cortical regions displaying a reduced activity of acetylcholinesterase and high-affinity choline uptake sites as a consequence of cholinergic lesion, whereas AMPA and kainate binding sites were significantly increased in these regions *(43,55)*. The immunolesion-induced increases in the amplitude of hippocampal NMDA-mediated EPSP have been concluded to reflect impairments in postsynaptic NMDA receptors, such as gating properties of associated channels *(56)*. Muscimol binding to GABA-A receptors was increased in the caudal portions of frontal and parietal cortices, as well as occipital and temporal cortex as compared to the corresponding brain regions from vehicle-injected control rats. Binding levels of benzodiazepine receptors and α_1-adrenoceptor binding sites were not affected by the lesion in any of the cortical regions studied *(43)*, whereas the levels of α- and β-

adrenoceptor binding were decreased in a number of cortical regions and hippocampal formation after lesion. The serotonin 2A (5-HT$_{2A}$) binding was markedly reduced in cortical regions displaying a reduced activity of acetylcholinesterase; 5HT$_{1A}$ receptor binding was transiently reduced in some anterior cortical regions, but not in the hippocampal areas following immunolesion *(57)*.

Reductions in the binding level of cortical receptors following lesion could be caused by either a loss of receptor sites if located on degenerating terminals or a downregulation of receptor function if there is any enhanced neuronal activity of the corresponding transmitter system. Lesion-induced increases in receptor binding may be considered upregulation of receptor sites, which is assumed to compensate for reduced presynaptic input of the corresponding transmitter. Therefore, the cholinergic lesion-induced differential changes in receptor binding reflect an important modulatory role of the cholinergic input in cortical noncholinergic transmitter systems, which may also contribute to the cognitive deficits in Alzheimer's disease. This was emphasized in a study demonstrating that GABA-ergic, serotonergic, and glutamatergic receptor modulation differentially affect posttrial memory processing in the hippocampus *(58)*.

When comparing the immunolesion data with corresponding changes in postmortem material from patients with Alzheimer's disease, the same sort of alterations in NMDA, AMPA, and kainate, α_2- and 5-HT$_{2A}$ receptor subtypes were observed *(59,60)*, suggesting that the cortical receptor changes in patients with Alzheimer's disease are secondary to the cholinergic deficits. The data available on β-adrenoceptors in cortical areas from Alzheimer brains are controversial, demonstrating both increase and decrease in cortical and hippocampal β-receptor binding compared to age-matched controls *(61,62)*. Taken together, these findings support both a glutamatergic and an aminergic strategy, which might have therapeutic potential in treating Alzheimer's disease, and demonstrate that cholinergic immunolesion by 192 IgG-sap exhibits a valuable tool to produce specific cholinergic deficits in rats as a model to study the effect of treatment with various drugs.

It has long been assumed that dysfunction of cholinergic neurotransmission may also contribute to the noncognitive behavioral abnormalities in Alzheimer's disease, including psychosis, depression, anxiety, overactivity, sleep disturbances, and hyperphagia; for review, *see* ref. 5. The differential receptor changes observed after cholinergic immunolesion thus may also play a role in mediating the noncognitive dysfunctions in Alzheimer's disease.

CHRONIC NGF TREATMENT INDUCES RECOVERY OF CORTICAL CHOLINERGIC MARKERS AFTER PARTIAL CHOLINERGIC IMMUNOLESION

Although the changes in markers of the neocortical cholinergic system found in brains of patients with Alzheimer's disease are also accompanied by alterations in other cortical transmitter systems like glutamate, noradrenaline, or serotonin, clinical and pharmacological research has predominantly focused on enhancing central nervous cholinergic neurotransmission by cholinomimetics with the expectation of improving cognitive function. Drugs to enhance cortical cholinergic neurotransmission are still the only therapeutic strategy to treat the cognitive deficits of Alzheimer's disease. Although the second generation of centrally acting acetylcholinesterase inhibitors (e.g., donepezil, rivastigmine, galanthamine) have better pharmacological profiles than the first trials with tacrine, the efficacy in improving cognitive function and behavioral deficits in patients with Alzheimer's disease is modest and is not evident in a substantial minority of patients; for review, *see* ref. 5.

As the effect of intracerebroventricular application of 192 IgG-sap on cholinergic neurodegeneration is dose dependent, the extent of cholinergic cell loss in rat basal forebrain can properly be adjusted by injecting doses of the cholinergic immunotoxin that produce submaximal effects *(63)*. Such partial destruction of cholinergic basal forebrain neurons should more properly mimic the situation in Alzheimer's disease and may be an appropriate tool to test for novel therapeutic strategies to compensate for the reduced cholinergic activity. It is well-known that NGF plays an important role in maintaining functions of cholinergic basal forebrain neurons.

To explore the beneficial effects of NGF on cholinergic neuronal maintenance and protection and to avoid the drawbacks of using injections or minipumps for long-term NGF treatment, intracerebral transplantation of NGF-secreting cells have been offered as an alternative. Intraventricular transplantation of NGF-secreting fibroblasts for 8 wk has been found to recover choline acetyltransferase activity in the basal forebrain and high-affinity choline uptake and density of acetylcholinesterase-positive fibers in the cerebral cortex and hippocampus following partial cholinergic immunolesion of basal forebrain *(63)*. The remaining cholinergic cells following partial immunolesion displayed a higher intracellular staining for NGF-like immunoreactivity, and the cell size increased by up to 25% compared with unoperated controls *(63)*.

Similar to findings in human brain tissue from patients with Alzheimer's disease *(64,65)*, increased cortical and hippocampal NGF levels have also been observed in rats cholinergically lesioned by 192 IgG-sap *(14)*. Moreover, chronic cholinergic drug treatment of rats subjected to basal forebrain cholinergic lesion by 192 IgG-sap provided further evidence that cortical and hippocampal NGF proteins, but not mRNA levels, are controlled by cholinergic activity *(14)*.

Transplants of NGF-secreting fibroblasts directly into the somatosensory cortex have been described to restore stimulus-evoked activity in barrel cortex of basal forebrain-lesioned rats *(66)*. Intraventricular injections of NGF to cholinergic-lesioned rats resulted in significantly improved functional responses in the barrel cortex without any increase in cholinergic innervation of the cerebral cortex *(67)*, suggesting that NGF may also act directly on cortical neurons to restore lesion-impaired functional activity *(66)*. Transplants of ex vivo transduced, clonal NGF-secreting immortalized neural progenitor cells bilaterally into the nucleus basalis and septum of middle-aged rats prevented the development of cholinergic neuron atrophy and cognitive impairment during aging *(68)*.

Although the beneficial effects of NGF on neuronal maintenance and rescue from damage appeared promising for the therapeutic potential of NGF, the intracerebroventricular administration of NGF to patients with Alzheimer's disease *(69)* and to rodents *(70)* produced a number of unwanted side effects. This may partly be because of the diversity of cells that respond to NGF signaling. For review, *see* the work of Sofroniew et al. *(71)*. However, a study provided evidence that NGF, when infused intraparenchymally to rats with complete unilateral fornix transections, rescued basal forebrain cholinergic neurons, but did not induce any adverse effects at least over a 2-wk infusion period *(72)*.

The development of transgenic mice that express a neutralizing anti-NGF recombinant antibody *(73)* added further evidence that failure in NGF signaling contributes to cholinergic neurodegeneration. These anti-NGF mice, in which the levels of antibodies are three orders of magnitude higher in adult than in newborn mice *(74)*, demonstrated age-dependent Alzheimer-like neurodegenerative pathology, including formation of amyloid plaques, hyperphosphorylated tau, and neurofibrillary tangles in cortex and hippocampus *(73)*. Aged anti-NGF mice also displayed extensive neuronal loss throughout the cortex, cholinergic deficits in the basal forebrain, and behavioral deficits *(73)*.

CHOLINERGIC IMMUNOLESION AND APP

Besides amyloid plaques and neurofibrillary tangles, the loss of cortical and hippocampal function as a result of basal forebrain cholinergic degeneration is a consistent feature of Alzheimer's disease. There has been much debate whether these lesions are interrelated or take place independently *(75)*.

A number of in vitro experiments demonstrated that the processing and metabolism of the APP (which contains the amyloidogenic sequence found in senile plaques) are controlled by activation of various neurotransmitter receptors coupled to protein kinase C, including M1-muscarinic cholinergic, glutamatergic, and serotonergic receptors *(12,76,77)*. The regulation of APP processing is receptor subtype specific: Activation of M1 or M3 but not M2 or M4 muscarinic receptor subtypes stimulates the nonamyloidogenic pathway of APP processing, but inhibits β-amyloid formation *(76,78–80)*. Thus, cholinergic degenerations in the basal forebrain of patients with Alzheimer's disease that lead to cholinergic neocortical hypoactivity and reduced stimulation of postsynaptic cholinergic receptors might be responsible for altered APP processing.

To prove this hypothesis, a number of cholinergic lesion paradigms, including cholinergic immunolesion by 192 IgG-sap, have been employed to study the effect of cholinergic input on synthesis *(81)*, expression *(7,8,14,82,83)*, and processing of cortical APP *(14,84)*. Indeed, the loss of cholinergic innervation has been found to alter APP expression. In the cholinergic-denervated cortex produced by the injection of excitotoxins into either the rat nucleus basalis magnocellularis or fimbria fornix transection, increased synthesis of both APP mRNA and APP protein has been observed *(81)*.

Using selective cholinergic immunolesion by 192 IgG-sap, elevated APP immunoreactivity in neocortical and hippocampal regions that demonstrated reduced acetylcholinesterase staining were observed in a regional and laminar-specific pattern *(8,9)*. Similarly, Western analyses performed in cerebral cortical and hippocampal tissue preparations from cholinergic-lesioned rats 12 mo after 192 IgG-sap application demonstrated slightly increased APP levels compared to controls *(10,11)*. The cholinergic lesion-induced enhancement in cerebral cortical APP level correlated with the cognitive deficits in water maze testing of rats with 192 IgG-sap lesion *(10,11)*.

Selective cholinergic immunolesion of the medial septal area produced a reduction in APP mRNA in several subfields of the hippocampal formation *(83)*. Similarly, lesion of the entire basal forebrain cholinergic system by intracerebroventricular administration of 192 IgG-sap resulted in modest reductions in APP695 mRNA 30 d or more after lesion *(7)*; the level of total APP mRNA was not significantly altered in rats with 192 IgG-sap lesions *(7,14)*. However, the pattern of APP mRNA isoforms (ratio APP770:751:695) in 192 IgG-sap-treated rats transiently changed to a lower abundance of APP770 and APP751 vs APP695 compared to control data, already detectable 7 d after lesion but decreasing up to 30 d postlesion. Beyond 90 d after lesion, the APP isoform pattern exhibited ratios similar to controls *(14)*.

The cholinergic lesion-induced alterations in APP protein level might also indicate abnormal processing of APP. Indeed, in just 2 wk after selective cholinergic immunolesion the membrane-bound APP detected in cholinergic-denervated cerebral cortical membrane fractions was strikingly enhanced; the level of the soluble secreted form of APP assayed in the supernatant of the same tissue preparation was significantly decreased compared to normal rats *(14)*. These changes in membrane-bound and secreted APP strongly correlated with the activity of cortical choline acetyltransferase, thus clearly demonstrating a cholinergic regulation of cortical APP processing in vivo, which may at least partly contribute the pathogenesis of Alzheimer's disease. Thus, enhancement of cortical cholinergic neurotransmission by pharmacological manipulations should interfere with cortical APP processing by favoring the nonamyloidogenic pathway.

Indeed, treatment of rats with muscarinic receptor agonists resulted in decreased APP levels in neocortex and hippocampus and increased levels of secreted APP in cerebrospinal fluid (CSF) *(10)*, indicating that treatment with muscarinic receptor agonists leads to enhanced processing of APP by α-secretase. It is interesting to note that cholinergic-immunolesioned rats also responded to muscarinic receptor agonist treatment by a dramatic reduction in hippocampal APP level *(10)*. The cholinergic lesion-induced increases of secreted APP level in CSF could be reversed by cholinergic augmentation with phenserine, a cholinesterase inhibitor, and administration of the muscarinic antagonist scopolamine to sham-lesioned rats led to an increase in the CSF levels of secreted APP similar to that observed in cholinergic-lesioned animals *(84)*. Nicotine also has been found to modify APP processing in rats by reducing the formation of potentially amyloidogenic products *(85)*. Chronic nicotine treatment reduced β-amyloidosis in the brain of a mouse model of Alzheimer's disease *(86)*.

Taken together, these observations strongly support that the processing of APP can be pharmacologically modulated.

Cholinergic neurons are one of the major sources of APP in the rat basal forebrain *(87)*. Similarly, a high expression of the β-secretase (BACE1) mRNA has also been observed in cholinergic basal forebrain nuclei by nonradioactive *in situ* hybridization *(88)*, but the functional importance of this coexpression still remains to be clarified. Selective cholinergic immunolesion, however, resulted in an upregulation of BACE1 immunoreactivity in reactive astrocytes detectable throughout the hippocampal formation 14 d following intracerebroventricular application of 192 IgG-sap *(89)*. Similar glial upregulation of BACE1 was observed in other experimental paradigms producing gliosis/inflammation in the brain *(89)*, suggesting a role of BACE1 in the initiation or maintenance of inflammatory processes in the brain.

CHOLINERGIC DYSFUNCTION AND GLUCOSE METABOLISM

Besides the morphological alterations, Alzheimer's disease is associated with a markedly impaired cerebral glucose metabolism as detected by reduced cortical [^{18}F]desoxyglucose utilization in positron emission tomography of patients with Alzheimer's disease (*see* Pietrini et al. *[90]* and references therein). It is detected by altered activities of key glycolytic enzymes, as well as pyruvate and oxoglutarate dehydrogenases in the brains of patients with Alzheimer's disease *(91)*, by reduced densities in cortical glucose transporter subtypes (GLUT1 and GLUT3) *(92–94)*, as well as by disturbances in the insulin signaling transduction cascade *(95–97)*.

As glucose also serves as a substrate for the synthesis of acetylcholine, the impaired cerebral glucose metabolism in Alzheimer brains has been assumed to contribute to the loss of basal forebrain cholinergic function *(98)*. This suggestion was based on a number of pharmacological, biochemical, and behavioral studies demonstrating that glucose affects brain cholinergic neurotransmission, and that the memory-enhancing effect of glucose may result from enhanced cortical acetylcholine synthesis or its release, which in turn may modulate muscarinic acetylcholine receptors known to be critically involved in memory *(99–104)*. Conversely, the basal forebrain cholinergic system plays a role in cerebral cortical blood flow mediated by activation of cholinergic receptors and NO-related mechanisms and may affect glucose utilization in the cerebral cortex *(105–112)*.

However, studies in transgenic Alzheimer-like mice also provided evidence that long-lasting high β-amyloid burden may affect both cortical cholinergic neurotransmission (*see*, e.g., refs. *113* and *114* and references therein). High APP burden also impairs cerebral cortical glucose metabolism by reducing glycolytic activity in β-amyloid plaque-associated neurons along with concomitant upregulation in reactive, plaque-surrounding astrocytes *(115)*, thus hinting to an interrelationship between cholinergic dysfunction, impaired glucose metabolism, and β-amyloid plaque deposition in Alzheimer's disease.

The mechanisms underlying the specific degeneration of basal forebrain cholinergic neurons in Alzheimer's disease are still largely unknown. The fact that acetyl-coenzyme A (CoA) is required for both energy generation and acetylcholine synthesis may render cholinergic cells particularly vulnerable and susceptible to particular pathological signals. Alternatively, cholinergic deficits may also affect acetyl-CoA and energy metabolism in cholinoceptive cortical target regions that may stimulate further neuronal cell death and represent a mechanism underlying the changes in cerebral glucose metabolism in patients with Alzheimer's disease *(116)*.

Indeed, cortical cholinergic denervation produced by a single intracerebroventricular application of the cholinergic immunotoxin 192 IgG-sap in adult rats resulted in a 39% decrease of acetyl-CoA level in synaptosomal mitochondria, which was accompanied by a 74% increase in the synaptoplasmic fraction already detectable 7 d following lesion *(117)*. Levels of acetyl-CoA and CoASH assayed in the fraction of whole brain mitochondria from lesioned cortex were 61 and 48%, respectively (higher compared to controls), providing evidence that the loss of cholinergic cortical input may contribute to changes in the energy metabolism in cholinoceptive noncholinergic cells *(117)*.

Moreover, cortical cholinergic depletion by intracerebroventricular application of 192 IgG-sap resulted also in a transient increase of the phosphofructokinase activity peaking on day 7 postlesion in cortical areas *(118)*. In parallel, an increased steady-state mRNA level of phosphofructokinase was determined by reverse transcription (RT)/real-time polymerase chain reaction (PCR) and *in situ* hybridization. In contrast, Western blot analysis and quantitative PCR revealed no changes in the phosphofructokinase isoenzyme pattern after immunolesion *(118)*.

Similar transient changes following basal forebrain cholinergic lesions have been reported for a number of other glucose metabolic parameters. Transient increases in D-glucose-displaceable [^{3}H]cytochalasin-B binding to the total population of glucose transporter in cortical regions displaying reduced acetylcholinesterase activity were observed within 7 d after cholinergic immunolesion and peaking around 30 d postlesion *(119)*. Western analysis revealed that the changes in total glucose transporter binding were caused by changes in the GLUT3 subtype only; the levels of GLUT1 and GLUT3 mRNA (Northern analysis) were not affected by cholinergic immunolesion *(119)*. Following fimbria–fornix transection, changes in phosphofructokinase activity and [^{3}H]cytochalasin-B binding to glucose transporter have been reported also to be of transient nature only *(120)*.

In vivo [^{14}C]deoxyglucose uptake was transiently increased in cholinergically denervated cortical regions by intracerebroventricular 192 IgG-sap and was highest between 3 and 7 d after lesion *(119)*, which correlates well with the lesion-induced increase of GLUT3 transporters. The cholinergic lesion-induced transient upregulation of cortical glucose transporters and deoxyglucose uptake reflects an increased glucose demand in regions depleted of acetylcholine, suggesting functional links between cortical cholinergic activity and glucose metabolism. However, these changes did not result in any alterations of the overall rate of total glucose degradation in the cerebral cortex of cholinergic-immunolesioned rats as assayed by [^{14}C]D-glucose degradation in tissue homogenates *(119)*.

Following nucleus basalis magnocellularis ablation, the regional cerebral metabolic rate of glucose [rCMR(glc)] was initially reduced in cholinergically denervated cortex, but almost normalized to control values 1 to 2 wk after the lesion without any recovery of choline acetyltransferase activity *(107,109,112)*. Similarly, 7 and 21 d after unilateral lesioning of cholinergic basal forebrain neurons by 192 IgG-sap, there was decreased rCMR(glc) in a number of cortical and subcortical regions *(120)*. However, long-term selective lesion of basal forebrain cholinergic cells by bilateral intraventricular injection of 192 IgG-sap induced sustained reductions in hippocampal and cortical rCMR(glc), which correlated with lesion-induced cognitive impairments, further supporting the hypothesis of the cholinergic influence on cortical glucose metabolism and cognition *(106)*.

In contrast, Orzi et al. *(110)* failed to observe any recovery of the rCMR(glc) up to 2 wk after lesion of the nucleus basalis magnocellularis by kainic acid. These differences might be because of the different specificity and selectivity of the lesion paradigms used to produce basal forebrain cholinergic cell loss.

Under physiological conditions, cerebral blood flow and cortical utilization of glucose are tightly coupled to neuronal activity and energy demand (*see* ref. *121*; for review *see* ref. *122*), but under conditions of cholinergic dysfunction the cerebral blood flow has been reported to be uncoupled from glucose utilization *(11,110)*.

Whereas lesions of the basal forebrain cholinergic system have reduced cerebral glucose uptake *(10)*, activations of the cholinergic system by electrical stimulation or injection of L-glutamate into the nucleus basalis *(121)* by application of muscarinic or nicotinic agonists *(123,124)* or cholinesterase inhibition *(125)* have increased cerebral cortical glucose uptake. These data clearly demonstrated that alterations in the activity of cortical cholinergic input may control glucose metabolism of cholinoceptive cortical cells. It has been speculated that glucose itself may be the signal for regulating the expression of glycolytic enzymes *(126)*, but muscarinic cholinergic *(123)*, as well as nicotinic cholinergic *(124)* receptor-mediated mechanisms might also be involved as well as other proglycolytic neurotransmitter systems *(122)*.

CHOLINERGIC IMMUNOLESION-INDUCED INFLAMMATORY RESPONSES

There is increasing evidence that persistent inflammatory events in the central nervous system may contribute to neurodegenerative processes *(127)*. In particular, inflammatory processes have been suggested to play a role in the degeneration of basal forebrain cholinergic cells in Alzheimer's disease *(128–132)*. This is emphasized by observations of increased levels of inflammatory cytokines such as interleukin (IL)-1, IL-6, and tumor necrosis factor-α in Alzheimer brains *(133–135)*.

Detailed knowledge of mechanisms of cytokine-related cytotoxicity in neurodegeneration is fundamental to derive strategies against progressive inflammation-mediated neuronal injury. To elucidate the role of pro- and anti-inflammatory cytokines in brain inflammatory processes, adequate experimental paradigms are required to simulate various aspects of neuroinflammation in neurodegenerative events. The cholinergic immunotoxin 192 IgG-sap has been employed to study neuroinflammatory events occurring during the course of cholinergic cell loss in the basal forebrain. The basal forebrain cholinergic neurodegeneration by intracerebroventricular 192 IgG-sap starts not earlier than 3 d after injection and is complete 7 d after treatment *(38,42,47)*. This neurodegeneration is accompanied by a striking reactive glial response in the lesion site, which is of transient nature only. Seven days postlesion, the highest level of activated microglia *(41,47)* was observed, whereas the number of lesion-induced reactive astrocytes was highest between 15 and 30 d following injection *(136,137)*.

Using sensitive semiquantitative RT-PCR, *in situ* hybridization, and immunocytochemistry, the expression of both mRNA and protein of IL-1β and IL-6 in the basal forebrain was not found to be induced in activated microglia or reactive astrocytes by cholinergic neurodegeneration *(136–138)*, whereas reduced activities of the neuronal NO synthase in select cholinoceptive neocortical and hippocampal neurons have been observed following cholinergic immunolesion *(29)*. As the total amount of cortical neuronal NO synthase protein was not affected by basal forebrain cholinergic lesion, it has been suggested that the ratio of catalytically active and inactive cortical neuronal NO synthase is driven by basal forebrain cholinergic input, presumably via M1-muscarinic cholinergic receptors *(29)*.

Leukemia inhibitory factor (LIF, previously designated cholinergic differentiation factor) is well known to promote cholinergic gene expression in several neuronal populations *(139)*. In adult intact rat brain, LIF mRNA has exclusively been found in neurons. In particular, LIF mRNA is constitutively expressed in both cholinergic and GABA-ergic neurons in rat basal forebrain, suggesting a role for LIF in the function of these mature neurons *(136)*.

Intracerebroventricular infusion of LIF has maintained choline acetyltransferase expression in vivo in rats subjected to axotomy of medial septal neurons *(141)*. Degeneration of basal forebrain cholinergic cells by the cholinergic immunotoxin 192 IgG-sap did not induce any expression of LIF mRNA in glial cells, activated at the lesion site, but a decrease in the number of cells expressing LIF within the basal forebrain nuclei occurred, which should have been caused by the immunotoxin-mediated degeneration of cholinergic neurons *(31)*.

In contrast to basal forebrain cholinergic immunolesion, proinflammatory cytokine expression has been induced in a number of other lesion paradigms, including trimethyl tin treatment, trauma, and ischemia *(141–143)*, as well as kainic acid injection *(144)* and rabies infection *(145)*.

Microglial activation in response to pathological stimuli is characterized by increased migratory activity and potential cytotoxic action on injured neurons during later stages of neurodegeneration *(146)*. Phagocytosis of neurons, as well as neuronal regeneration, requires the interaction of microglial cells with degenerating axons and neuronal somata, which is known to be mediated by the expression of cell adhesion molecules *(147,148)*. Adhesion molecules functionally represent cell surface receptors that enable cell–cell and cell–extracellular matrix interactions. Particularly, the intercellular adhesion molecule 1 (ICAM-1) and its ligand, the leukocyte function-associated antigen 1 (LFA-1), have been suggested to play important roles in the recruitment, migration, and retention of microglial cells to sites of tissue damage *(149,150)*. ICAM-1 is a member of the immunoglobulin supergene family, and its expression is markedly upregulated by inflammatory mediators *(151)*. In vitro studies have shown that both neuronal and glial cells are capable of expressing ICAM-1 in response to various proinflammatory cytokines and toxins *(152)*.

Pathological expression of cell adhesion molecules and functional impairments in related signal transduction mechanisms have been suggested as a key factor in the development of several neurodegenerative disorders *(153)*. Notably, in Alzheimer's disease a differentially increased expression of ICAM-1, observed in β-amyloid-containing brain tissue, is assumed to contribute to the progression of the neuronal cell loss *(154)*. A β-amyloid-plaque-associated upregulation of ICAM-1 has also been observed in transgenic Tg2576 mice with Alzheimer plaque pathology *(113)*.

To elucidate any functional role of adhesion molecules in cholinergic neurodegenerative events, the cellular expression pattern of ICAM-1 and LFA-1 was studied during the time-course of cholinergic cell loss induced by a single intracerebroventricular application of 192 IgG-sap. A gradual loss of choline acetyltransferase-immunoreactive cells starting 3 d, but nearly complete 7 d, after injection of the toxin has been observed; it was accompanied by a striking appearance of activated microglial cells in the lesioned areas *(30)*. Four days following injection of 192 IgG-sap, ICAM-1 immunoreactivity was predominantly observed in choline acetyltransferase-positive neurons and partly in activated microglia in the basal forebrain nuclei; LFA-1 expression at this time-point was restricted to neurons *(30)*. However, 7 d after cholinergic basal forebrain lesion, only a few shrunken neuronal somata were immunoreactive for ICAM-1 and LFA-1, and activated microglial cells demonstrated strong immunoreactivity for ICAM-1 and LFA-1 in the lesioned forebrain areas. These differential cell-specific upregulations of cell adhesion molecules during the course of cholinergic neurodegeneration in the basal forebrain suggested that ICAM-1 and LFA-1 may act as intercellular recognition signals by which degenerating cholinergic neurons actively participate in the sequence of events leading to their targeting and elimination by phagocytotic microglia *(30)*.

CONCLUDING REMARKS

The interrelationship among cortical cholinergic dysfunction, β-amyloid formation and deposition, impaired glucose metabolism, and local inflammatory upregulation and noncognitive behavioral abnormalities in Alzheimer's disease is still poorly understood. Selective and specific lesion of cholinergic basal forebrain neurons by intracerebroventricular injection of the immunotoxin 192 IgG-sap is a useful animal approach to mimic cortical cholinergic dysfunction and to study the mechanisms by which impaired cortical cholinergic input may drive some pathological neurochemical sequelae of Alzheimer's disease, including processing of APP, energy metabolism, and noncholinergic cortical neurotransmission. Further, the cholinergic immunolesion paradigm should be of particular value to elaborate and test therapeutic strategies compensating for the reduced cortical cholinergic input.

SUMMARY

The basal forebrain cholinergic system is known to play an important role in normal cognitive function, and cortical cholinergic dysfunction has been implicated in cognitive deficits that occur in Alzheimer's disease and other dementing disorders. To characterize the role of the central cholinergic system in vivo, lesion paradigms are required that selectively and specifically destroy cholinergic neurons. A monoclonal antibody to the low-affinity NGF receptor 192 IgG coupled to the cytotoxin saporin has been described as an efficient and selective immunotoxin for the NGF-receptor-bearing cholinergic neurons in rat basal forebrain.

This chapter summarized the usefulness of 192 IgG-sap as a powerful tool for producing an animal model with selective and specific basal forebrain cholinergic lesions in rats that can be applied to mimic basal forebrain cholinergic system-associated sequelae of Alzheimer's disease, including changes in noncholinergic cortical neurotransmission, processing of the APP, and inflammation, as well as glucose metabolism. This animal approach should also be particularly valuable for elaboration and testing of therapeutic strategies designed to compensate for the reduced cortical cholinergic input.

REFERENCES

1. Bartus RT, Dean RL, Beer B, Lippa AS. The cholinergic hypothesis of geriatric memory dysfunction. Science 1982;217:408–414.
2. Coyle JT, Price DL, DeLong MR. Alzheimer's disease: a disorder of cortical cholinergic innervation. Science 1983;219:1184–1190.
3. Bartus RT. On neurodegenerative diseases, models, and treatment strategies: lessons learned and lessons forgotten a generation following the cholinergic hypothesis. Exp Neurol 2000;163:495–529.
4. Francis PT, Palmer AM, Snape M, Wilcock GK. The cholinergic hypothesis of Alzheimer's disease: a review of progress. J Neurol Neurosurg Psychiatry 1999;66:137–147.
5. Palmer AM. Pharmacotherapy of Alzheimer's disease: progress and prospects. Trends Pharmacol Sci 2002;23:426–433.
6. Bierer LM, Haroutunian V, Gabriel S, et al. Neurochemical correlates of dementia severity in Alzheimer's disease: relative importance of the cholinergic deficits. J Neurochem 1995;64:749–760.
7. Apelt J, Schliebs R, Beck M, Roßner S, Bigl V. Expression of amyloid precursor protein mRNA isoforms in rat brain is differentially regulated during postnatal maturation and by cholinergic activity. Int J Dev Neurosci 1997;15:95–112.
8. Leanza G. Chronic elevation of amyloid precursor protein expression in the neocortex and hippocampus of rats with selective cholinergic lesions. Neurosci Lett 1998;257:53–66.
9. Lin L, LeBlanc CJ, Deacon TW, Isacson O. Chronic cognitive deficits and amyloid precursor protein elevation after selective immunotoxin lesions of the basal forebrain cholinergic system. Neuroreport 1998;9:547–552.
10. Lin L, Georgievska B, Mattsson A, Isacson O. Cognitive changes and modified processing of amyloid precursor protein in the cortical and hippocampal system after cholinergic synapse loss and muscarinic receptor activation. Proc Natl Acad Sci USA 1999;96:12,108–12,113.

11. Lin L, Georgievska B, Mattsson A, Browne SE, Isacson O. In vivo regulation of amyloid precursor protein processing by mucarinic receptor activation and regional reductions in glucose utilization in rats with cholinergic deficits. Soc Neurosci Abstr 1999;25:2054.

12. Nitsch RM, Deng M, Growdon JH, Wurtman RJ. Serotonin 5-HT$_{2a}$ and 5-HT$_{2c}$ receptors stimulate amyloid precursor protein ectodomain secretion. J Biol Chem 1996;271:4188–4194.

13. Muller DM, Mendla K, Farber SA, Nitsch RM. Muscarinic M1 receptor agonists increase the secretion of the amyloid precursor protein ectodomain. Life Sci 1997;60:985–991.

14. Roßner S, Wortwein G, Gu Z, et al. Cholinergic control of nerve growth factor in adult rats: evidence from cortical cholinergic deafferentation and chronic drug treatment. J Neurochem 1997;69:947–953.

15. Roßner S, Ueberham U, Schliebs R, Perez-Polo JR, Bigl V. The regulation of amyloid precursor protein metabolism by cholinergic mechanisms and neurotrophin receptor signaling. Prog Neurobiol 1998;56:541–569.

16. Härtig W, Bauer A, Brauer K, et al. Functional recovery of cholinergic basal forebrain neurons under disease conditions: old problems, new solutions? Rev Neurosci 2002;13:95–165.

17. Schliebs R, Roßner S, Bigl V. Immunolesion by 192 IgG-saporin of rat basal forebrain cholinergic system: a useful tool to produce cortical cholinergic dysfunction. Progr Brain Res 1996;109:253–264.

18. Krügel U, Bigl V, Eschrich K, Bigl M. Deafferentation of the septo-hippocampal pathway in rats as model of the metabolic events in Alzheimer's disease. Int J Dev Neurosci 2001;19:263–277.

19. Bigl V, Schliebs R. Simulation of cortical cholinergic deficits—a novel experimental approach to study pathogenetic aspects of Alzheimer's disease. J Neural Transm 1998;54(suppl):237–247.

20. Wrenn CC, Wiley RG. The behavioral functions of the cholinergic basal forebrain: lessons from 192 IgG-saporin. Int J Dev Neurosci 1998;16:595–602.

21. Wiley RG, Kline RII IV. Neuronal lesioning with axonally transported toxins J Neurosci Methods 2000;103:73–82.

22. Wenk GL, Harrington CA, Tucker DA, Rance NE, Walker LC. Basal forebrain neurons and memory: a biochemical, histological, and behavioral study of differential vulnerability to ibotenate and quisqualate. Behav Neurosci 1992;106:909–923.

23. Hanin I. Cholinergic toxins and Alzheimer's disease. Ann NY Acad Sci 1992;648:63–70.

24. Wiley RG. Neural lesioning with ribosome-inactivating proteins: suicide transport and immunolesioning. Trends Neurosci 1992;15:285–290.

25. Barefoot HC, Baker HF, Ridley RM. Synergistic effects of unilateral immunolesions of the cholinergic projections from the basal forebrain and contralateral ablations of the inferotemporal cortex and hippocampus in monkeys. Neuroscience 2000;98:243–251.

26. Berger-Sweeney J, Stearns NA, Murg SL, Floerke-Nashner LR, Lappi DA, Baxter MG. Selective immunolesions of cholinergic neurons in mice: effect on neuroanatomy, neurochemistry, and behavior. J. Neurosci 2001;21:8164–8173.
27. Tremere LA, Pinaud R, Grosche J, Härtig W, Rasmusson DD. Antibody for human p75LNTR identifies cholinergic basal forebrain non-primate species. Neuroreport 2000;11:2177–2183.
28. McGaughy J, Everitt BJ, Robbins TW, Sarter M. The role of cortical cholinergic afferent projections in cognition: impact of new selective immunotoxins. Behav Brain Res 2000;115:251–263.
29. Hartlage-Rübsamen M, Schliebs R. Rat basal forebrain cholinergic lesion affects neuronal nitric oxide synthase in cholinoceptive hippocampal and neocortical target regions. Brain Res 2001;889:155–164.
30. Hartlage-Rübsamen M, Schliebs R. Sequential upregulation of cell adhesion molecules in degenerating rat basal forebrain cholinergic neurons and in phagocytic microglial cells. Brain Res 2001;897:20–26.
31. Lemke R, Hartlage-Rübsamen M, Schliebs R. Differential injury-dependent glial expression of interleukins-1alpha,beta and interleukin-6 in rat brain. Glia 1999;27:75–87.
32. Wiley RG, Oeltmann TN, Lappi DA. Immunolesioning: selective destruction of neurons using immunotoxin to rat NGF receptor. Brain Res 1991;562:149–153.
33. Gage FH, Batchelor P, Chen KS, et al. NGF receptor reexpression and NGF-mediated cholinergic neuronal hypertrophy in the damaged adult neostriatum. Neuron 1989;2:1177–1184.
34. Yan Q, Johnson EM Jr. Immunohistochemical localization and biochemical characterization of nerve growth factor receptor in adult rat brain. J Comp Neurol 1989;290:585–598.
35. Thomas LB, Book AA, Schweitzer JB. Immunohistochemical detection of a monoclonal antibody directed against the NGF receptor in basal forebrain neurons following intraventricular injection. J Neurosci Methods 1991;37:37–45.
36. Berger-Sweeney J, Heckers S, Mesulam MM, Wiley RG, Lappi DA, Sharma M. Differential effects on spatial navigation of immunotoxin-induced cholinergic lesions of the medial septal area and nucleus basalis magnocellularis. J Neurosci 1994;14:4507–4519.
37. Book AA, Wiley RG, Schweitzer JB. Specificity of 192 IgG-saporin for NGF receptor-positive cholinergic basal forebrain neurons in the rat. Brain Res 1992;590:350–355.
38. Heckers S, Ohtake T, Wiley RG, Lappi DA, Geula C, Mesulam MM. Complete and selective cholinergic denervation of rat neocortex and hippocampus but not amygdala by an immunotoxin against the p75 NGF receptor. J Neurosci 1994;14:1271–1289.
39. Rossner S, Perez-Polo JR, Wiley RG, Schliebs R, Bigl V. Differential expression of immediate early genes in distinct layers of rat cerebral cortex after selective immunolesion of the forebrain cholinergic system. J Neurosci Res 1994;38:282–293.

40. Roßner S, Schliebs R, Perez-Polo JR, Wiley RG, Bigl V. Differential changes in cholinergic markers from selected brain regions after specific immunolesion of rat cholinergic basal forebrain system. J Neurosci Res 1995;40:31–43.

41. Roßner S, Härtig W, Schliebs R, et al. 192 IgG-saporin immunotoxin-induced loss of cholinergic cells differentially activates microglia in rat basal forebrain nuclei. J Neurosci Res 1995;41:335–346.

42. Roßner S, Schliebs R, Härtig W, Bigl V. 192 IgG-saporin-induced selective lesion of cholinergic basal forebrain system: neurochemical effects on cholinergic neurotransmission in rat cerebral cortex and hippocampus. Brain Res Bull 1995;38:371–381.

43. Roßner S, Schliebs R, Bigl V. 192 IgG-saporin-induced immunotoxic lesions of cholinergic basal forebrain system differentially affect glutamatergic and GABAergic markers in cortical rat brain regions. Brain Res 1995;696:165–176.

44. Leanza G, Nilsson OG, Wiley RG, Bjorklund A. Selective lesioning of the basal forebrain cholinergic system by intraventricular 192 IgG-saporin: behavioural, biochemical and stereological studies in the rat. Eur J Neurosci 1995;7:329–343.

45. Lee MG, Chrobak JJ, Sik A, Wiley RG, Buzsaki G. Hippocampal theta activity following selective lesion of the septal cholinergic system. Neuroscience 1994;62:1033–1047.

46. Wenk GL, Stoehr JD, Quintana G, Mobley S, Wiley RG. Behavioral, biochemical, histological, and electrophysiological effects of 192 IgG-saporin injections into the basal forebrain of rats. J Neurosci 1994;14:5986–5995.

47. Seeger G, Hartig W, Rossner S, et al. Electron microscopic evidence for microglial phagocytic activity and cholinergic cell death after administration of the immunotoxin 192 IgG-saporin in rat. J Neurosci Res 1997;48:465–476.

48. Book AA, Wiley RG, Schweitzer JB. 192 IgG-saporin: I. Specific lethality for cholinergic neurons in the basal forebrain of the rat. J Neuropathol Exp Neurol 1994;53:95–102.

49. Potter PE, Gaughan C, Assouline Y. Lesion of septal-hippocampal neurons with 192 IgG-saporin alters function of M1 muscarinic receptors. Neuropharmacology 1999;38:579–586.

50. Sorger D, Schliebs R, Kampfer I, et al. In vivo [^{125}I]-iodobenzovesamicol binding reflects cortical cholinergic deficiency induced by specific immunolesion of rat basal forebrain cholinergic system. Nucl Med Biol 2000;27:23–31.

51. Bickel U, Kewitz H. Colocalization of choline acetyltransferase and nerve growth factor receptor in the rat basal forebrain. Dementia 1990;1:146–150.

52. Woolf NJ, Gould E, Butcher LL. Nerve growth factor receptor is associated with cholinergic neurons of the basal forebrain but not the pontomesencephalon. Neuroscience 1989;30:143–152.

53. Butt AE, Bowman TD. Transverse patterning reveals a dissociation of simple and configural association learning abilities in rats with 192 IgG-saporin lesions of the nucleus basalis magnocellularis. Neurobiol Learn Mem 2002;77:211–233.

54. Pizzo DP, Thal LJ, Winkler J. Mnemonic deficits in animals depend upon the degree of cholinergic deficit and task complexity. Exp Neurol 2002;177:292–305.
55. Nicolle MM, Shivers A, Gill TM, Gallagher M. Hippocampal *N*-methyl-D-aspartate and kainate binding in response to entorhinal cortex aspiration or 192 IgG-saporin lesions of the basal forebrain. Neuroscience 1997;77:649–659.
56. Jouvenceau A, Dutar P, Billard JM. Alteration of NMDA receptor-mediated synaptic responses in CA1 area of the aged rat hippocampus: contribution of GABAergic and cholinergic deficits. Hippocampus 1998;8:627–637.
57. Heider M, Schliebs R, Rossner S, Bigl V. Basal forebrain cholinergic immunolesion by 192 IgG-saporin: evidence for a presynaptic location of subpopulations of α 2- and β-adrenergic as well as 5-HT$_{2A}$ receptors on cortical cholinergic terminals. Neurochem Res 1997;22:957–966.
58. Farr SA, Flood JF, Morley JE. The effect of cholinergic, GABAergic, serotonergic, and glutamatergic receptor modulation on posttrial memory processing in the hippocampus. Neurobiol Learn Mem 2000;73:150–167.
59. Kalaria RN, Andorn AC. Adrenergic receptors in aging and Alzheimer's disease: decreased α 2-receptors demonstrated by [^{3}H]p-aminoclonidine binding in prefrontal cortex. Neurobiol Aging 1991;12:131–136.
60. Nordberg A. Neuroreceptor changes in Alzheimer disease. Cerebrovasc Brain Metab Rev 1992;4:303–328.
61. Kalaria RN, Andorn AC, Tabaton M, Whitehouse PJ, Harik SI, Unnerstall JR. Adrenergic receptors in aging and Alzheimer's disease: increased β 2-receptors in prefrontal cortex and hippocampus. J Neurochem 1989;53:1772–1781.
62. Shimohama S, Taniguchi T, Fujiwara M, Kameyama M. Changes in β-adrenergic receptor subtypes in Alzheimer-type dementia. J Neurochem 1987;48:1215–1221.
63. Roßner S, Yu J, Pizzo K, et al. Effects of intraventricular transplantation of NGF-secreting cells on cholinergic basal forebrain neurons after partial immunolesion. J. Neurosci Res 1996;45:40–56.
64. Crutcher KA, Scott SA, Liang S, Everson WV, Weingartner J. Detection of NGF-like activity in human brain tissue: increased levels in Alzheimer's disease. J Neurosci 1993;13:2540–2550.
65. Hellweg R, Gericke CA, Jendroska K, Hartung HD, Cervos-Navarro J. NGF content in the cerebral cortex of non-demented patients with amyloid-plaques and in symptomatic Alzheimer's disease. Int J Dev Neurosci 1998;16:787–794.
66. Rahimi O, Juliano SL. Transplants of NGF-secreting fibroblasts restore stimulus-evoked activity in barrel cortex of basal-forebrain-lesioned rats. J Neurophysiol 2001;86:2081–2096.
67. Rahimi O, Eslin DE, Hill GF II, Juliano SL. Nerve growth factor increases stimulus-evoked metabolic activity in acetylcholine-depleted barrel cortex. Somatosens Mot Res 1999;16:151–162.
68. Martinez-Serrano A, Björklund A. Ex vivo growth factor gene transfer to the basal forebrain in presymptomatic middle-aged rats prevents the development of cholinergic neuron atrophy and cognitive impairment during aging. Proc Natl Acad Sci USA 1998;95:1858–1863.

69. Eriksdotter-Jönhagen M, Nordberg A, Amberla K, et al. Intracerebroventricular infusion of nerve growth factor in three patients with Alzheimer's disease. Dement Geriatr Cogn Disord 1998;9:246–257.
70. Winkler J, Ramirez GA, Thal LJ, Waite JJ. Nerve growth factor (NGF) augments cortical and hippocampal cholinergic functioning after p75NGF receptor-mediated deafferentation but impairs inhibitory avoidance and induces fear-related behaviors. J Neurosci 2000;20:834–844.
71. Sofroniew MV, Howe CL, Mobley WC. Nerve growth factor signaling, neuroprotection, and neural repair. Annu Rev Neurosci 2001;24:1217–1281.
72. Tuszynski MH. Intraparenchymal NGF infusions rescue degenerating cholinergic neurons. Cell Transplant 2000;9:629–636.
73. Capsoni S, Ugolini G, Comparini A, Ruberti F, Berardi N, Cattaneo A. Alzheimer-like neurodegeneration in aged antinerve growth factor transgenic mice. Proc Natl Acad Sci USA 2000;97:6826–6831.
74. Ruberti F, Capsoni S, Comparini A, et al. Phenotypic knock-out of nerve growth factor in adult transgenic mice reveals severe deficits in basal forebrain cholinergic neurons, cell death in the spleen, and skeletal muscle dystrophy. J Neurosci 2000;20:2589–2601.
75. Roberson MR, Harrell LE. Cholinergic activity and amyloid precursor protein metabolism. Brain Res Rev 1997;30:50–69.
76. Nitsch RM, Slack BE, Wurtman RJ, Growdon JH. Release of Alzheimer amyloid precursor derivatives stimulated by activation of muscarinic acetylcholine receptors. Science 1992;258:304–307.
77. Lee RK, Wurtman RJ, Cox AJ, Nitsch RM. Amyloid precursor protein processing is stimulated by metabotropic glutamate receptors. Proc Natl Acad Sci USA 1995;92:8083–8087.
78. Farber SA, Nitsch RM, Schulz JG, Wurtman RJ. Regulated secretion of beta-amyloid precursor protein in rat brain. J Neurosci 1995;15:7442–7451.
79. Hung AY, Haass C, Nitsch RM, et al. Activation of protein kinase C inhibits cellular production of the amyloid beta-protein. J Biol Chem 1993;268:22,959–22,962.
80. Jacobsen JS, Spruyt MA, Brown AM, et al. The release of Alzheimer's disease beta amyloid peptide is reduced by phorbol treatment. J Biol Chem 1994;269:8376–8382.
81. Wallace W, Ahlers ST, Gotlib J, et al. Amyloid precursor protein in the cerebral cortex is rapidly and persistently induced by loss of subcortical innervation. Proc Natl Acad Sci USA 1993;90:8712–8716.
82. Harkany T, Abraham I, Timmermann W, et al. β-amyloid neurotoxicity is mediated by a glutamate-triggered excitotoxic cascade in rat nucleus basalis. Eur J Neurosci 2000;12:2735–2745.
83. Ramirez MJ, Heslop KE, Francis PT, Rattray M. Expression of amyloid precursor protein, tau and presenilin RNAs in rat hippocampus following deafferentation lesions. Brain Res 2001;907:222–232.
84. Haroutunian V, Greig N, Pei XF, et al. Pharmacological modulation of Alzheimer's β-amyloid precursor protein levels in the CSF of rats with forebrain cholinergic system lesions. Mol Brain Res 1997;46:161–168.

85. Lahiri DK, Utsuki T, Chen D, et al. Nicotine reduces the secretion of Alzheimer's beta-amyloid precursor protein containing β-amyloid peptide in the rat without altering synaptic proteins. Ann NY Acad Sci 2002;965:364–372.
86. Nordberg A, Hellstrom-Lindahl E, Lee M, et al. Chronic nicotine treatment reduces β-amyloidosis in the brain of a mouse model of Alzheimer's disease (APPsw). J Neurochem 2002;81:655–658.
87. Harkany T, Varga C, Grosche J, et al. Distinct subtypes of nucleus basalis neurons exhibit similar sensitivity to excitotoxicity. Neuroreport 2002;13:767–772.
88. Bigl M, Apelt J, Luschenkina EA, Lange-Dohna C, Rossner S, Schliebs R. Expression of beta-secretase mRNA in transgenic mouse brain with Alzheimer plaque pathology. Neurosci Lett 2000;292:107–110.
89. Hartlage-Rübsamen M, Zeitschel U, Apelt J, et al. Astrocytic expression of the Alzheimer's disease β-secretase (BACE1) is stimulus-dependent. Glia 2003;41:169–179.
90. Pietrini P, Alexander GE, Furey ML, Hampel H, Guazzelli M. The neurometabolic landscape of cognitive decline: in vivo studies with positron emission tomography in Alzheimer's disease. Int J Psychophysiol 2000;37:87–98.
91. Bigl M, Brückner MK, Arendt T, Bigl V, Eschrich K. Activities of key glycolytic enzymes in the brains of patients with Alzheimer's disease. J Neural Transm 1999;106:499–511.
92. Harr SD, Simonian NA, Hyman BT. Functional alterations in Alzheimer's disease: decreased glucose transporter 3 immunoreactivity in the perforant pathway terminal zone. J Neuropathol Exp Neurol 1995;54:38–41.
93. Mooradian AD, Chung HC, Shah GN. GLUT-1 expression in the cerebra of patients with Alzheimer's disease. Neurobiol Aging 1997;18:469–474.
94. Simpson IA, Chundu KR, Davies-Hill T, Honer WG, Davies P. Decreased concentrations of GLUT1 and GLUT3 glucose transporters in the brains of patients with Alzheimer's disease. Ann Neurol 1994;35:546–551.
95. Frölich L, Blum-Degen D, Bernstein HG, et al. Brain insulin and insulin receptors in aging and sporadic Alzheimer's disease. J Neural Transm 1998;105:423–438.
96. Frölich L, Blum-Degen D, Riederer P, Hoyer S. A disturbance in the neuronal insulin receptor signal transduction in sporadic Alzheimer's disease. Ann NY Acad Sci 1999;893:290–293.
97. Hoyer S. The brain insulin signal transduction system and sporadic (type II) Alzheimer disease: an update. J Neural Transm 2002;109:341–360.
98. Meier-Ruge WA, Bertoni-Freddari C. Pathogenesis of decreased glucose turnover and oxidative phosphorylation in ischemic and trauma-induced dementia of the Alzheimer type. Ann NY Acad Sci 1997;826:229–241.
99. Durkin TP, Messier C, de Boer P, Westerink BH. Raised glucose levels enhance scopolamine-induced acetylcholine overflow from the hippocampus: an in vivo microdialysis study in the rat. Behav Brain Res 1992;49:181–188.
100. Kopf SR, Baratti CM. Effects of posttraining administration of glucose on retention of a habituation response in mice: participation of a central cholinergic mechanism. Neurobiol Learn Mem 1996;65:253–260.

101. Kopf SR, Baratti CM. Memory-improving actions of glucose: involvement of a central cholinergic muscarinic mechanism. Behav Neural Biol 1994;62:237–243.
102. Lawson CJ, Homewood J, Taylor AJ. The effects of l-glucose on memory in mice are modulated by peripherally acting cholinergic drugs. Neurobiol Learn Mem 2002;77:17–28.
103. Ragozzino ME, Pal SN, Unick K, Stefani MR, Gold PE. Modulation of hippocampal acetylcholine release and spontaneous alternation scores by intrahippocampal glucose injections. J Neurosci 1998;18:1595–15601.
104. Stone WS, Rudd RJ, Gold PE. Glucose attenuation of atropine-induced deficits in paradoxical sleep and memory. Brain Res 1995;694:133–138.
105. Blin J, Ivanoiu A, Coppens A, et al. Cholinergic neurotransmission has different effects on cerebral glucose consumption and blood flow in young normals, aged normals, and Alzheimer's disease patients. Neuroimage 1997;6:335–343.
106. Browne SE, Lin L, Mattsson A, Georgievska B, Isacson O. Selective antibody-induced cholinergic cell and synapse loss produce sustained hippocampal and cortical hypometabolism with correlated cognitive deficits. Exp Neurol 2001;170:36–47.
107. DeMicheli E, Lamour Y, Bassant MH, Soncrant TT. Sustained cortical metabolic responsivity to physostigmine after nucleus basalis magnocellularis ablation in rats. Brain Res 1993;615:80–86.
108. Katsumi Y, Hayashi T, Oyanagi C, et al. Glucose metabolism in the rat frontal cortex recovered without the recovery of choline acetyltransferase activity after lesioning of the nucleus basalis magnocellularis. Neurosci Lett 2000;280:9–12.
109. Lamour YA, Holloway HW, Larson DM, Soncrant TT. The effect of lesions of the nucleus basalis magnocellularis on local brain glucose utilization in the rat: time course. Neurodegeneration 1993;2:41–50.
110. Orzi F, Diana G, Casamenti F, Palombo E, Fieschi C. Local cerebral glucose utilization following unilateral and bilateral lesions of the Nucleus basalis magnocellularis in the rat. Brain Res 1988;462:99–103.
111. Ouchi Y, Fukuyama H, Ogawa M, et al. Cholinergic projection from the basal forebrain and cerebral glucose metabolism in rats: a dynamic PET study. J Cereb Blood Flow Metab 1996;16:34–41.
112. Soncrant TT, Holloway HW, Horwitz B, Rapoport SI, Lamour YA. Effect of nucleus basalis magnocellularis ablation on local brain glucose utilization in the rat: functional brain reorganization. Eur J Neurosci 1992;4:653–662.
113. Apelt J, Leßig, Schliebs R. β-amyloid-associated expression of intercellular adhesion molecule-1 (ICAM-1) in brain cortical tissue of transgenic Tg2576 mice. Neurosci Lett 2002;329:111–115.
114. Klingner M, Apelt J, Kumar A, et al. Alterations in cholinergic and non-cholinergic neurotransmitter receptor densities in transgenic Tg2576 mouse brain with β-amyloid plaque pathology. Int J Dev Neurosci 2003;21:357–369.
115. Bigl M, Apelt J, Eschrich K, Schliebs R. Cortical glucose metabolism is altered in aged transgenic Tg2576 mice that demonstrate Alzheimer plaque pathology. J Neural Transm 2003;110:77–94.

116. Szutowicz A. Aluminum, NO and nerve growth factor neurotoxicity in cholinergic neurons. J Neurosci Res 2001;66:1009–1018.
117. Tomaszewicz M, Roßner S, Schliebs R, Cwikowska J, A. Szutowicz A. Changes in cortical acetyl-CoA metabolism after selective basal forebrain cholinergic degeneration by 192 IgG-saporin. J Neurochem 2003;87:318–324.
118. Zeitschel U, Schliebs R, Roßner S, Bigl V, Eschrich K, Bigl M. Changes in activity and expression of phosphofructokinase in different rat brain region after basal forebrain cholinergic lesion. J Neurochem 2002;83:371–380.
119. Mehlhorn G, Loffler T, Apelt J, et al. Glucose metabolism in cholinoceptive cortical rat brain regions after basal forebrain cholinergic lesion. Int J Dev Neurosci 1998;16:675–690.
120. Bassant MH, Poindessous-Jazat F, Schmidt BH. Sustained effect of metrifonate on cerebral glucose metabolism after immunolesion of basal forebrain cholinergic neurons in rats. Eur J Pharmacol 2000;387:151–162.
121. Sato A, Sato Y. Cholinergic neural regulation of regional cerebral blood flow. Alzheimer Dis Assoc Disord 1995;9:28–38.
122. Heininger K. Unifying hypothesis of Alzheimer's disease. IV. Causation and sequence of events. Rev Neurosci 2000;11:213–328.
123. Husain K, Ansari RA. Influence of cholinergic and adrenergic blocking drugs on hyperglycemia and brain glycogenolysis in diazinon-treated animals. Can J Physiol Pharmacol 1988;66:1144–1147.
124. Duelli R, Staudt R, Maurer MH, Kuschinsky W. Local transport kinetics of glucose during acute and chronic nicotine infusion in rat brains. J Neural Transm 1998;105:1017–1028.
125. Peterson C. Tetrahydroaminoacridine increases acetylcholine synthesis and glucose oxidation by mouse brain slices in vitro. Neurosci Lett 1990;115:274–278.
126. Marie S, Diaz-Guerra MJ, Miquerol L, Kahn A, Iynedjian PB. The pyruvate kinase gene as a model for studies of glucose-dependent regulation. J Biol Chem 1993;268:23,881–23,890.
127. Perry VH, Bolton SJ, Anthony DC, Betmouni S. The contribution of inflammation to acute and chronic neurodegeneration. Res Immunol 1998;149:721–725.
128. Akiyama H, Barger S, Barnum S, et al. Inflammation and Alzheimer's disease. Neurobiol Aging 2000;21:383–421.
129. Lüth HL, Apelt J, Ihunwo A, Schliebs R. Degeneration of β-amyloid-associated cholinergic structures in transgenic APP_{SW} mice. Brain Res 2003;977:16–22.
130. McGeer PL, McGeer EG, Yasojima K. Alzheimer disease and neuroinflammation. J Neural Transm 2000;59(suppl):53–57.
131. Wenk GL, Willard LB. The neuronal mechanisms underlying cholinergic cell death within the basal forebrain. Int J Dev Neurosci 1998;16:729–735.
132. Willard LB, Hauss-Wegrzyniak B, Wenk GL. Pathological and biochemical consequences of acute and chronic neuroinflammation within the basal forebrain cholinergic system of rats. Neuroscience 1999;88:193–200.

133. Bauer J, Strauss S, Schreiter-Gasser U, et al. Interleukin-6 and α-2-macroglobulin indicate an acute-phase state in Alzheimer's disease cortices. FEBS Lett 1991;285:111–114.

134. Griffin WST, Sheng JG, Roberts GW, Mrak RE. Interleukin-1 expression in different plaque types in Alzheimer's disease: significance in plaque evolution. J Neuropathol Exp Neurol 1995;54:276–281.

135. McGeer EG, McGeer PL. The importance of inflammatory mechanisms in Alzheimer's disease. Exp Gerontol 1998;33:371–378.

136. Lemke R, Hartig W, Roßner S, Bigl V, Schliebs R. Interleukin-6 is not expressed in activated microglia and in reactive astrocytes in response to lesion of rat basal forebrain cholinergic system as demonstrated by combined in situ hybridization and immunocytochemistry. J Neurosci Res 1998;51:223–236.

137. Lemke R, Gadient R A, Patterson PH, Bigl V, Schliebs R. Leukemia inhibitory factor (LIF) mRNA-expressing neuronal subpopulations in rat basal forebrain, Neurosci Lett 1997;229:69–71.

138. Hartlage-Rübsamen M, Lemke R, Schliebs R. Interleukin-1beta, inducible nitric oxide synthase, and nuclear factor-κB are induced in morphologically distinct microglia after rat hippocampal lipopolysaccharide/interferon-gamma injection. J Neurosci Res 1999;57:388–398.

139. Murphy M, Dutton R, Koblar S, Cheema S, Bartlett P. Cytokines which signal through the LIF receptor and their actions in the nervous system. Prog Neurobiol 1997;52:355–378.

140. Cheema SS, Arumugam D, Murray SS, Bartlett PF. Leukemia inhibitory factor maintains choline acetyltransferase expression in vivo. Neuroreport 1998;9:363–366.

141. Arvin B, Neville LF, Barone FC, Feuerstein GZ. The role of inflammation and cytokines in brain injury. Neurosci Biobehav Rev 1996;20:445–452.

142. Gadient RA, Otten UH. Interleukin-6 (IL-6)—a molecule with both beneficial and destructive potentials. Prog Neurobiol 1997;52:379–390.

143. Gruol DL, Nelson TE. Physiological and pathological roles of interleukin-6 in the central nervous system. Mol Neurobiol 1997;15:307–339.

144. Minami M, Kuraishi Y, Satoh M. Effects of kainic acid on messenger RNA levels of IL-1 β, IL-6, TNF α and LIF in the rat brain. Biochem Biophys Res Commun 1991;176:593–598.

145. Marquette C, Van Dam AM, Ceccaldi PE, Weber P, Haour F, Tsiang H. Induction of immunoreactive interleukin-1 beta and tumor necrosis factor-α in the brains of rabies virus infected rats. J Neuroimmunol 1996;68:45–51.

146. Kreutzberg GW. Microglia: a sensor for pathological events in the CNS. Trends Neurosci 1996;19:312–318.

147. Brown HC, Perry VH. Differential adhesion of macrophages to white and grey matter in an in vitro assay. Glia 1998;23:361–373.

148. Kloss CU, Werner A, Klein MA, et al. Integrin family of cell adhesion molecules in the injured brain: regulation and cellular localization in the normal and regenerating mouse facial motor nucleus. J Comp Neurol 1999;411:162–178.

149. Hailer NP, Bechmann I, Heizmann S, Nitsch R. Adhesion molecule expression on phagocytic microglial cells following anterograde degeneration of perforant path axons. Hippocampus 1997;7:341–349.
150. Jones LS, Grooms SY. Normal and aberrant functions of integrins in the adult central nervous system. Neurochem Int 1997;31:587–595.
151. Springer TA. Adhesion receptors of the immune system. Nature 1990;346: 425–434.
152. Lee SJ, Benveniste EN. Adhesion molecule expression and regulation on cells of the central nervous system. J Neuroimmunol 1999;98:77–88.
153. Cotman CW, Hailer NP, Pfister KK, Soltesz I, Schachner M. Cell adhesion molecules in neural plasticity and pathology: similar mechanisms, distinct organizations? Prog Neurobiol 1998;55:659–669.
154. Verbeek MM, Otte-Holler I, Wesseling P, Ruiter DJ, de Waal RM. Differential expression of intercellular adhesion molecule-1 (ICAM-1) in the A β-containing lesions in brains of patients with dementia of the Alzheimer type. Acta Neuropathol (Berl) 1996;91:608–615.

5

192 IgG-Saporin-Induced Partial Cortical Cholinergic Deafferentation as a Model for Determining the Interactions Between Brain Aging and Neurodevelopmental Defects in the Cortical Cholinergic Input System

Martin Sarter and John P. Bruno

INTRODUCTION

The anti-p75-immunotoxin 192 immunoglobulin G-saporin (192 IgG-sap) has been instrumental in testing the hypothesis that the integrity of the cortical cholinergic input system is necessary for the mediation of a wide range of attentional functions and capacities *(1–10)*. As discussed elsewhere *(11)*, attentional functions represent a crucial set of cognitive variables that contribute to the efficacy of learning and recalling of declarative information. Thus, impairments in attentional abilities rapidly yield escalating impairments in learning and memory. Different types of dysregulation of cortical cholinergic transmission have been hypothesized to mediate the diverse attentional impairments that are characteristic of major neuropsychiatric disorders and that contribute to the manifestation of the main cognitive symptoms of these disorders *(12–16)*.

The relationships between the degeneration of basal forebrain cholinergic neurons and the onset and progression of dementia have remained a matter of debate, although some aspects of this debate have been extensively substantiated. Specifically, the status of cortical cholinergic inputs predicts the cognitive status of patients with senile dementia unlike any other measure of cortical integrity, including the density of senile plaques *(17–24)*.

From: *Molecular Neurosurgery With Targeted Toxins*
Edited by: R. G. Wiley and D. A. Lappi © Humana Press Inc., Totowa, NJ

The role of the cortical cholinergic input system in dementia has been questioned primarily on the basis of psychopharmacological evidence. For example, the fact that the acute administration of muscarinic receptor antagonists to healthy humans does not reproduce the entire spectrum of impaired cognitive functions observed in Alzheimer's disease (AD; *25,26*) has been interpreted as reflecting a rather limited role of the cholinergic system in AD. However, an acute drug effect cannot model decades of escalating decline, and a proper psychopharmacological model in fact would need to assess the effects of chronically administered muscarinic antagonists. It can be safely predicted that such a treatment would cause a devastating and comprehensive decline in cognitive functions, even more so in aged subjects *(27)*.

A second major critique has been based on the narrow therapeutic potential of cholinesterase inhibitors which, likewise, has been interpreted as reflecting the limited involvement of the cholinergic system in the cognitive decline in AD. However, as discussed elsewhere *(13,28)*, there are many fundamental reasons to predict the restricted beneficial cognitive effects of these drugs, including the facts that they further dissociate postsynaptic cholinergic signaling from presynaptic cholinergic activity and that muscarinic receptor signal transduction cascades are disrupted in AD *(29–31)*. Studies continue to substantiate the relationship between decreases in cortical cholinergic innervation and cognitive decline *(17,32)*.

Based largely on the finding that, in patients with mild cognitive impairments, basal forebrain cholinergic neurons exhibit a strikingly reduced level of expression of trkA receptors *(33–35)*, hypotheses have emerged that describe the accelerating decline of the basal forebrain cortical cholinergic input system as a result of disruption of earlier trophic factor support and of reciprocal interactions between a declining cholinergic system and other converging, age-related cellular and vascular processes, including the processing and metabolism of amyloid precursor protein, and the regulation of the microvascular system *(36–48)*.

An important component of this major hypothesis refers to the age-related reregulation of (residual) cortical cholinergic inputs. Neurochemical and behavioral experiments have indicated that the regulation and function of the residual cortical cholinergic input system are robustly altered by the aging process. Specifically, in the aging brain, residual cortical cholinergic inputs no longer respond to activating behavioral or neurochemical manipulations and thus are no longer capable of mediating demands on attentional processing.

These hypotheses were tested by assessing the regulation and function of the (residual) cortical cholinergic input system in aging animals suffering from a limited loss of cortical cholinergic inputs produced by intrabasalis or intracortical *(49)* infusions of 192 IgG-sap. Thus, the usefulness of the immunotoxin as a research tool has been extended to produce an initial and approximate model of the early decline in the integrity of the cortical cholinergic input system, and this model permits study of the mechanisms that accelerate the decline in the regulation of a compromised cortical cholinergic input system during aging *(50)*.

ATTENUATION OF REACTIVITY OF RESIDUAL CORTICAL CHOLINERGIC INPUTS IN AGED ANIMALS

There is surprisingly little knowledge about the regulation and activity of residual cortical cholinergic inputs in AD or in animals modeling the declining integrity of this system. However, such information is important and of obvious relevance for drug treatment strategies focusing on the augmentation or reactivation of cholinergic transmission. For example, residual cholinergic neurons may exhibit up- or downregulated release and transporter mechanisms *(23,51–55)*, the activity of the hydrolyzing acetylcholine (ACh) esterases may be differently regulated following partial cholinergic deafferentation *(56,57)*, or residual cholinergic neurons may be subject to disproportionate inhibitory control and thus remain relatively inactive or unresponsive to activating stimuli *(58)*. Moreover, aging is expected to modulate further the regulation and activity of residual cholinergic neurons.

In young-mature rats, the available data do not indicate that the regulation of residual cortical cholinergic inputs is radically different from the regulation of the intact neuronal system. Fadel et al. *(59)* used the immunotoxin to produce an approx 50% loss of cortical cholinergic inputs. Although, as would be expected, basal cortical ACh efflux was robustly decreased, behavioral and pharmacological stimuli resulted in increases in extracellular cortical ACh levels that, in terms of changes from baseline, were similar to those observed in intact animals.

This situation changes as such animals age. Using a design similar to our prior study *(59)*, Fadel et al. compared the regulation of residual cholinergic neurons in rats 4–7 and 24–28 mo old *(60)*. As shown in Fig. 1, basal ACh efflux was similarly reduced in young and aged rats, reflecting the comparable degree of cortical cholinergic deafferentation.

A combined pharmacological and behavioral stimulus was used to assess the reactivity of the cortical cholinergic system in young and aged, sham-operated and deafferented animals. Specifically, animals were trained to associate darkness with the presentation of palatable food; this complex stimulus increases cortical ACh efflux by about 100% *(61,62)*. In addition,

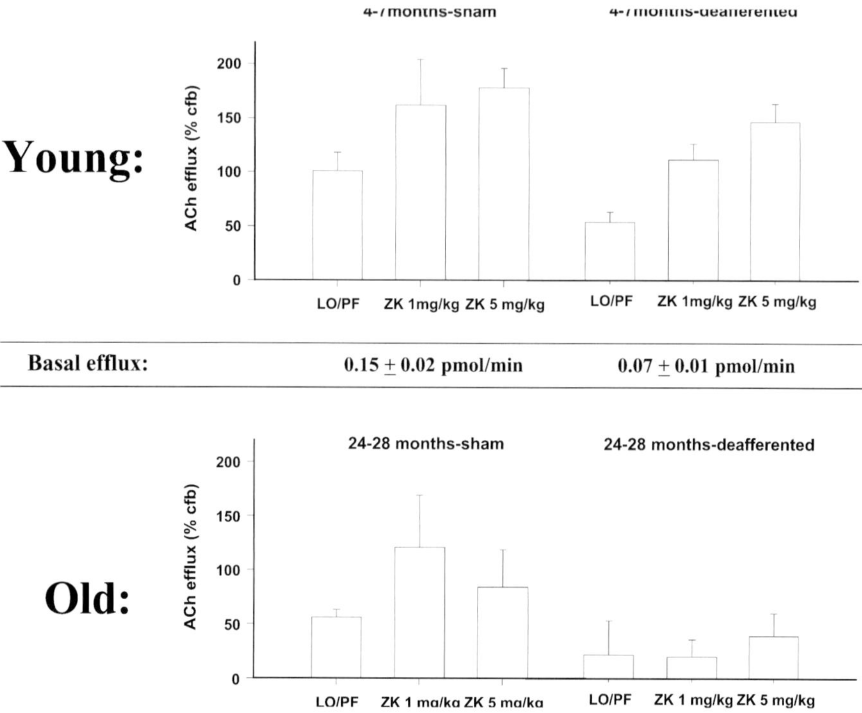

Fig. 1. Regulation of activity of residual cortical cholinergic inputs in young and aged animals. As described in detail in the study of Fadel et al. *(60)*, the density of cortical cholinergic inputs was decreased by infusions of 192 IgG-sap into the basal forebrain of young and aged animals. The decrease in basal acetylcholine (ACh) efflux as a result of the lesion was identical in young and aged rats (absolute levels are indicated in the box in the middle of the figure). To test the responsivity of the residual cortical cholinergic input system in young and aged rats, a combined behavioral and pharmacological stimulus was administered. This stimulus consisted of turning off the lights in the test room, which was previously conditioned to the presentation of palatable food (LO/PF), and the systemic administration of two doses of a weak negative γ-aminobutyric acid modulator, the β-carboline ZK 93426 (ZK; 1 and 5 mg/kg). As indicated in the upper left graph, in young, sham-operated animals, the combined stimulus produced a 150% increase in ACh efflux of over baseline (cfb = change from baseline). Although the effects of the stimulus appeared dampened in aged, sham-operated animals (lower left), they were not significantly different from those in young rats. Likewise, in young and deafferented animals, and in terms of changes from their lower baseline, the stimulus was statistically as effective in increasing ACh efflux from residual cortical cholinergic inputs as in intact, young animals (upper right). However, in aged and deafferented animals, the residual cortical cholinergic input system remained completely unresponsive to the combined behavioral and pharmacological stimulus.

animals were treated systemically with two doses of a weak negative γ-aminobutyric acid (GABA) modulator, the β-carboline ZK 93426, which further augments the behavior-induced increase in cortical ACh efflux *(62)*.

As shown in Fig. 1, ACh efflux in young, sham-operated animals was increased by this combined behavioral and pharmacological stimulus by about 160% over baseline. Similar to several previous studies using in vivo microdialysis *(50)*, aged, sham-operated rats responded similarly to this stimulus. Likewise, and although Fig. 1 appears to indicate a dampened response, the stimulus was equally effective in young/deafferented animals. However, in aged/deafferented animals, cortical ACh efflux did not respond to these activating manipulations (Fig. 1). To reiterate, the degree of these animals' cortical cholinergic deafferentation was similar to that in young animals, as indicated by neurochemical and histochemical measures, but the residual cholinergic system of aged animals apparently was reregulated fundamentally, rendering it completely unresponsive to the behavioral and pharmacological stimuli used in our experiments.

Obviously, results based on one set of stimuli may not readily generalize to another set of behavioral or pharmacological stimuli. However, other studies likewise suggested that changes in the regulation of residual cholinergic neurons remain limited in young animals. For example, only limited alterations in behavior-induced increases in ACh efflux, vesamicol-binding, and other measures indicating the dynamic activity of residual cholinergic transmission after partial deafferentation were found in young-mature rats *(1,63–65)*.

The mechanisms mediating the dysregulation of residual cortical cholinergic inputs in aged animals have remained unsettled. Inspired by the finding that basal forebrain lesions increase the activity of cortical GABA-ergic terminals *(66)* and that aged cholinergic neurons are more effectively inhibited by positive GABA modulators *(67)*, the effects of the $GABA_A$-receptor antagonist bicuculline, administered locally into the cortex through the dialysis probe, were assessed to test the possibility that an increased GABA-ergic inhibition of residual cholinergic terminals occurred in aged animals. The data from this experiment did not indicate that bicuculline produces a greater increase in ACh release in aged animals and thus did not support this hypothesis *(68)*.

However, it is also possible that such an indirect pharmacological approach does not offer the sensitivity necessary to demonstrate age-related differences in the GABA-ergic regulation of (residual) cholinergic terminals. Furthermore, our efforts to measure directly the cortical GABA release in young and aged rats, using in vivo microdialysis, did not yield conclusive findings, possibly partly because of the general complexities associated with the determination of neuronally released amino acid neurotransmitters using the microdialysis method *(69)*.

Although, as mentioned, the evidence in support of robust effects of age on the activity and reactivity of cortical cholinergic inputs has remained limited *(50)*, some data indicated clear consequences of aging. In particular, in aged rats, depolarization of cortical terminals by administering potassium (in vivo through the dialysis probe or in vitro) produced substantially lower levels of extracellular ACh levels in aged compared to young rats *(70–73)*. On the other hand, cortical perfusion of atropine produced much higher levels of ACh efflux than perfusion with potassium, and the effects of atropine did not differ between young and aged animals *(70)*; therefore, the basis for the differential effects of potassium do not appear to be caused by a limited capacity of aged cholinergic synapses to store and release ACh.

Obviously, multiple cellular mechanisms could account for the age-related differences in the effects of potassium, including changes in calcium-buffering capacities *(74)*. Furthermore, the abnormal regulation of residual cholinergic neurons may be caused by alterations in cortical efferent projections that feedback, via long-loop multisynaptic circuits, to the basal forebrain. Alterations in such long-loop circuits may be a result of interactions with the age-related disruption of muscarinic receptor signaling *(75,76)*. The potency of any or several of these mechanisms could increase as a result of partial deafferentation, yielding an unresponsive residual cortical cholinergic input system.

Although the underlying mechanisms mediating the age-related decrease in the responsivity of residual cholinergic neurons remain to be determined, this finding may add to the validity of 192 IgG-sap-induced loss of cholinergic neurons as a model for the decline in this particular neuronal system in AD. The available evidence is limited and mixed *(51,52,54)*, but choline transport into cortical synaptosomes and cortical ACh synthesis appear to be reduced in patients with AD *(23,77)*. Thus, the determination of the mechanisms that mediate the attenuated reactivity of residual cholinergic neurons in aged subjects will be important in understanding the accelerated cognitive decline in AD.

ATTENTION PERFORMANCE OF PARTIALLY DEAFFERENTED AGING ANIMALS

The findings described here predict that, in animals with partial loss of the cortical cholinergic inputs, the cognitive functions that depend on the integrity of this system will decline as the animals age because aging attenuates the excitability of the residual cholinergic system. As mentioned, attentional processes and capacities have been extensively demonstrated as impaired as a function of the degree of loss of cortical cholinergic inputs.

Thus, rats were trained in a sustained attention task, the performance of which was previously demonstrated as impaired following 192 IgG-sap-induced lesions of the cortical cholinergic input system *(2,3,78,79)*, and to produce an increase in cortical ACh efflux that was not observed in animals performing various procedures designed to control for the effects of the motivational procedures and sensorimotor activity *(80–82)*. Following acquisition of this task, an intentionally limited loss of cortical cholinergic inputs (42–63%) was produced using the immunotoxin in half of the animals, and all animals remained on task throughout their life (for details, *see* ref. *83*). The limited deafferentation remained—to reiterate, intentionally— too small to produce acute effects on performance. In fact, the performance of lesioned and sham-lesioned rats did not differ until the rats reached 31 mo of age, approx 85% of their life-span. The impairment in performance in deafferented animals manifested as a very robust augmentation in the performance decrement within a session (Fig. 2).

The nature of this "vigilance decrement" supported a rather specific interpretation in terms of impairments in sustained attention. Moreover, and importantly, the size of this effect resembled the effects of almost-complete cortical cholinergic deafferentation in young animals. Thus, this finding can be interpreted, similar to the conclusions from the neurochemical studies described above, as reflecting the attenuation of the reactivity of the residual neurons in aged animals. The performance of the animals further declined as they aged; however, increased mortality rates and confounding effects on secondary measures of performance rendered these data less interpretable.

Despite the robust interactions between aging and deafferentation observed in this study, these findings may in fact underestimate the true impact of aging on a residual cortical cholinergic input system. Because these animals remained on task throughout their life, this continued practice, including the potentially beneficial effects on continued attentional practice on cholinergic function, may have limited the manifestation of age-related consequences of the prior deafferentation.

SUMMARY

Longitudinal studies assessing the interactions between aging and preexisting abnormalities in the integrity or regulation of relevant neuronal systems are rare despite their obvious heuristic power, and despite their irreplaceable role for testing ontogenetic theories about brain aging *(48)*.

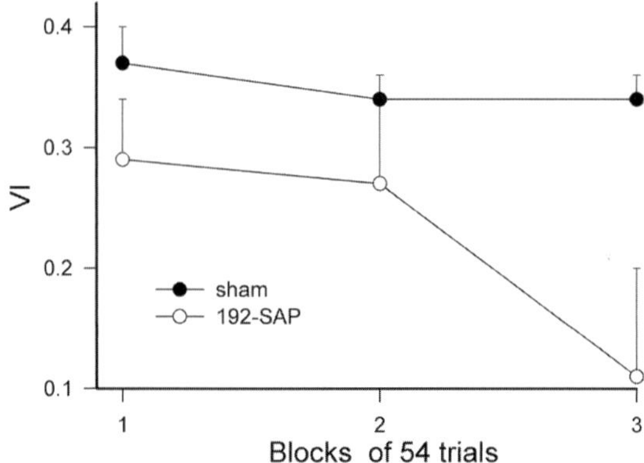

Fig. 2. Age-related effects of partial cortical cholinergic deafferentation on the performance of rats in a sustained attention task. Young animals were trained in this task, and about 50% of the cortical cholinergic inputs were destroyed using the immunotoxin. Animals remained on task throughout their lifespan. The limited deafferentation did not, intentionally, produce acute effects on performance. The figure shows the performance of the animals when they reached 31 mo of age (about 85% of their lifespan). VI depicts an overall measure of performance that is calculated on the basis of the relative number of hits and correct rejections (for details, *see* ref. *83*). Block (abscissa) refers to three successive blocks of 54 trials each, for a total of 162 trials that formed a daily test session. At 31 mo of age, previously deafferented animals exhibited a steep decline in performance over trials, termed a *vigilance decrement*. This decline is hypothesized to reflect the attenuated responsivity of residual cholinergic neurons in aged animals (*see* Fig. 1).

The use of the immunotoxin to assess the long-term and age-related consequences of early limitations in the integrity of the cortical cholinergic input system represents an obviously crude and early approach that will have to be replaced by more subtle and more valid manipulations of the development and maturation of the cortical cholinergic input system, such as, for example, the early-life disruption of its trophic factor support.

Minimally, the data generated by experiments that assessed the age-related neuronal and behavioral/cognitive consequences of 192 IgG-sap-induced partial cortical cholinergic deafferentation demonstrated that aging results in a dramatic dysregulation of the residual neuronal system. The alternative to approaches that focus on the examination of such interactions between early abnormalities in the regulation of neuronal systems that mediate crucial aspects of cognitive functions and aging would be to conceptualize pathological brain aging as primarily driven by major neuropathological events that manifest abruptly at higher ages. However, the available data increasingly do not support such a view *(50,84)*. The immunotoxin 192 IgG-sap has and will remain a crucial instrument in the exploration of the developmental variables that cause an age-related decline in the integrity and regulation of the cortical cholinergic input system.

ACKNOWLEDGMENT

Our research was supported by the Public Health Service (AG65244, NS37026, MH63114, MH57436, and K02 MH01072).

REFERENCES

1. McGaughy J, Dalley JW, Morrison CH, Everitt BJ, Robbins TW. Selective behavioral and neurochemical effects of cholinergic lesions produced by intrabasalis infusions of 192 IgG-saporin on attentional performance in a five-choice serial reaction time task. J Neurosci 2002;22:1905–1913.
2. McGaughy J, Kaiser T, Sarter M. Behavioral vigilance following infusions of 192 IgG-saporin into the basal forebrain: selectivity of the behavioral impairment and relation to cortical AChE-positive fiber density. Behav Neurosci 1996;110:247–265.
3. McGaughy J, Sarter M. Sustained attention performance in rats with intracortical infusions of 192 IgG-saporin-induced cortical cholinergic deafferentation: effects of physostigmine and FG 7142. Behav Neurosci 1998;112:1519–1525.
4. McGaughy J, Everitt BJ, Robbins TW, Sarter M. The role of cortical cholinergic afferent projections in cognition: impact of new selective immunotoxins. Behav Brain Res 2000;115:251–263.
5. Baxter MG, Bucci DJ, Holland PC, Gallagher M. Impairments in conditioned stimulus processing and conditioned responding after combined selective removal of hippocampal and neocortical cholinergic input. Behav Neurosci 1999;113:486–495.
6. Bucci DJ, Holland PC, Gallagher M. Removal of cholinergic input to rat posterior parietal cortex disrupts incremental processing of conditioned stimuli. J Neurosci 1998;18:8038–8046.
7. Everitt BJ, Robbins TW. Central cholinergic systems and cognition. Annu Rev Psychol 1997;48:649–684.
8. Sarter M, Givens B, Bruno JP. The cognitive neuroscience of sustained attention: where top-down meets bottom-up. Brain Res Rev 2001;35:146–160.
9. Sarter M, Bruno JP. Cortical cholinergic inputs mediating arousal, attentional processing and dreaming: differential afferent regulation of the basal forebrain by telencephalic and brainstem afferents. Neuroscience 2000;95:933–952.
10. Turchi J, Sarter M. Cortical acetylcholine and processing capacity: effects of cortical cholinergic deafferentation on crossmodal divided attention in rats. Cogn Brain Res 1997;6:147–158.
11. Sarter M, Bruno JP, Givens B. Attentional functions of cortical cholinergic inputs: what does it mean for memory? Neurobiol Learn Mem 2003;80:245–256.

12. Sarter M, Turchi J. Age- and dementia-associated impairments in divided attention: psychological constructs, animal models, and underlying neuronal mechanisms. Dement Geriatr Cogn Disord 2002;13:46–58.
13. Sarter M, Bruno JP. Abnormal regulation of corticopetal cholinergic neurons and impaired information processing in neuropsychiatric disorders. Trends Neurosci 1999;22:67–74.
14. Sarter M, Bruno JP, Turchi J. Basal forebrain afferent projections modulating cortical acetylcholine, attention, and implications for neuropsychiatric disorders. Ann NY Acad Sci 1999;877:368–382.
15. Sarter M, Bruno JP. Cortical acetylcholine, reality distortion, schizophrenia, and Lewy body dementia: too much or too little cortical acetylcholine? Brain Cogn 1998;38:297–316.
16. Sarter M. Neuronal mechanisms of the attentional dysfunctions in senile dementia and schizophrenia: two sides of the same coin? Psychopharmacol (Berl) 1994;114:539–550.
17. Pappas BA, Bayley PJ, Bui BK, Hansen LA, Thal LJ. Choline acetyltransferase activity and cognitive domain scores of Alzheimer's patients. Neurobiol Aging 2000;21:11–17.
18. Procter AW. Neurochemical correlates of dementia. Neurodegeneration 1996;5:403–407.
19. Palmer AM. Neurochemical studies of Alzheimer's disease. Neurodegeneration 1996;5:381–391.
20. Baskin DS, Browning JL, Pirozzolo FJ, Korporaal S, Baskin JA, Appel SH. Brain choline acetyltransferase and mental function in Alzheimer disease. Arch Neurol 1999;56:1121–1123.
21. Lehericy S, Hirsch EC, Cervera-Pierot P, et al. Heterogeneity and selectivity of the degeneration of cholinergic neurons in the basal forebrain of patients with Alzheimer's disease. J Comp Neurol 1993;330:15–31.
22. Giannakopoulos P, Hof PR, Michel JP, Guimon J, Bouras C. Cerebral cortex pathology in aging and Alzheimer's disease: a quantitative survey of large hospital-based geriatric and psychiatric cohorts. Brain Res Rev 1997;25:217–245.
23. Sims NR, Bowen DM, Allen SJ, et al. Presynaptic cholinergic dysfunction in patients with dementia. J Neurochem 1983;40:503–509.
24. Hanyu H, Asano T, Sakurai H, Tanaka Y, Takasaki M, Abe K. MR analysis of the substantia innominata in normal aging, Alzheimer disease, and other types of dementia. AJNR Am J Neuroradiol 2002;23:27–32.
25. Beatty WW, Butters N, Janowsky DS. Patterns of memory failure after scopolamine treatment: implications for cholinergic hypotheses of dementia. Behav Neural Biol 1986;45:196–211.
26. Kopelman MD, Corn TH. Cholinergic "blockade" as a model for cholinergic depletion. A comparison of the memory deficits with those of Alzheimer-type dementia and the alcoholic Korsakoff syndrome. Brain 1988;111:1079–1110.
27. Molchan SE, Martinez RA, Hill JL, et al. Increased cognitive sensitivity to scopolamine with age and a perspective on the scopolamine model. Brain Res Rev 1992;17:215–226.

28. Sarter M, Bruno JP. Mild cognitive impairment and the cholinergic hypothesis: a very different take on recent data. Ann Neurol 2002;52:384–385.
29. Greenwood AF, Powers RE, Jope RS. Phosphoinositide hydrolysis, G alpha q, phospholipase C, and protein kinase C in post mortem human brain: effects of post mortem interval, subject age, and Alzheimer's disease. Neuroscience 1995;69:125–138.
30. Jope RS, Song L, Powers RE. Cholinergic activation of phosphoinositide signaling is impaired in Alzheimer's disease brain. Neurobiol Aging 1997;18:111–120.
31. Fowler CJ, Garlind A, O'Neill C, Cowburn RF. Receptor-effector coupling dysfunctions in Alzheimer's disease. Ann NY Acad Sci 1996;786:294–304.
32. Minger SL, Esiri MM, McDonald B, et al. Cholinergic deficits contribute to behavioral disturbance in patients with dementia. Neurology 2000;55:1460–1467.
33. Chu Y, Cochran EJ, Bennett DA, Mufson EJ, Kordower JH. Down-regulation of trkA mRNA within nucleus basalis neurons in individuals with mild cognitive impairment and Alzheimer's disease. J Comp Neurol 2001;437:296–307.
34. Mufson EJ, Lavine N, Jaffar S, Kordower JH, Quirion R, Saragovi HU. Reduction in p140-TrkA receptor protein within the nucleus basalis and cortex in Alzheimer's disease. Exp Neurol 1997;146:91–103.
35. Mufson EJ, Ma SY, Cochran EJ, et al. Loss of nucleus basalis neurons containing trkA immunoreactivity in individuals with mild cognitive impairment and early Alzheimer's disease. J Comp Neurol 2000;427:19–30.
36. Auld DS, Kar S, Quirion R. Beta-amyloid peptides as direct cholinergic neuromodulators: a missing link? Trends Neurosci 1998;21:43–49.
37. Chen KS, Nishimura MC, Armanini MP, Crowley C, Spencer SD, Phillips HS. Disruption of a single allele of the nerve growth factor gene results in atrophy of basal forebrain cholinergic neurons and memory deficits. J Neurosci 1997;17:7288–7296.
38. de la Torre JC, Stefano GB. Evidence that Alzheimer's disease is a microvascular disorder: the role of constitutive nitric oxide. Brain Res Rev 2000;34:119–136.
39. Holtzman DM, Lee S, Li Y, et al. Expression of neuronal-NOS in developing basal forebrain cholinergic neurons: regulation by NGF. Neurochem Res 1996;21:861–868.
40. Isacson O, Seo H, Lin L, Albeck D, Granholm AC. Alzheimer's disease and Down's syndrome: roles of APP, trophic factors and ACh. Trends Neurosci 2002;25:79–84.
41. Kalaria RN. Small vessel disease and Alzheimer's dementia: pathological considerations. Cerebrovasc Dis 2002;13(suppl 2):48–52.
42. Mufson EJ, Counts SE, Ginsberg SD. Gene expression profiles of cholinergic nucleus basalis neurons in Alzheimer's disease. Neurochem Res 2002;27:1035–1048.
43. Mufson EJ, Kroin JS, Sendera TJ, Sobreviela T. Distribution and retrograde transport of trophic factors in the central nervous system: functional implications for the treatment of neurodegenerative diseases. Prog Neurobiol 1999;57:451–484.

44. Roßner S. Cholinergic immunolesions by 192 IgG-saporin—a useful tool to stimulate pathogenic aspects of Alzheimer's disease. Int J Dev Neurosci 1997;15:835–850.

45. Rossner S, Ueberham U, Schliebs R, Perez-Polo JR, Bigl V. The regulation of amyloid precursor protein metabolism by cholinergic mechanisms and neurotrophin receptor signaling. Prog Neurobiol 1998;56:541–569.

46. Snowdon DA. Aging and Alzheimer's disease: lessons from the Nun Study. Gerontologist 1997;37:150–156.

47. Sofroniew MV, Howe CL, Mobley WC. Nerve growth factor signaling, neuroprotection, and neural repair. Annu Rev Neurosci 2001;24:1217–1281.

48. Sarter M, Bruno JP. Developmental origins of the age-related decline in cortical cholinergic function and in associated cognitive abilities. Neurobiol Aging 2004;25:1127–1139.

49. Holley LA, Wiley RG, Lappi DA, Sarter M. Cortical cholinergic deafferentation following the intracortical infusion of 192 IgG-saporin: a quantitative histochemical study. Brain Res 1994;663:277–286.

50. Sarter M, Bruno JP. Age-related changes in rodent cortical acetylcholine and cognition: main effects of age vs age as an intervening variable. Brain Res Rev 1998;27:143–156.

51. Efange SM, Garland EM, Staley JK, Khare AB, Mash DC. Vesicular acetylcholine transporter density and Alzheimer's disease. Neurobiol Aging 1997;18:407–413.

52. Pascual J, Fontan A, Zarranz JJ, Berciano J, Florez J, Pazos A. High-affinity choline uptake carrier in Alzheimer's disease: implications for the cholinergic hypothesis of dementia. Brain Res 1991;552:170–174.

53. Bowen DM, Allen SJ, Benton JS, et al. Biochemical assessment of serotonergic and cholinergic dysfunction and cerebral atrophy in Alzheimer's disease. J Neurochem 1983;41:266–272.

54. Bissette G, Seidler FJ, Nemeroff CB, Slotkin TA. High affinity choline transporter status in Alzheimer's disease tissue from rapid autopsy. Ann NY Acad Sci 1996;777:197–204.

55. Sihver W, Gillberg PG, Svensson AL, Nordberg A. Autoradiographic comparison of [^{3}H](–)nicotine, [^{3}H]cytisine and [^{3}H]epibatidine binding in relation to vesicular acetylcholine transport sites in the temporal cortex in Alzheimer's disease. Neuroscience 1999;94:685–696.

56. Fishman EB, Siek GC, MacCallum RD, Bird ED, Volicer L, Marquis JK. Distribution of the molecular forms of acetylcholinesterase in human brain: alterations in dementia of the Alzheimer type. Ann Neurol 1986;19:246–252.

57. Atack JR, Perry EK, Bonham JR, Perry RH. Molecular forms of acetylcholinesterase and butyrylcholinesterase in human plasma and cerebrospinal fluid. J Neurochem 1987;48:1845–1850.

58. Salehi A, Lucassen PJ, Pool CW, Gonatas NK, Ravid R, Swaab DF. Decreased neuronal activity in the nucleus basalis of Meynert in Alzheimer's disease as suggested by the size of the Golgi apparatus. Neuroscience 1994;59:871–880.

59. Fadel J, Moore H, Sarter M, Bruno JP. Trans-synaptic stimulation of cortical acetylcholine release after partial 192 IgG-saporin-induced loss of cortical cholinergic afferents. J Neurosci 1996;16:6592–6600.
60. Fadel J, Sarter M, Bruno JP. Age-related attenuation of stimulated cortical acetylcholine release in basal forebrain-lesioned rats. Neuroscience 1999;90:793–802.
61. Moore H, Sarter M, Bruno JP. Bidirectional modulation of cortical acetylcholine efflux by infusion of benzodiazepine receptor ligands into the basal forebrain. Neurosci Lett 1995;189:31–34.
62. Moore H, Sarter M, Bruno JP. Bidirectional modulation of stimulated cortical acetylcholine release by benzodiazepine receptor ligands. Brain Res 1993;627:267–274.
63. Raulli RE, Arendash G, Crews FT. Effects of nBM lesions on muscarinic-stimulation of phosphoinositide hydrolysis. Neurobiol Aging 1989;10:191–197.
64. Holley LA, Miller JA, Chmielewski PA, Dudchenko P, Sarter M. Interactions between the effects of basal forebrain lesions and chronic treatment with MDL 26,479 on learning and markers of cholinergic transmission. Brain Res 1993;610:181–193.
65. Wenk GL, Mobley SL. Choline acetyltransferase activity and vesamicol binding in Rett syndrome and in rats with nucleus basalis lesions. Neuroscience 1996;73:79–84.
66. Abdulla FA, Calaminici MR, Raevsky VV, Sinden JD, Gray JA, Stephenson JD. An iontophoretic study of the effects of alpha-amino-hydroxy-5-methyl-4-isoxazole propionic acid lesions of the nucleus basalis magnocellularis on cholinergic and GABAergic influences on frontal cortex neurones of rats. Exp Brain Res 1994;98:441–456.
67. Griffith WH, Murchison DA. Enhancement of GABA-activated membrane currents in aged Fischer 344 rat basal forebrain neurons. J Neurosci 1995;15:2407–2416.
68. Bruno JP, Herzog CD, Nowak KA, Sarter M. Age-related alterations in potassium-stimulated cortical acetylcholine efflux: potential role of GABA-ergic transmission. Soc Neurosci Abstr 2002;28:238–239.
69. Del Arco A, Segovia G, Fuxe K, Mora F. Changes in dialysate concentrations of glutamate and GABA in the brain: an index of volume transmission mediated actions? J Neurochem 2003;85:23–33.
70. Moore H, Stuckman S, Sarter M, Bruno JP. Potassium, but not atropine-stimulated cortical acetylcholine efflux, is reduced in aged rats. Neurobiol Aging 1996;17:565–571.
71. Herzog CD, Nowak KA, Sarter M, Bruno JP. Microdialysis without acetylcholinesterase inhibition reveals an age-related attenuation in stimulated cortical acetylcholine release. Neurobiol Aging 2003;24:861–863.
72. Takei N, Nihonmatsu I, Kawamura H. Age-related decline of acetylcholine release evoked by depolarizing stimulation. Neurosci Lett 1989;101:182–186.
73. Meyer EM, Crews FT, Otero DH, Larsen K. Aging decreases the sensitivity of rat cortical synaptosomes to calcium ionophore-induced acetylcholine release. J Neurochem 1986;47:1244–1246.

74. Griffith WH, Jasek MC, Bain SH, Murchison D. Modification of ion channels and calcium homeostasis of basal forebrain neurons during aging. Behav Brain Res 2000;115:219–233.

75. Narang N, Joseph JA, Ayyagari PV, Gerber M, Crews FT. Age-related loss of cholinergic-muscarinic coupling to PLC: comparison with changes in brain regional PLC subtypes mRNA distribution. Brain Res 1996;708:143–152.

76. Wellman CL, Pelleymounter MA. Differential effects of nucleus basalis lesions in young adult and aging rats. Neurobiol Aging 1999;20:381–393.

77. Rylett RJ, Ball MJ, Colhoun EH. Evidence for high affinity choline transport in synaptosomes prepared from hippocampus and neocortex of patients with Alzheimer's disease. Brain Res 1983;289:169–175.

78. McGaughy J, Sarter M. Effects of ovariectomy, 192 IgG-saporin-induced cortical cholinergic deafferentation, and administration of estradiol on sustained attention performance in rats. Behav Neurosci 1999;113:1216–1232.

79. McGaughy J, Decker MW, Sarter M. Enhancement of sustained attention performance by the nicotinic acetylcholine receptor agonist ABT-418 in intact but not basal forebrain-lesioned rats. Psychopharmacology (Berl) 1999;144:175–182.

80. Arnold HM, Burk JA, Hodgson EM, Sarter M, Bruno JP. Differential cortical acetylcholine release in rats performing a sustained attention task vs behavioral control tasks that do not explicitly tax attention. Neuroscience 2002;114:451–460.

81. Himmelheber AM, Sarter M, Bruno JP. Increases in cortical acetylcholine release during sustained attention performance in rats. Cogn Brain Res 2000;9:313–325.

82. Himmelheber AM, Sarter M, Bruno JP. Operant performance and cortical acetylcholine release: role of response rate, reward density, and non-contingent stimuli. Cogn Brain Res 1997;6:23–36.

83. Burk JA, Herzog CD, Porter MC, Sarter M. Interactions between aging and cortical cholinergic deafferentation on attention. Neurobiol Aging 2002;23:467–477.

84. Petersen RC, Smith GE, Waring SC, Ivnik RJ, Tangalos EG, Kokmen E. Mild cognitive impairment: clinical characterization and outcome. Arch Neurol 1999;56:303–308.

6

Exploring the Role of Acetylcholine in Primate Cognition Using Me20.4 IgG-Saporin

Rosalind M. Ridley and Harry F. Baker

INTRODUCTION

"Do not go gentle into that good night,
Old age should burn and rave at close of day;
Rage, rage against the dying of the light."
Dylan Thomas, 1914–1953

Two factors led to the emergence of the "cholinergic hypothesis of geriatric memory dysfunction" *(1)*: evidence that cholinergic blockade in human volunteers leads to impaired acquisition of new information *(2,3)* and the demonstration of loss of cortical cholinergic activity and loss of cholinergic cell bodies in the basal forebrain of patients dying with Alzheimer's disease *(4–6)*. It has been proposed that it is the loss of the rising cholinergic pathways from the basal forebrain to the cortex (including the hippocampus) that is responsible for the amnesia seen in dementing illnesses *(6)*. This view has been challenged (e.g., in ref. *7*). Cholinergic antagonists also block transmission at cholinergic neurons intrinsic to many subcortical areas and block transmission in the cholinergic projections to noncortical areas; this may affect memory, either directly or via an influence on arousal and attention. Furthermore, studies with rats did not produce a correlation between the magnitude of cholinergic loss in the basal forebrain across various nonimmunotoxic lesion techniques and learning or performance impairments *(8)*.

From: *Molecular Neurosurgery With Targeted Toxins*
Edited by: R. G. Wiley and D. A. Lappi © Humana Press Inc., Totowa, NJ

However, although these early studies did not establish a role for the basal forebrain cholinergic projections in learning, they did not establish a specific role for it in any other cognitive function because none of the lesion methods used were specific to the cholinergic system. It remains a possibility that the behavioral tasks used in these various studies were inappropriate rather than that these studies demonstrated, unequivocally, that basal forebrain acetylcholine is not involved in any aspect of learning and memory.

Clinical observation has also been unable to determine a specific role for acetylcholine in mnemonic function. Degeneration of many neuronal systems and other pathological changes are found in the brains of patients dying with Alzheimer's disease *(9–11)* and any of these may have contributed to a wide range of cognitive impairments, including memory loss. Although loss of cholinergic markers measured postmortem does correlate with dementia scores premortem *(12,13)*, other aspects of pathology, such as cortical neurofibrillary tangle density and loss of pyramidal cells also correlate with severity of symptoms *(14–16)*.

Patients with Alzheimer's disease show impairment on acquisition of long-term memories and on tests of recent memory *(17)*. Aged monkeys show impairments on a wide range of memory tests, including repeated-trial learning (long-term memory tasks) *(18,19)* and tests of recent memory *(20)*. Thus, either acetylcholine is involved in a wide range of memory functions (and probably other cognitive functions as well) or, if only some of the memory deficits in Alzheimer's disease and aging are caused by cholinergic loss, other memory deficits must be caused by other pathology.

The enhancement of cholinergic neurotransmission using cholinesterase inhibitors (e.g., donepezil) is currently a licensed treatment for the memory impairments of Alzheimer's disease *(21)*. This method is only moderately successful. Efficacy is limited because cholinesterase inhibitors act by preventing the breakdown of acetylcholine and can therefore only be of value when some acetylcholine is still present, and dose is limited by the occurrence of undesirable autonomic side effects and other toxicity. Drugs that specifically target cholinoceptive receptors in neural circuits involved in learning and memory may be much more effective. Such drugs would not compensate directly for loss of noncholinergic neurons in Alzheimer's disease, but if the loss of the rising cholinergic projections does contribute to memory impairment, then it will be necessary to address this loss with effective treatment. Furthermore, there is evidence that immunotoxic cholinergic lesions induce β-amyloid deposition *(22)*, and that cholinergic agonists suppress the production of the β-amyloid precursor peptide *(23)*, suggesting that prolonged cholinergic support may retard pathogenic mechanisms as well as provide cognitive enhancement in Alzheimer's disease.

Developing both cholinergic and noncholinergic drug treatments requires an understanding of the neural circuitry involved in memory formation and the neurotransmitter relationships within these circuits. The immunotoxin Me20.4 immunoglobulin G-saporin (IgG-sap) can be used to produce precisely targeted lesions of the cholinergic system in primates, and these animals can be tested on a range of memory tasks. This model can be used to explore the functional relationship between the various parts of the rising cholinergic projections and the neurons and receptors with which they interact, and can be used to assess the efficacy of potential therapeutic agents in diseases which involve the cholinergic system or these target neuronal circuits.

WHY USE PRIMATES?

The experiments described in this chapter used primates. They were bred in the United Kingdom, and their use is governed by UK Home Office regulations. The majority of the experiments were done using New World common marmosets (*Callithrix jacchus*), but one experiment was carried out using Old World rhesus monkeys *(Macaca mulatta)*. Marmosets can be trained on a variety of repeated-trial object-reward association tasks in the Wisconsin General Test Apparatus (WGTA), and many of the experiments using immunotoxins have compared the effects of immunotoxic lesions of parts of the rising cholinergic system with the effects of surgical removal or excitotoxic destruction of the target area of those projections. So, the effects of lesions of the basal forebrain cholinergic projections have been compared with the effects of suction ablations of the inferotemporal (IT) cortex, which cause impairment on visual object-reward association tasks *(24)*; or with excitotoxic lesions of the hippocampus or fornix transections, both of which cause impairment on conditional learning *(25,26)*.

The cognitive abilities of the marmoset are adequate for performance of these types of task, which probably depend on the use of declarative (as opposed to procedural) memory, although the extent to which performance of these tasks is dependent on memory for events (cf. episodic memory in humans) or memory for facts (cf. semantic memory in humans) is more difficult to determine *(27,28)*. Macaque monkeys can be trained on a wider range of tasks in the WGTA (or its automated versions), especially tasks for which each stimulus is only presented once. These tasks marmosets find difficult to master. There is also a general consensus regarding which of the types of task that the macaques can master, assess recognition memory, episodic memory, or factual memory. It is therefore appropriate to use macaque monkeys to assess the contribution of the cholinergic system to these components of declarative memory, all of which are impaired in the denser forms of amnesia in humans.

THE ANATOMY OF THE CHOLINERGIC SYSTEM IN OLD WORLD AND NEW WORLD PRIMATES

The rising cholinergic projections of the Old World macaque brain have been classified and mapped by Mesulam and colleagues *(29,30)*. Groups Ch1–Ch4 form a continuous band that runs from the medial septum, through the vertical limb of the diagonal band of Broca (VDB); the horizontal limb of the diagonal band; the nucleus basalis of Meynert (NBM) in the substantia innominata; behind the anterior commissure, in the medial medullary lamella between the internal and external components of the globus pallidus; and in the lateral medullary lamella between the globus pallidus and the putamen. Groups Ch5–Ch6 project from the pedunculopontine nucleus to the thalamus, Ch7 projects from the medial habenula to the interpeduncular nucleus, and Ch8 projects from the parabigeminal nucleus to the superior colliculus. The same pattern of cholinergic neurons has been demonstrated in the New World marmoset brain using choline acetyltransferase (ChAT) staining *(31)*. Neurons of groups Ch1–Ch4 project to all cortical areas and receive cortical afferents from more restricted areas, including frontal and limbic cortex *(32,33)*. Basal forebrain cholinergic cells also receive subcortical afferents from all the midbrain catecholamine projections *(34,35)*.

CHOLINERGIC IMMUNOTOXINS IN PRIMATES

Immunolesioning of the rat cholinergic system has been carried out using the immunotoxin 192 IgG-sap *(36)*. The antibody 192 IgG recognizes the low-affinity neurotrophin receptor protein p75, which is found *inter alia* on cholinergic cells in rats. This antibody does not recognize the homologue of p75 in primates, but the monoclonal antibody ME20.4 IgG raised against human p75 can be used in nonhuman primates. ME20.4 IgG has been shown, by double-labeling experiments with antibodies against ChAT, to be a reliable marker for cholinergic basal forebrain cells in humans *(37,38)*, cebus monkeys *(39)*, and marmosets *(40)*. The p75 receptor protein is a member of the tumor necrosis factor family *(41)* and binds neurotrophins, especially nerve growth factor *(42)*. Immunohistochemical staining using the ME20.4 IgG antibody has shown that, in the marmoset, the cells of the rising cholinergic projections of the basal forebrain are strongly reactive to this antibody; the adjacent cholinergic interneurons of the basal ganglia are less reactive *(40)*. In the macaque, the cholinergic cells of the basal forebrain are very reactive to ME20.4 IgG; the cholinergic interneurons of the basal ganglia are even less reactive to ME20.4 IgG (personal observation). The immunotoxin ME20.4 IgG-saporin is an effective toxin for the basal forebrain cholinergic system in macaque monkeys *(43,44)* and marmosets

(40). It is available commercially from Advanced Targeting Systems (San Diego, CA). The toxin can be injected directly into the area containing cholinergic cell bodies. The effectiveness of this method can be demonstrated by immunohistological staining of the cell bodies using antibodies to p75 receptor protein (*see* Fig. 1), by histochemical enzyme staining for acetylcholinesterase (AChE) in the target area of the cholinergic projections (*see* Fig. 2) or by radioenzymatic assay of ChAT in brain samples from the target area. Figure 3 shows correlations between learning disability and the magnitude of cholinergic lesions in marmosets and macaques. It is also possible to inject the toxin into the target areas. The toxin is taken up by the cholinergic terminals and transported back to the cholinergic cell bodies, which then die.

The basal forebrain cholinergic cells are not confined within a tightly delineated nucleus. Even in areas with large numbers of p75-positive cells, such as the part of the Ch4 cluster below the anterior commissure, these cells are found in an open "lattice" structure. Very thin bands of p75-positive neurons are found in the medullary lamellae, and small clusters or even isolated neurons can be found in the white matter of the anterior commissure, internal capsule, and anterior fornix. This means that an effective lesion can only be achieved using a specifically targeted immunotoxin that leaves the adjacent noncholinergic cells largely intact.

COGNITIVE TESTING IN PRIMATES

Pharmacological Studies

In assessing the role of basal forebrain acetylcholine in mnemonic functions in primates it is useful to consider background evidence based on the effects of cholinergic drugs. Aged monkeys showed improved recent memory performance when treated with the cholinesterase inhibitor physostigmine *(45)*. After administration of the cholinergic blocking agent scopolamine, normal monkeys were impaired on acquisition of information into long-term memory *(46,47)* and on tests of recent memory *(48,49)*.

This suggests that acetylcholine does not have a specific role in one of the classical divisions of memory (e.g., short-term or long-term memory), but rather that it makes a pertinent contribution to many forms of memory (and possibly wider aspects of cognition), and/or that different components of the cholinergic system contribute to different memory functions. Monkeys with lesions of the basal forebrain, compared to control monkeys, are differentially sensitive to scopolamine on tasks involving either acquisition into long-term memory *(50,51)* or recent memory *(52,53)*. This observation is important because demented and elderly patients also showed enhanced sensitivity to scopolamine in cognitive functioning *(54,55)*.

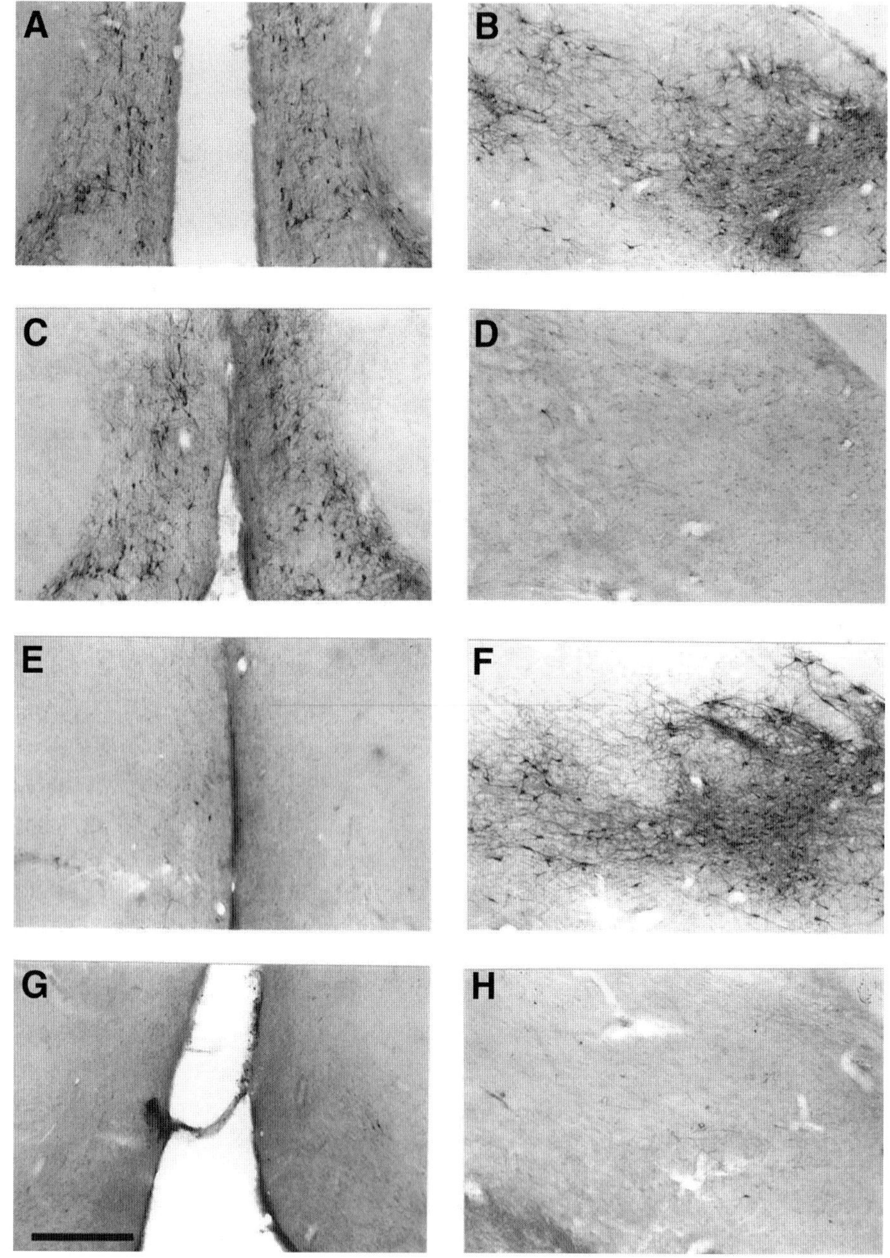

Fig. 1

In marmosets *(47)*, scopolamine impaired acquisition of repeated-trial, object-reward association tasks. It did not affect retention of previously well-learned object-reward tasks when given just before retention testing or immediately after learning the original discrimination. This shows that cholinergic blockade does not affect brain mechanisms involved in retrieval and does not induce forgetting. However, if these monkeys learned an object-reward association under scopolamine and were then tested, without drug, on the reversal of that object-reward association 24 h later, they showed impaired retention of the task (evidenced by chance performance compared to worse-than-chance performance by the control marmosets at the start of reversal testing; *see* Fig. 4A). This result indicated that information learned under scopolamine to the same criterion of performance, and therefore requiring more acquisition trials, was not consolidated into long-term memory as securely as information acquired under saline.

On the other hand, when tested on reversal, under scopolamine, on tasks previously learned without drug, monkeys showed good retention (evidenced by worse-than-chance performance at the start of reversal learning) but were impaired at completing the reversal tasks (*see* Fig. 4B). These results demonstrated that scopolamine affects acquisition but not retrieval or maintenance of long-term memories. It is most unlikely that a nonmnemonic effect of this dose of scopolamine, such as an effect on arousal or attention would produce, simultaneously, impaired acquisition and unimpaired retrieval and performance of the demands of the task. This finding makes it pertinent to ask whether the basal forebrain has a specific role in the acquisition of long-term memories. The question is relevant to understanding age-related memory decline. Aged macaques were also impaired on reversal learning and displayed the same pattern of good retention of the first reward contingency, but poor acquisition of the new reward contingency *(46,56)*.

Fig. 1. *(from opposite page)* ME20.4 IgG immunostaining indicates the loss of p75-positive neurons confined to the area of the immunotoxic lesion *(63)*. **(A)** vertical limb of the diagonal band of Broca (VDB) in unlesioned marmoset; **(B)** nucleus basalis of Meynert (NBM) in unlesioned marmoset (note p75-positive neurons); **(C)** VDB in marmoset with NBM lesion; **(D)** NBM in marmoset with NBM lesion (note loss of p75-positive neurons in NBM only); **(E)** VDB in marmoset with VDB lesion; **(F)** NBM in marmoset with VDB lesion (note loss of p75-positive neurons in VDB only); **(G)** VDB in marmoset with VDB and NBM lesion; **(H)** NBM in marmoset with VDB and NBM lesion (note loss of p75-positive neurons in both NBM and VDB). Bar = 0.5 mm.

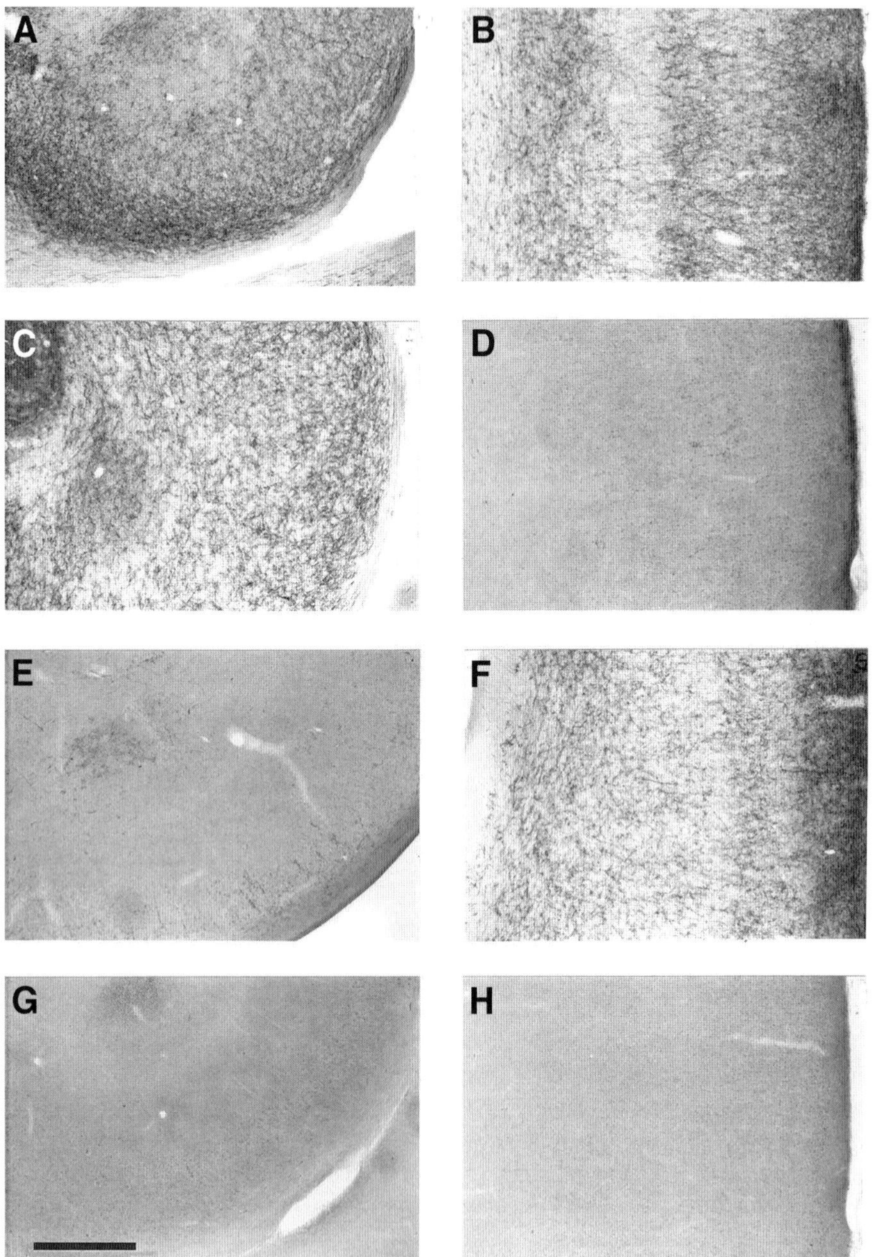

Fig. 2

Scopolamine had a greater effect on acquisition of a conditional task than on acquisition of single-pair, object-reward association tasks *(57)*. This conditional task was also specifically sensitive to lesions of the hippocampus *(26)*. This suggests that, in line with the general view of the importance of the hippocampus in long-term declarative memory formation, it is the cholinergic projections to the medial temporal lobe structures rather than to the neocortex that are particularly involved in this type of memory. This makes it possible that the reason why a low dose of scopolamine exacerbates the effect of lesions of the NBM is because the neocortex and hippocampus interact in these memory functions rather than that scopolamine blocks residual cholinergic activity in the target areas following NBM lesions.

Lesion Studies Using Excitotoxins

Some studies were undertaken using excitotoxins to lesion the basal forebrain in monkeys before immunotoxins were available. Excitotoxic lesions of the basal forebrain in macaques differentially impaired response times to unattended stimuli but did not affect performance on a variety of memory tasks *(53)*. On the other hand, Irle and Markowitsch *(58)* found broad and sustained learning and memory impairments on tests of both long-term and recent memory tasks in squirrel monkeys with excitotoxic lesions of the NBM. Excitotoxic lesions of the VDB in marmosets produced impairments specific to learning (and relearning) repeated-trial, conditional tasks *(59,60)*.

Excitotoxic lesions are only specific to the cholinergic system insofar as they are anatomically targeted to areas containing cholinergic cells, but the dependence of the cognitive impairment on the cholinergic component of the lesion can be demonstrated by its amelioration by cholinergic agonists and its exacerbation by cholinergic antagonists. Although it could be argued

---

Fig. 2. *(From opposite page)* Acetylcholinesterase staining indicates the loss of cholinergic nerve terminals in the target areas of the projections from the immunotoxic-lesioned areas *(63)*. (**A**) CA1 in unlesioned marmoset; (**B**) temporal neocortex in unlesioned marmoset (note similar levels of cholinergic innervation in **A** and **B**); (**C**) CA1 in marmoset with nucleus basalis of Meynert (NBM) lesion; (**D**) temporal neocortex in marmoset with NBM lesion (note loss of cholinergic innervation in temporal neocortex only); (**E**) CA1 in marmoset with vertical limb of the diagonal band of Broca (VDB) lesion; (**F**) temporal neocortex in marmoset with VDB lesion (note loss of cholinergic innervation in CA1 only); (**G**) CA1 in marmoset with VDB and NBM lesion; (**H**) temporal neocortex in marmoset with VDB and NBM lesion (note loss of cholinergic innervation in both CA1 and temporal neocortex). Bar = 0.5 mm.

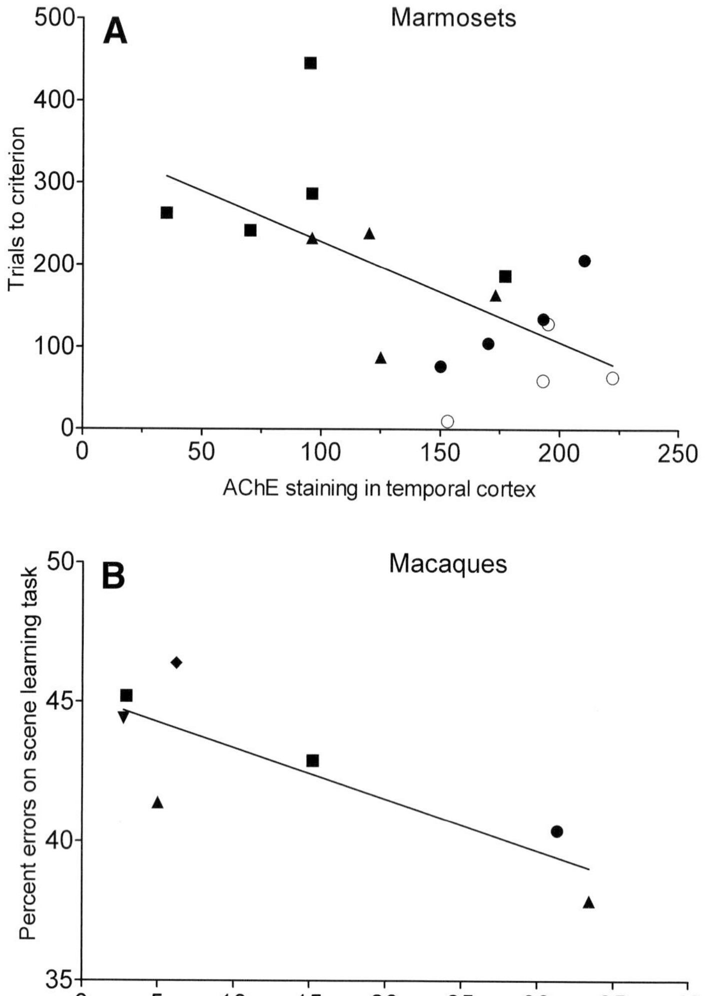

Fig. 3. A correlation between learning impairment and cholinergic loss is seen in marmosets and rhesus macaques with immunotoxic lesions of the basal forebrain. **(A)** Correlation between the number of trials to criterion on visual discrimination learning tasks (mean of two colored and one black object discriminations) and the level of acetylcholinesterase staining in temporal cortex (based on optical density measures of fixed regions on histological slides). Marmosets were either uninjected controls (○) or had been injected bilaterally in the nucleus basalis of Meynert (NBM) with ME20.4 IgG-sap with different amounts per hemisphere (● 0.35 μg; ▲ 0.7 μg; ■ 1.4 μg) *(66)*. Correlation: $r = 0.6087$, $p < 0.01$. **(B)** Correlation

that cholinergic agonists might improve performance in animals with cognitive impairment of any origin, this is not the case. On equivalent tasks, a cholinergic agonist did not improve learning in monkeys with excitotoxic lesions of the body of the hippocampus *(61)*, although it did improve learning in monkeys with excitotoxic lesions of the cholinergic projections to the hippocampus *(59)*. A cholinergic agonist did not improve learning in monkeys with structural lesions to the output pathways and subcortical input pathways to the temporal lobes *(62)*, but it did improve learning in monkeys with excitotoxic lesions of the cholinergic projections to the temporal lobe *(51)*. Monkeys with excitotoxic lesions of the basal forebrain were affected by administration of scopolamine at a dose that did not affect performance in normal monkeys *(50–53)*.

An interesting feature of the work of Voytko et al. *(53)* is that the effect of the basal forebrain lesion on response time to unattended stimuli in the attention task was evident without additional scopolamine (and was not tested under scopolamine), whereas the effect on memory was only evident as a differential sensitivity to scopolamine. As discussed above, scopolamine may be adding to the cholinergic dysfunction in the NBM, or it may be acting in another place (e.g., the hippocampus), which makes a contribution to memory formation that is synergistic to the contribution of the NBM.

Immunolesions in the VDB, NBM, or Both in Marmosets

Immunotoxic lesions of the cholinergic projections from the VDB to the hippocampus and entorhinal cortex in marmosets produced substantial impairments on learning conditional tasks but not on learning object-reward association tasks in the WGTA (*see* Fig. 5A,B) *(61,63)*. Two types of conditional tasks have been tested. In the visuospatial task, the monkeys learn, over the course of many trials in several daily test sessions, that reward is to be found under the left-presented object of a pair of identical objects but under the right-presented object of a different pair of identical objects. In the visuovisual conditional task, the monkeys learn that reward is to be found

---

Fig. 3 *(From opposite page)* between percentage errors on the scene-learning task and the percentage p75-positive neurons remaining in lesioned NBM plus vertical limb of the diagonal band of Broca (VDB) (based on computerized cell counts relative to cell counts in noninjected hemisphere). All macaques received injections of ME20.4 IgG-sap unilaterally into the NBM plus VDB (plus ipsilateral fornix transection) followed, after 6 wk, by contralateral IT ablation. Amounts of saporin per hemisphere were as follows: ● 2.7 µg, $n = 1$; ▲ 5.4 µg, $n = 2$; ■ 10.8 µg, $n = 2$; ◆ 15.2 µg, $n = 1$; ▼ 27.0 µg, $n = 1$ *(44)*. Correlation: $r = 0.8277, p < 0.05$.

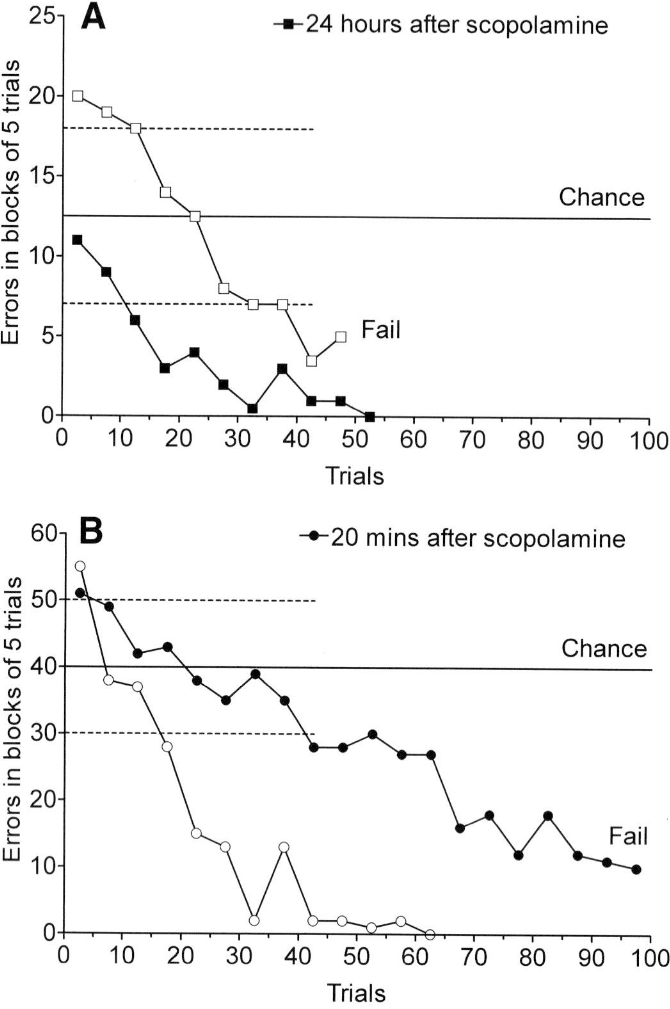

Fig. 4. Learning curves showing the effect of scopolamine on retention and acquisition during reversal of visual discriminations (47). (**A**) Graphs show errors in blocks of five trials by five marmosets. Chance = 12.5 errors; dotted lines indicate limits of chance when all five marmosets were performing. ■ 24 h after 0.06 mg/kg scopolamine; □ 24 h after saline, which had been given 20–30 min before original learning of each object-reward association. Marmosets tested 24 h after learning under scopolamine show impaired retention of the original reward association, as evidenced by chance performance at the beginning of reversal learning, whereas marmosets tested 24 h after learning under saline showed good retention, evidenced by worse-than-chance performance at the beginning of reversal learning. Marmosets tested 24 h after learning under scopolamine did not show impaired acquisition of the reversed object-reward association. (**B**) Graphs show errors in blocks of five

under one object from a pair of different objects when both objects are presented on one background but under the other object when both objects are presented on a different background. Specific impairment was also seen on these conditional tasks, but not on object-reward association tasks, after excitotoxic lesions confined to the hippocampus *(25,64)*. Impairments on a Y-maze task equivalent to the conditional visuospatial and visuovisual tasks were also seen after excitotoxic hippocampal lesions in rats *(65)*. This shows that there is a close relationship in the pattern of impairments seen after lesions of a subset of cells of the basal forebrain and their target area.

Immunotoxic lesions of the NBM did not lead to impairment on the conditional visuospatial task (*see* Fig. 5A), but a significant impairment was seen on single-pair, object-reward association tasks given as the first few tasks after NBM surgery (*see* Fig. 5B) *(63)*. Scores on subsequent relearning and new learning of single-pair, object-reward association tasks were generally elevated, indicating some impairment, but comparisons with control animals were not significant. In another study, the marmosets that had received the largest dose of immunotoxin were significantly impaired on the mean score on relearning and new learning of several single-pair, object-reward association tasks, although comparison with control animals on individual tasks was only significant on two new learning tasks *(66)*. The effects of NBM lesions therefore were neither large nor sustained. This lesioned group, however, showed impairment in response to a dose of scopolamine that was too low to affect performance in control animals.

Subsequent assessment of the effects of suction ablations of one of the main target areas of the NBM, the IT cortex, in marmosets indicated that shortly after surgery they were severely impaired on relearning of single-pair, object-reward association tasks but were not significantly impaired on subsequent individual single pair, object reward association tasks given either consecutively or concurrently. These marmosets, like macaque monkeys with anterior IT lesions *(67)*, were impaired when required to reach

---

Fig. 4 (*From opposite page*) trials by four marmosets across reversal of four different object-reward associations first learned 24 h previously. Chance = 40 errors; dotted lines indicate limits of chance when all four marmosets were performing. Scopolamine (●, 0.06 mg/kg) or saline (○) were given intramuscularly 20–30 min before testing on reversal. Marmosets treated with either saline or scopolamine showed good retention of the previous object-reward association, as evidenced by worse-than-chance performance at the beginning of reversal learning. Marmosets treated with scopolamine showed impaired acquisition of the reversed reward association.

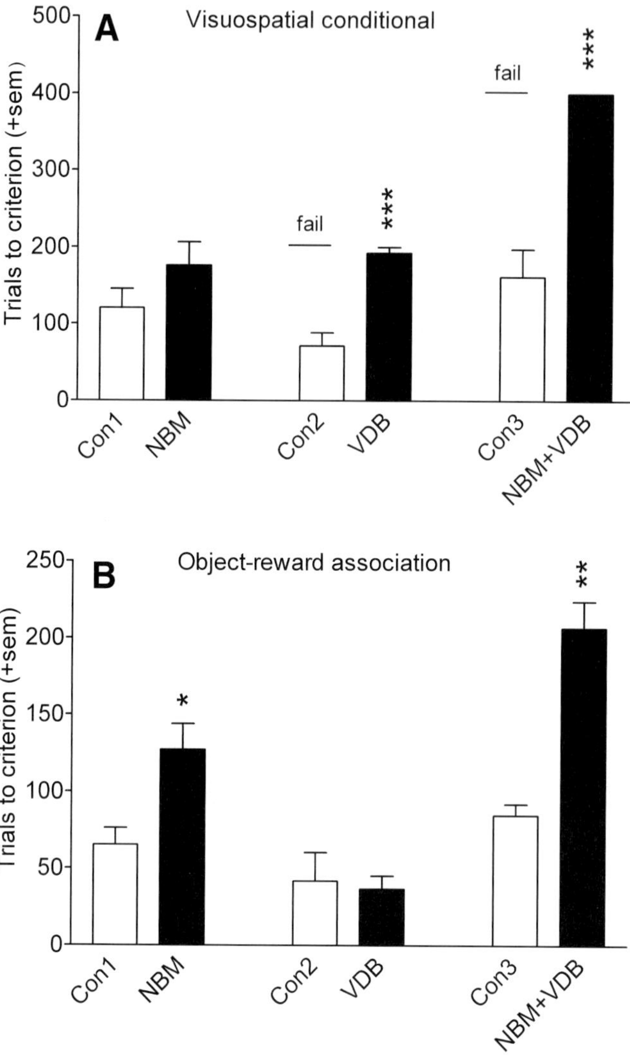

Fig. 5. Comparison of effects of immunotoxic lesions of the nucleus basalis of Meynert (NBM), the vertical limb of the diagonal band of Broca (VDB), or NBM plus VDB on visual discrimination learning or visuospatial conditional learning in marmosets. These data show that lesions that included the NBM produced impairment on visual discrimination learning; lesions that included the VDB produced impairment on visuospatial conditional learning. **(A)** Pooled data from first example of visuospatial conditional learning from refs. *61* and *63*. Con1 = 11 unoperated monkeys; NBM = 11 monkeys with bilateral immunotoxic lesions of the NBM *(61,63)*. Con2 = five unoperated monkeys; VDB = five monkeys with bilateral immunotoxic lesions of the VDB *(63)*. Con3 = six unoperated monkeys;

one criterion over consecutive trials across all the different component tasks of a concurrent object-reward association test. Marmosets with bilateral NBM lesions had been tested on a version of concurrent discrimination *(66)* but in a manner not strictly comparable to the concurrent task given to marmosets with IT ablation.

More detailed analysis of the effects of IT lesion in macaques suggested that the function of IT may be more perceptual than mnemonic, and that impairment will only be found when discriminating between certain specific stimuli *(68,69)*. A similar pattern of task-specific impairments can be seen in the learning scores for individual tasks given to marmosets with NBM lesions suggesting that impaired perceptual analysis (and therefore perceptual memory) may result from NBM lesions.

Combination of Immunolesions and Other Lesions in Marmosets and Macaques

Neuroanatomic studies (e.g., refs. *70–73*) indicated that suction ablations of the IT cortex will substantially reduce the input of visual information to the medial temporal lobe, including the hippocampus. Immunotoxic lesions of the projections to IT may prevent the processing of information in IT, but unmodified visual information may be sent on to the medial temporal lobe structures. It is therefore appropriate to assess the effect of combined lesions of the NBM plus VDB on object-reward association learning and to compare this with the effect of bilateral IT ablation (compare Fig. 5B with Fig. 6B). Immunotoxic lesions of the NBM plus VDB produced significant and persistent impairments on acquisition of repeated-trial, single-pair, object-reward associations *(61,63)*.

Fig. 5 *(From opposite page)* NBM + VDB = five monkeys with bilateral immunotoxic lesions of both the NBM and the VDB *(61)*. Testing was curtailed at 200 trials for monkeys with VDB lesions and 400 trials for monkeys with NBM and VDB lesions. No control monkeys or monkeys with NBM lesions were curtailed within the criterion set in their experiment. ***$p < 0.01$, Mann–Whitney U test. **(B)** Pooled data from the first postoperative examples of colored and black object discriminations from refs. *61* and *63*. Con1 = 11 unoperated monkeys; NBM = 11 monkeys with bilateral immunotoxic lesions of the NBM *(61,63)*. Con2 = five unoperated monkeys; VDB = five monkeys with bilateral immunotoxic lesions of the VDB *(63)*. Con3 = six unoperated monkeys; NBM+VDB = five monkeys with bilateral immunotoxic lesions of both the NBM and the VDB *(61)*. *$p < 0.05$; **$p < 0.01$, Mann–Whitney U test.

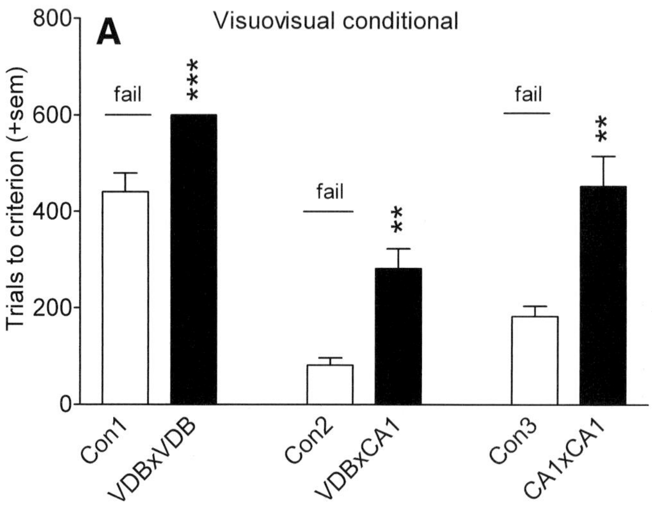

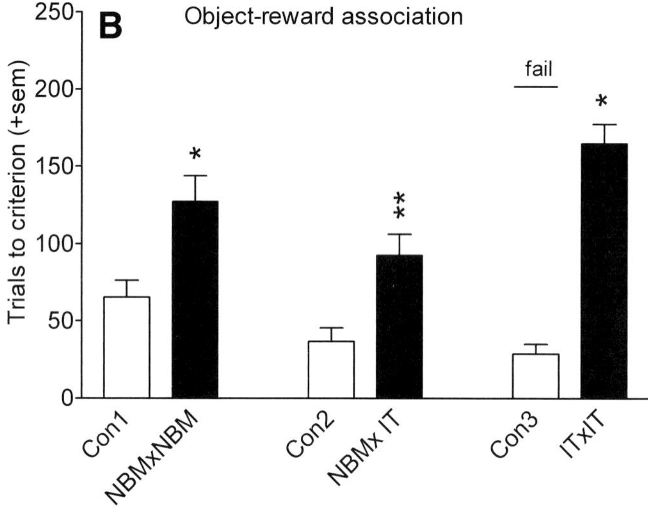

Fig. 6. Comparison of the effects of bilateral lesions of a basal forebrain projection area, its target area, or crossed unilateral lesions of the projection and target areas. Learning scores for control groups differed between experiments because of different training history and because different objects and different backgrounds were used. Control and lesioned monkeys in each comparison had the same conditions of testing. Testing was curtailed at 600 trials for monkeys with vertical limb of the diagonal band of Broca (VDB) × VDB or CA1 × CA1 lesions and 400 trials for monkeys with VDB × CA1 lesions. No control monkeys were curtailed within the criterion set for their experiment. These data show that lesions of the projection area, crossed unilateral lesions of the projection area plus the target area, or bilateral

A study of crossed unilateral lesions of the hippocampus in one hemisphere and IT cortex in the other suggested that the hippocampus interacts with IT during the acquisition of single-pair, object-reward associations *(74)*. Furthermore, immunotoxic VDB lesions produced a small exacerbation of the concurrent object-reward association impairment found after IT ablations *(24)*. A contribution of the cholinergic projection to the hippocampus on repeated-trial tasks in monkeys with compromised temporal neocortical function was also demonstrated by the severely deleterious effect on concurrent learning of adding a fornix transection to transection of the fiber tracts (including cholinergic fibers) in the amygdala and temporal stem *(75)* even though fornix transection alone has little effect on this type of task *(76)*. (This result also argues against the claim that performance on the concurrent task requires the interaction of IT cortex with the caudate nucleus rather than the hippocampus [77].)

A further way of examining the proposition that the cholinergic projections support the functions of the target areas is to assess the effect of crossed unilateral lesions of the cholinergic projection in one hemisphere and the target area in the other. Because unilateral target area lesions rarely produce substantial impairment, an impairment after crossed lesions would imply that the cholinergic projection had disabled the target area in the hemisphere opposite to the ablated target area. Furthermore, impairment can be attrib-

---

Fig. 6 *(From opposite page)* lesions of the target area produced similar effects on learning. **(A)** First example of visuovisual conditional learning from refs. *60, 64,* and *79*. Con1 = four unoperated monkeys; VDB × VDB = four monkeys with bilateral excitotoxic lesions of the VDB *(60)*. Con2 = six unoperated monkeys; VDB × CA1 = six monkeys with crossed unilateral immunotoxic VDB lesions and excitotoxic CA1 lesions *(79)*. Con3 = seven unoperated monkeys; CA1 × CA1 = seven monkeys with bilateral excitotoxic lesions of CA1 *(64)*. Testing was curtailed at 600 trials for monkeys with VDB × VDB or CA1 × CA1 lesions and 400 trials for monkeys with VDB × CA1 lesions. No control monkeys were curtailed within the criterion set for their experiment. **$p < 0.01$; ***$p < 0.001$, Mann–Whitney U test. **(B)** Mean of colored and black object discriminations from refs. *24, 61, 63,* and *78*. Con1 = 11 unoperated monkeys; nucleus basalis of Meynert (NBM) × NBM = 11 monkeys with bilateral immunotoxic lesions of the NBM *(61,63)*. Con2 = six unoperated monkeys; NBM × inferotemporal (IT) = six monkeys with crossed unilateral immunotoxic NBM lesions and unilateral IT ablations *(78)*. Con3 = five unoperated monkeys; IT × IT = five monkeys with bilateral IT ablation *(24)*. Testing was curtailed at 200 trials for monkeys with IT × IT ablations. No control monkeys were curtailed. *$p < 0.05$; **$p < 0.01$, Mann–Whitney U test.

uted solely to dysfunction of the area implicated bilaterally rather than to any extraneous damage associated with either unilateral lesion.

Barefoot et al. *(63)* found that monkeys with crossed unilateral lesions of the NBM and IT cortex were impaired on single-pair, object-reward associations (*see* Fig. 6B), although as in the case of bilateral NBM lesions, the impairment ameliorated with time. Impairment however was reinstated when an immunotoxic VDB lesion was added to the hemisphere with the NBM lesion. This suggested that the original amelioration of impairment was caused by the hippocampus fulfilling some of the functions normally carried out by the IT cortex.

In a further study, Barefoot et al. *(78)* found impairment on single-pair, object-reward associations when a unilateral NBM lesion was made in monkeys that had already received a hippocampal lesion in that hemisphere and a VDB-plus-IT lesion in the other hemisphere. This again suggested that learning impairments are found only when the neocortex and medial temporal lobe structures are disabled bilaterally.

As argued previously, IT ablations disrupt the visual input to the hippocampus, so the appropriate cholinergic lesion to compare with ablations of IT cortex may be a combined NBM-plus-VDB lesion. Crossed unilateral lesion of the NBM and VDB in one hemisphere and IT in the other hemisphere produce substantial impairment on acquisition of repeated-trial, single-pair discriminations (*see* Fig. 7A). Furthermore, because a similar impairment was found when an NBM lesion was combined with either an excitotoxic lesion of the hippocampus *(79)* or a VDB lesion in the same hemisphere *(78)*, it is unlikely that the latter effect was caused by the spread of immunotoxin between the NBM and the VDB producing a more effective lesion of both areas.

The visuovisual conditional task has been used to assess the relationship between the VDB and its target area, the medial temporal lobe. Crossed unilateral immunotoxic lesions of the VDB and excitotoxic lesion of one part of the medial temporal lobe system, the CA1 area of the hippocampus, produce impairment on acquisition of the visuovisual conditional task, as do bilateral excitotoxic lesion of the VDB or CA1 (*see* Fig. 6A).

Only one study assessed the cognitive effects of immunotoxic lesions of the basal forebrain in macaques *(44)*. The same immunotoxin (ME20.4 IgG-saporin) was used for macaques and marmosets at concentrations that ranged from 0.05 µg/µL to 0.5 µg/µL for macaques and 0.1 µg/µL to 0.2 µg/µL for marmosets. Because the macaque brain is much larger than the marmoset brain, 54 injection sites, necessitating 22 needle penetrations, were made in one hemisphere in the macaque brain, whereas only six penetrations were

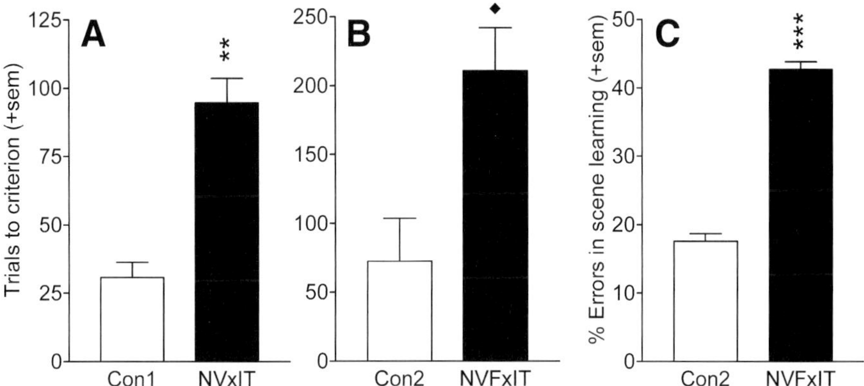

Fig. 7. Comparison of the effects of immunotoxic lesions of the nucleus basalis of Meynert (NBM) and vertical limb of the diagonal band of Broca (VDB) in combination with ablation of the contralateral inferotemporal (IT) cortex in marmosets and rhesus monkeys. Impairment seen after crossed unilateral lesions can be attributed to those parts of the brain that are dysfunctional bilaterally. This lesion produces impairment on acquisition of information in different types of memory task. **(A)** Trials to criterion for visual discrimination learning (mean of two colored and two black object discriminations) in marmosets. Con1 = six unoperated control marmosets; NV × IT = six marmosets with ME20.4 IgG-sap unilateral lesions in the NBM and VDB and contralateral IT ablations. $**p < 0.01$, Mann–Whitney U test *(78)*. **(B)** Trials to criterion on concurrent visual discrimination learning with computer-generated colored alphanumeric objects in rhesus monkeys. Con2 = two rhesus monkeys with saline injections in NBM and VDB, ipsilateral fornix transection, and contralateral IT ablations. NVF × IT = seven rhesus monkeys with ME20.4-sap injections in NBM and VDB, ipsilateral fornix transection, and contralateral IT ablations *(44)*. ◆ $p < 0.05$, one-tailed *t*-test. **(C)** Percentage errors in scene learning with computer-generated, alphanumeric, whole-screen scenes. Con2 = two rhesus monkeys with saline injections in NBM-plus-VDB, ipsilateral fornix transection, and contralateral IT ablations. NVF × IT = seven rhesus monkeys with ME20.4 IgG-sap injections in NBM and VDB, ipsilateral fornix transection, and contralateral IT ablations *(44)*. $***p < 0.001$, two-tailed *t*-test.

made in the marmoset brain to cover both the NBM and the VDB. Injections of immunotoxin at concentrations of 0.1 µg/µL to 0.5 µg/µL in the macaque brain and more than 0.2 µg/µL in the marmoset brain were associated with some cavitation of the tissue. However, an absolute amount of toxin had to be delivered to an area to produce a substantial lesion, and a low concentration may necessitate a larger volume of toxin or a larger number of needle penetrations, both of which can produce cavitation in the brain. Nonetheless, impairment on scene learning by macaques was correlated with the degree of cholinergic cell loss (*see* Fig. 3B) but not with the degree of cavitation.

Stereotaxic surgery is more difficult in the macaque brain than in that of the marmoset because of the larger size and greater variation in size between macaques. The exposure of the anterior commissure afforded by the unilateral fornix transection in this experiment assisted in the stereotaxic placements in the macaque. The stereotaxic atlas for the marmoset *(80)* is excellent for coordinates up to 10 mm from the intraural line. (The main body of the NBM lies at 9.5 mm AP, whereas the VDB lies at 10.5–11.5 mm AP). However, this atlas was constructed using marmosets that weighed about 280 g. This was normal for marmosets born before 1980, but marmosets born in captivity now routinely reach an adult weight of more than 350 g and may reach 450 g without obesity. Birth weight has also risen considerably, and an increase in adult brain size is to be anticipated. Some correction may therefore now be advisable for coordinates distant from the intraural line in larger individuals.

A bilateral immunotoxic lesion would have been difficult to perform in macaques, but it was feasible to study the effects of a unilateral immunotoxic lesion with an IT ablation in the other hemisphere. Macaques first received immunotoxic lesions using ME20.4 IgG-sap in the VDB and NBM and unilateral fornix transection in one hemisphere. This did not result in significant learning impairment. In a second surgery, they received an IT ablation in the opposite hemisphere and were then found to be impaired on the limited-trial, visuospatial scene memory task (*see* Fig. 7C) and on the repeated-trial, concurrent, object-reward association task (*see* Fig. 7B).

Previous work had shown that unilateral IT ablation did not produce impairment on the scene memory task *(81)*.

In the scene memory task, monkeys had to respond, on each trial, to alphanumeric figures presented in the same position in each trial against complex visual backgrounds on a computer screen. The spatial and contextual background in this task made it easy for control monkeys to learn the task in just a few trials. In the concurrent object-reward association task, the objects were small alphanumeric figures presented in variable positions against a black background. This task required repeated presentation of the objects for learning to be completed. The impairment on learning the scene memory task was correlated with the degree of cholinergic cell loss rather than general tissue loss in the immunolesioned hemisphere (*see* Fig. 3B). The lesioned monkeys had difficulty learning which alphanumeric figure was correct in the scene memory task, but they had no difficulty responding to the figures rather than to other places on the complex-patterned background. This suggests that they did not have difficulty attending to perceptual aspects of the task and did not suffer from general agnosia.

From this, it can be supposed that the impairment on the concurrent object-reward association task was also not caused by a perceptuo-attentional loss or an agnosia and was therefore mnemonic. Furthermore, one of these monkeys was tested on retention of a concurrent task and showed no impairment, indicating that these monkeys had an impairment on acquisition rather than retrieval, further strengthening the argument that these monkeys did not have a general performance difficulty.

The unilateral fornix transection on the side of the immunotoxic lesion would have deprived the hippocampus and entorhinal cortex of its cholinergic input. Two control monkeys received an IT ablation in one hemisphere and a unilateral fornix transection and saline, rather than immunotoxin, injections into the basal forebrain in the opposite hemisphere. These monkeys showed only a moderate impairment on both of the memory tasks, indicating that the immunotoxic lesion in the other monkeys was responsible for the increased magnitude of the impairment on the limited-trial scene memory and the repeated-trial, concurrent object-reward association task in these monkeys. These results are important in several respects.

1. They demonstrate that the basal forebrain cholinergic system is involved in memory in macaques, the nonhuman primate species in which most neuropsychological tests have been carried out.
2. They demonstrate that impairment is seen on a limited-trial task (indeed, substantial learning can be seen on the second trial of each scene problem by control animals, so this task has formal similarities to the trial-unique tasks used to assess aspects of single-event [episodic] memory). This relates to the early studies of trial-dependent and trial-unique tests of recent memory in aged macaques and macaques treated with scopolamine or physostigmine and suggests that the effects seen in those early studies were caused by effects in the cholinergic system of the basal forebrain rather than elsewhere.
3. Impairment on the repeated-trial, concurrent object-reward task supports the observation (discussed previously) that basal forebrain acetylcholine contributes to the acquisition of long-term memories and to the performance of tests of recent memory. (Points 2 and 3 together suggest that loss of acetylcholine in elderly patients will contribute to a loss of cognitive abilities that will be manifest as a loss of acquisition of memories for everyday events and a difficulty in learning new facts, e.g., about new technology.)
4. Because the control monkeys had unilateral transection of the fornix (where the fornix carries most of the cholinergic projection from the VDB), most of the additional mnemonic effect of the immunotoxin injections would have been caused by the lesion of the NBM rather than of the VDB. These results there-

fore showed a contribution of the NBM to learning and memory even though the impairments were demonstrated in monkeys with additional lesions of the VDB and fornix.

5. On the other hand, monkeys with lesions of the amygdala and temporal stem (which transect the cholinergic projections from the NBM) were less impaired on scene learning than monkeys with lesions of the amygdala, temporal stem, and fornix even though fornix transection alone produced only a mild impairment on this task *(75)*. These results, for a test of an episodic type of memory, parallel the effects of lesions in marmosets in which (as discussed above) severe and persistent impairment on the acquisition of long-term memories was seen in animals with NBM-plus-VDB lesions even though lesions of the VDB alone did not produce impairment on this type of task and NBM lesions produced a milder and transient effect.

6. Impairment on both the scene memory task and the concurrent object-reward association task following bilateral surgical transection of the anterior temporal stem, amygdala, and fornix *(75)* suggested that, because this lesion transects the cholinergic input from the NBM and VDB to the entire temporal lobe, it may have been the loss of this input, rather than the loss of efferents from the medial temporal lobe, that was responsible for this severe learning impairment. Monkeys with this triple lesion were not impaired on retention of a concurrent object-reward association set acquired prior to surgery *(75,82)*. Insofar as the effects of this lesion are caused by cholinergic loss in the temporal lobes, these results support the view that acetylcholine is involved in the acquisition of new memories and knowledge rather than retrieval of old memories. Impaired performance on retention tasks may be seen, however, when a degree of forgetting necessitates relearning on a retention task and when that relearning is subject to impairment. These results further suggest that impairment on the scene memory task and the concurrent object-reward association task is a model of the dense amnesia seen in patients with substantial damage to the temporal lobes and in patients with advanced dementia.

Combinations of Immunolesions and Pharmacological Manipulations

Animals with cholinergic immunolesions are good models for study of the interaction of the cholinergic system with other neurotransmitter systems. Francis and colleagues *(83,84)* formulated a description of the way in which the modulatory neurotransmitters interact with sensorimotor information-carrying neuronal pathways. Glutamatergic pyramidal cells form reciprocal connections in the neocortex and hippocampal formation and project to the striatum and other output pathways *(85)*.

Loss of pyramidal cells begins early in the course of Alzheimer's disease *(11)* and correlates with the severity of dementia *(15,16)*. These glutamatergic pyramidal cells are subject to cholinergic enhancement *(83)*, and a large number of pyramidal cells display immunoreactivity to both muscarinic and nico-

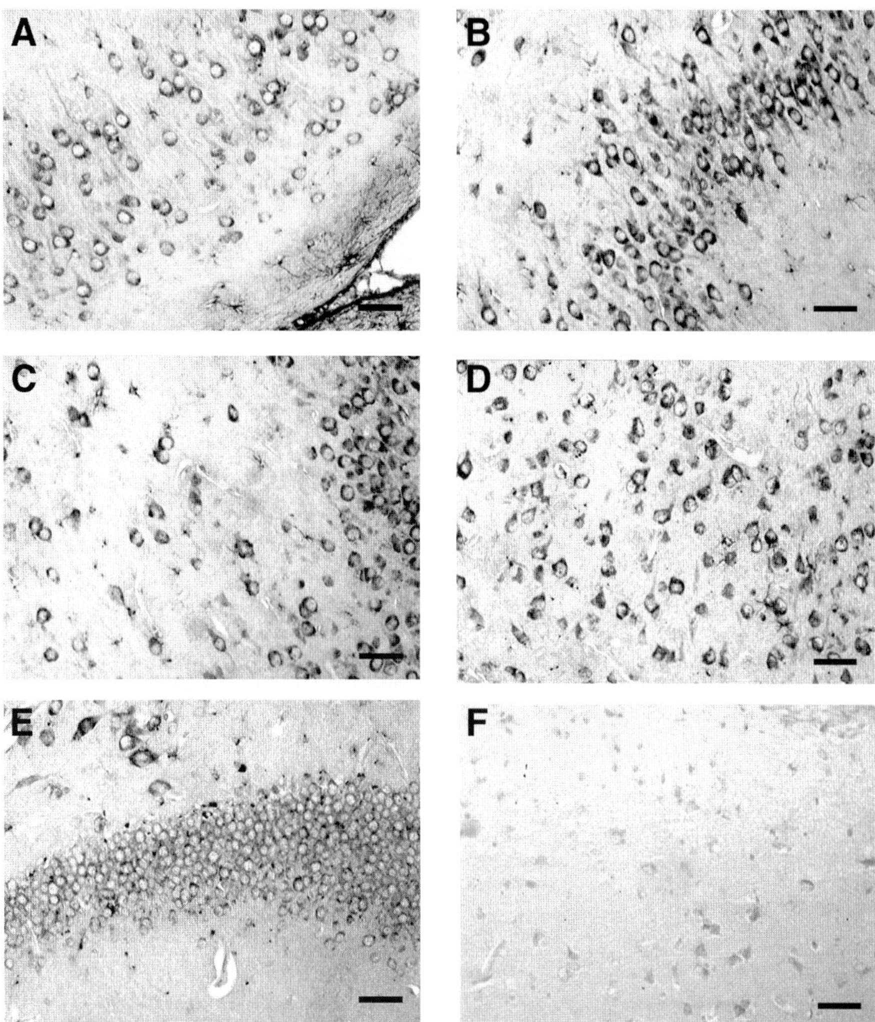

Fig. 8. Immunostaining for nicotinic acetylcholine receptor subunit α7 in pyramidal neurons in marmoset hippocampus in fields **(A)** CA1, **(B)** CA3, **(C)** CA4, and **(D)** subiculum. **(E)** There was no immunoreactivity in the granule cell layer of the dentate gyrus. **(F)** Control from CA4 field with no primary antibody. Bar = 50 μm.

tinic receptors *(86)*. Figure 8 shows nicotinic α7 immunostaining on pyramidal cells in the hippocampus in marmosets. From this, it can be supposed that the cholinergic system will exert its effects on cognitive function by its interaction with the glutamatergic pyramidal cell pathways.

Muscarinic Receptors

It was reported above that scopolamine, a muscarinic-blocking agent, affects object-reward association learning independent of any effect it may have on arousal or attention *(47)*. Experiments that looked at the effects of muscarinic agonists (arecoline or pilocarpine) or antagonists (scopolamine) in immunolesioned monkeys indicated that the cholinergic NBM cells exert effects on learning and memory via muscarinic receptors. Effects of excitotoxic lesions of the NBM on object-reward association learning were ameliorated by arecoline and reinstated by a low dose of scopolamine that was ineffective in nonlesioned monkeys *(51)*. It was also shown that immunotoxic lesions of the NBM produced impairment on object-reward association tasks that was both dependent on the lesion size and susceptible to differential exacerbation by scopolamine *(66)*. The effects on single-pair, object-reward associations of lesions of the NBM (together with lesions of the VDB or hippocampus) were alleviated by pilocarpine; the effects of lesions of the NBM plus VDB (but not lesions of the NBM plus hippocampus) on visuospatial tasks could also be alleviated by pilocarpine *(61)*. Impairments on visuospatial conditional learning after excitotoxic or immunotoxic lesions of the VDB alone were also ameliorated by pilocarpine *(59,61)*; this impairment was substantial and persistent, so attempts to exacerbate it with scopolamine were not made. These results demonstrate that basal forebrain acetylcholine affects learning via muscarinic receptors.

Nicotinic Receptors

An attempt has also been made to assess the involvement of nicotinic receptors in the role of acetylcholine in cognition in marmosets. We have tested the effect of a specific $\alpha 7$ nicotinic receptor agonist, AR-23465 (AstraZeneca) on acquisition of the visuospatial task by marmosets with combined immunotoxic lesion of the VDB and fornix transection. This combined lesion was used to maximize the depletion of acetylcholine in the hippocampus. Fornix transection severs all the cholinergic fibers that pass through it to the hippocampus and entorhinal cortex but does not remove the cholinergic projections to the rostral (uncal) hippocampus, which pass from the basal forebrain through an anterior ventral path *(87,88)*. The effects of fornix transection on the visuospatial task are ameliorated by pilocarpine *(26)*, indicating that it is the cholinergic fornical afferents to the hippocampus rather than noncholinergic hippocampal efferents in the fornix that contribute to performance of the visuospatial task. Immunotoxic lesions of the VDB will reduce the cholinergic projections through both the fornix and the anterior ventral path but are unlikely to produce a complete lesion.

Based on preliminary rodent work by AstraZeneca, we used a dose of 3 mg/kg AR-23465. This was well tolerated in marmosets. There were 14 marmosets (5 male and 9 female), aged about 2 yr (i.e., young adult) and weighing 370 ± 10 g, first trained to perform the visuospatial task. Then, eight marmosets received immunotoxic lesions of the VDB followed, in a separate surgical procedure, by bilateral fornix transection. The other six marmosets remained as unoperated controls. Testing resumed 1 wk after fornix transection (or rest for the unlesioned marmosets).

On the first task given postoperatively, the lesioned marmosets were significantly impaired on relearning the visuospatial task originally learned prior to surgery (24 ± 13 trials to criterion $\pm$ standard error of the mean [SEM] for unlesioned animals; 170 ± 16 trials for lesioned animals; $p < 0.001$). After the end of drug testing, the lesioned marmosets remained impaired on the mean learning scores for two new examples of this task (28 ± 9 for unlesioned animals; 77 ± 10 for lesioned animals; $p < 0.01$).

To assess the efficacy of nicotinic stimulation, the marmosets were tested on acquisition of four new examples of the visuospatial task. They were injected intramuscularly, 20 min before testing each day, with 3 mg/kg of AR-23465 or a control substance that had undergone the same pharmacological screening as AR-23465 (carried out by AstraZeneca) and had been found devoid of significant $\alpha 7$ or other pharmacological potency. Marmosets were injected each day with one drug until they had completed one example of the visuospatial task. Then, after a 3-d washout period, the marmosets were tested on the other drug on the next example of the visuospatial task, in a balanced design, so that each example and each example position (first, second, etc.) were tested in half the marmosets under one drug and the other half under the other drug.

The lesioned marmosets were not significantly impaired relative to unlesioned animals under either the $\alpha 7$ agonist (60 ± 17 for unlesioned animals; 126 ± 31 for lesioned animals; not significant [ns]) or the control substance (unlesioned 60 ± 25; lesioned 128 ± 30, ns). However, because performance in the lesioned marmosets did not differ between the $\alpha 7$ agonist and the control substance, there was no evidence that the $\alpha 7$ agonist exerted an effect on learning this task.

It is possible that the control substance had a pharmacological potency not detected in drug screening and that the α agonist shared this potency. It is also possible that the $\alpha 7$ agonist and the control substance both had a nonspecific deleterious effect on performance in the unlesioned marmosets (although learning scores were not significantly elevated relative to no drug), and this had obscured the effect of fornix transection on this task. A further possibility is that either substance had a very long-term effect, resulting in improved performance across many days. This however is unlikely because there was no significant difference between the effects of the drugs on the first tasks on which they were administered and subsequent tasks, and a 3-d washout period was inserted between test days under different substances.

Notwithstanding these difficulties, this experiment failed to demonstrate a beneficial effect of a nicotinic agonist in monkeys with lesions of the cholinergic projections to the hippocampus. This result was in contrast to the beneficial effects of muscarinic agonists (and the deleterious effects of muscarinic antagonists) described earlier.

Influence on Glutamate Cells

The Bowen–Francis hypothesis can be further investigated in monkeys by assessing the effect on memory of manipulations that alter both cholinergic and glutamatergic transmission. MK801 blocks the *N*-methyl-D-aspartate receptor of the glutamatergic corticocortical pyramidal cells. This drug, like scopolamine, impaired performance of recognition tasks in macaques *(89)*, and low doses of MK801 and scopolamine given together had a more than additive effect on performance of this task *(90)*. MK801 also impaired acquisition of conditional and single-pair, object-reward associations in marmosets *(91)*. A low dose of MK801 (which was ineffective when given alone) produced impairment on single-pair, object-reward association learning in monkeys with cholinergic lesions of the NBM but not the VDB (*see* Fig. 9); this dose of MK801 did not produce impairment on the visuospatial task in monkeys with NBM lesions *(63)*.

These results indicated that the interaction between acetylcholine and glutamate was task specific; a reasonable interpretation of this effect is that acetylcholine and glutamate are interacting directly in the tissue that critically sustains that function. It is interesting to note that this interaction applies to certain types of repeated-trial tasks, as well as trial-unique tasks, suggesting that the mode of influence of cholinergic modulation on glutamatergic pyramidal cells is the same throughout the cortex and hippocampus, with the effect on different tasks caused by the nature of the information carried in the pyramidal cells.

The glutamatergic pyramidal cells are also subject to inhibitory modulation by serotonin, via $5HT_{1A}$ receptors *(92)*. The $5HT_{1A}$ receptor antagonist WAY100635 improved learning ability in monkeys treated with MK801 *(93)* or with fornix transection *(94)*. Because the effect of fornix transection is also ameliorated by cholinergic agonists, the most plausible explanation of these results is that the cholinergic projections exert an excitatory effect,

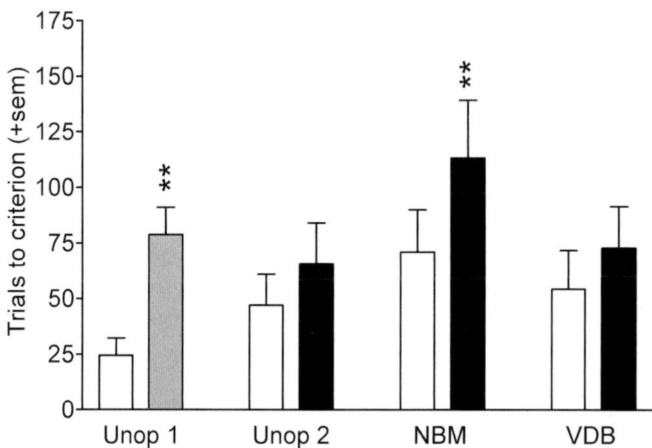

Fig. 9. Interaction between immunotoxic nucleus basalis of Meynert (NBM) lesion and glutamate blockade on visual discrimination learning*(63,91)*. Unop 1 = six monkeys treated with saline (open column) or 0.015 mg/kg MK801 (gray column) *(91)*. Unop 2 = five monkeys treated with saline (open column) or 0.006 mg/ kg MK801 (black column). NBM = six monkeys with bilateral immunotoxic NBM lesions treated with saline (open column) or 0.006 mg/kg MK801 (black column). Vertical limb of the diagonal band of Broca (VDB) = five monkeys with bilateral VDB lesions treated with saline (open column) or 0.006 mg/kg MK801 (black column) *(63)*. The higher dose of MK801 impaired learning. The lower dose of MK801 impaired learning only in monkeys that had NBM lesions. **$p < 0.01$, Mann–Whitney U test.

and serotonergic projections exert an inhibitory effect, on telencephalic glutamatergic transmission, and that the acquisition of memories is modulated by these oppositional factors.

WHAT IS THE ROLE OF BASAL FOREBRAIN ACETYLCHOLINE?

Anatomic Perspective

In the series of experiments described above, we showed that immunotoxic lesions of the basal forebrain cholinergic system in monkeys produce cognitive impairments that, when comparisons have been made, resemble those seen after lesions of the target areas. Crossed unilateral lesions of a cholinergic projection and its target area also produce effects equivalent to bilateral lesions of the target area. In monkeys with crossed unilateral lesions, because the only area of bilateral dysfunction is the target area, these experiments support the notion that the rising cholinergic projections perform a contributory function within the target area.

The effects of immunotoxic lesions are amenable to remediation by cholinergic agonist drugs, whereas the effects of comparable structural lesions of the target area are not. This indicates that the effects of the immunotoxic lesion are caused by cholinergic loss rather than some other damage. Monkeys with immunotoxic lesions are also more sensitive to cholinergic blocking agents (e.g., scopolamine) than are normal monkeys, but only on tasks sensitive to lesions of the relevant target area. This may mean that mild cholinergic blockade is acting within the target area of a subtotal cholinergic lesion so that greater dysfunction within the target area is produced. However, it is possible that mild cholinergic blockade, in an area of the brain with which the target area interacts, is producing an additive effect on cognition in immunolesioned monkeys. Scopolamine produces a greater effect on tasks sensitive to hippocampal than cortical dysfunction, and the hippocampus contributes to performance of some tasks primarily affected by lesions of neocortex. It is therefore possible that a low dose of scopolamine in monkeys with NBM lesions might increase impairment because of a loss of the contribution of the hippocampus to task performance. Nonetheless, these experiments indicate that the mental "product" of cholinergic activity is closely related to the mental product of the target area.

Psychological Perspective

In analyzing the role of the cholinergic system, tasks have been used that reflect the known, or presumed, functions of the target areas. Insofar as the target areas have different functions, the components of the cholinergic projections can be said to support different functions. So, if the hippocampus has a role in memory, the VDB may be said to support memory function. Similarly, perceptual and mnemonic functions of different parts of the neocortex will be supported by the part of the NBM that projects to those parts of neocortex.

In this respect, the question, What is the role of basal forebrain acetylcholine? cannot be answered by pointing to a single psychological product such as memory or attention. Indeed, it is absurd to attribute any psychological product to any specific part of the brain; those parts of the brain that keep the organism alive and awake contribute to the achievement of "vision" just as much as those parts of the brain traditionally regarded as part of "the visual system."

Learning impairments following immunotoxic lesions in monkeys were seen on repeated-trial tasks and on a limited-trial task (the scene memory task). Gaffan *(95)* argued that the scene memory task assesses episodic memory. From the point of view of psychological validity, the scene memory task requires that stimuli in the context of a spatially laid out background (i.e., events) are remembered after a very limited number of presentations. Such performance would benefit from episodic memory. Learning difficult repeated-trial tasks on the other hand resembles the acquisition of knowledge.

Comparison with clinical cases suggested that impairment may be seen on both trial-unique and repeated-trial learning in patients with amnesia *(96–98)*. Patients with fornix transection *(99)* or ischemic damage confined to the CA1 area of hippocampus *(100)* showed only moderately impaired memory, and this may be compared to the moderate impairment on only the scene memory task by macaques with fornix transection. Because fornix transection severs the cholinergic projections to the hippocampus and entorhinal cortex, the additional impairment seen in the macaques with immunotoxic lesions must have been mainly caused by the loss of the projections from the NBM.

Mishkin et al. *(101)* claimed that repeated-trial, object-reward association tasks assess the acquisition of procedural, habit-like skills. However, the well-known patient H.M. had difficulty on the concurrent object-reward association task *(96)*, but his lack of impairment on clear procedural tasks such as maze learning *(102)* confirms that repeated-trial tasks in the WGTA assess the acquisition of factual information referred to as semantic knowledge in humans and impaired in patients with degeneration in the temporal neocortex *(103)*. That loss of the cholinergic projections should cause impairment on tasks that assess both episodic and semantic memory is consistent with the symptoms of dementia that comprise a loss of acquisition of episodic memories in the early stages and broader semantic impairments in the later stages.

The visuospatial and visuovisual conditional tasks on which monkeys with immunotoxic lesions of the VDB were impaired do not, at face value, require the use of episodic memory because they are difficult tasks only acquired slowly after repeated presentations of the same stimuli. This suggests that the hippocampus may perform some more basic cognitive process that is a prerequisite of episodic memory in humans as well as other cognitive functions in humans and other animals. This way of looking at it allows contemplation of the functions of the hippocampus in an animal, such as a mouse, without assuming that the mouse is blessed with the same capacity for recollective episodic memory of previous events that is present in humans.

The distinctive common feature of the visuospatial and visuovisual tasks is that they are conditional tasks, that is, the correct choice between two stimuli is conditional on another piece of information. In this respect, these tasks are like those sensitive to hippocampal damage in rodents and that depend on spatial *(104)*, contextual *(105)*, configural *(106)*, or conditional information *(107)*. All of these require the integration of stimulus information with information from the background, the sum of the parts, or some other source; this integrative ability may be a prerequisite of the ability to integrate pieces of perceptual information into an event for recollection as an episodic memory. Viewed in this way, the cholinergic projection to the hippocampus contributes to episodic memory formation only insofar as it modulates the extent to which the hippocampus carries out this integrative function at any particular moment.

The single-pair, object-reward associations on which monkeys with immunotoxic lesions of the NBM were impaired require perceptual discrimination between the objects, as well as object-reward association. Although ablations of the IT cortex, including the perirhinal cortex, produce visual learning impairments, more detailed analysis of the nature of the deficit in each case suggests that the impairment lies in a perceptuomnemonic interface rather than in an isolated memory function *(68,108,109)*. It is argued below that acetylcholine modulates this function to contribute to whichever of the many aspects of visual input that occur every moment of conscious awareness so that they are noticed and remembered.

There are reasons for believing that the cholinergic system is concerned only with acquisition of new memories. Scopolamine treatment in humans impairs acquisition of long-term memories, but has much less effect on tests of primary memory *(17)*, and marmosets treated with scopolamine demonstrate simultaneous impaired learning and good retrieval *(47)*. Although immunotoxic cholinergic lesions in marmosets can produce impairment on relearning of tasks first learned prior to surgery, some normal forgetting may occur (as evidenced by learning scores greater than zero in control marmosets) such that some learning may be required for successful performance of these retention tasks.

In a comparison of lesions of the VDB, fornix, or hippocampus on conditional learning *(110)*, we found that lesions of the hippocampus produced maximal impairment on retention (from preoperative learning) and new learning, but no forgetting of material first learned, albeit with difficulty, after surgery. In the first case, information acquired by the hippocampus would have been removed by the surgery. In the latter case, learning must have been achieved outside the (absent) hippocampus and was presumably stored there as well. Fornix transection produced not only maximal impairment on new learning, but also some impairment on retention and some forgetting. The latter implies that encoding had been weak and subject to faster decay. In that study, lesions of the VDB, which also produced maximal impairment on new learning, had little effect on retention of information acquired prior to surgery but did produce a substantial amount of forgetting. This again is compatible with the notion of good retrieval of adequately encoded material but weak encoding of new material in the absence of hippocampal acetylcholine.

Neurophysiological Perspective

The major physiological effect of cholinergic stimulation is prolonged reduction of potassium conductance in the postsynaptic membrane, rendering the cholinoceptive cells more susceptible to other excitatory inputs *(111)*. Iontophoretic application of acetylcholine to neurons (in cat visual or somatosensory cortex) increases their responsiveness to preferred sensory trigger features; excitotoxic lesions of the NBM reduce that responsiveness *(112,113)*. Neurons in monkey basal forebrain (which are probably either cholinergic or functionally connected to cholinergic neurons) are particularly reactive to sensory inputs that are novel or of motivational, or task-related, significance *(114,115)*. This responsiveness is diminished when motivational significance is reduced by either satiety or task-determined extinction *(116,117)*.

This suggests that these cells are part of a recursive neuronal circuit that serves to enhance neural responses to sensory stimuli (which provide input to that circuit) according to the state and needs of the animal. In determining what an animal actually does, partially analyzed sensory information may trigger bottom-up attentional mechanisms sensitive to novelty, or motivational significance, and top-down mechanisms of directed attention depending on the demands of the task, including tasks set by the experimenter and those set by the animal's natural goal-directed behavior. The basal forebrain cholinergic system may play an important part in this mechanism of behavioral control by enhancing the activity of pyramidal cells so that the information that they carry contributes to behavior either at the time (a perceptual-attentional or response-selecting function) or in the future (a memory-forming function).

Cholinergic agonists increase and cholinergic antagonists decrease cortical arousal as measured by changes in electroencephalogram synchrony *(118)*, and cholinergic stimulation enhances long-term potentiation in hippocampal pyramidal cells *(119)*. Using the "subsequent memory" method, in which brain activity is compared during exposure to stimuli that are subsequently remembered relative to those that are not, Fell et al. *(120)* showed that memory-related activity occurred about 300 ms after visual input in anterior temporal neocortex, followed 200 ms later by memory-related activity in hippocampus. Although it is not known whether acetylcholine contributes to this effect, it does show that the target areas of both the NBM and VDB are involved sequentially in the encoding of "to-be-remembered" information.

Synthesis

The basal forebrain and brainstem cholinergic projections can be considered together with the other "rising" catecholamine projections (dopamine, serotonin, and noradrenaline) as part of an extended ascending reticular activating system *(121)*. All these systems are modulatory in their effect on the content of mental and motor activity, and yet they presumably have different functions. Some clues to the nature of the contribution made by acetylcholine can be found in the psychological nature of the impairments produced by cholinergic lesions and by neurophysiological effects of experimental manipulation of acetylcholine described above.

The NBM shows disproportionate enlargement in species with large brains, especially primates *(122)*. The concentration of cholinergic terminals in cerebral cortex is lowest in primary sensory cortex and becomes progressively denser through the perceptual association areas and on into paralimbic and limbic memory areas *(123)*. Postsynaptic cholinergic sensitivity in humans increases during childhood, is maximal during adulthood, and decreases in Alzheimer's disease but not in cognitively intact old people *(124)*. These three factors are consistent with basal forebrain acetylcholine having a role in cognitive processes that produce conscious perceptions and memories.

Neurophysiological studies indicate that the cholinergic system is particularly activated by stimuli that are motivationally significant. This suggests that the basal forebrain may play a part in determining *what* is attended to, remembered, and acted on. The Ch5–Ch6 neurons in the brainstem are part of a system that modulates arousal *(125)* and therefore make a contribution to *when* events in the outside world are attended to, remembered, and acted on. This distinction, however, may merely reflect different positions on a time continuum, with the most caudal parts of the cholinergic system contributing to the slow modulation of behavior by controlling the sleep/wake cycle and general arousal, the NBM contributing to the detection of perceptual regularities and their moderately slow conversion into factual knowledge, and the VDB contributing to the "once-only" conversion of a unique event into a specific episodic memory.

Easton and coworkers *(126–128)* suggested a model by which the neural correlates of arousal and motivation, from the rising monoamine systems, and frontal lobe mechanisms (which set goals and goal-directed attention) both control activity in the cholinergic system. The cholinergic cells of the basal forebrain receive input from the major rising monoamine systems *(34,35)*. Unilateral disruption of these monoamine systems by electrolytic lesion of the medial forebrain bundle (MFB) together with an IT lesion in the opposite hemisphere *(126–128)* produces learning impairments comparable to the learning impairments seen after crossed lesions are made of the basal forebrain cholinergic system and opposite IT cortex *(44)*. The inference to be drawn from this is that the MFB modulates the way in which the cholinergic system supports the function of the IT cortex.

In the same articles *(126–128)*, Easton and colleagues also reported that unilateral lesions of MFB and large, contralateral, frontal ablations produced the same learning impairments as those produced by crossed MFB lesions and IT ablations, or large bilateral frontal lesions. Here, it is argued that the frontal lobes set the goals that determine what is relevant to the animal in its ongoing interaction with the environment. Thus, arousal, motivation, and intention all impinge on the cholinergic system, which determines which of the many aspects of the sensory stream are strengthened so that they can control behavior and be chosen to form knowledge and memories. The model of Easton and Gaffan also suggests that the basal forebrain cholinergic projections will not be involved in the retrieval of old memories, and this is largely upheld by the observations described above. According to this model, because cholinergic activity is controlled by a variety of modulatory inputs, the model implies that what are remembered are not stimuli that are associated with reward, but stimuli that are important by virtue of their relationship to the animal's short-term and long-term goals. This means that it is not only nice things, but also unpleasant things and emotionally neutral but contextually important things that will be attended to and remembered.

An important feature of the preceding arguments is that the perceptual, attentional, and semantic and episodic memory functions discussed are all in the conscious, declarative domain. Perry et al. *(129)* widened the discussion by suggesting that cholinergic activity correlates well with states of consciousness. This may explain why in cases of severe perturbation of the cholinergic system such as the later stages of dementia and scopolamine overdose (zombieism), hallucinations and dissociated states of awareness, usually associated with complete amnesia for the dissociated state, may be observed.

ACKNOWLEDGMENTS

We thank Alison Graham for undertaking the α7 nicotinic immunostaining and for providing the micrographs used in Fig. 8. We thank David Gaffan for commenting on an early draft of this chapter. We are members of the MRC Center for Behavioral and Clinical Neuroscience in Cambridge.

REFERENCES

1. Bartus RT, Dean RL, Beer B. The cholinergic hypothesis of geriatric memory dysfunction. Science 1982;217:408–417.
2. Drachman DA, Leavitt J. Human memory and the cholinergic system. Arch Neurol 1974;30:113–121.
3. Crow TJ, Grove-White IG. An analysis of the learning deficit following hyoscine administration to man. Br J Pharmacol 1973;49:322–327.
4. Bowen DM, Smith CB, White P, Davison AN. Neurotransmitter-related enzymes and indices of hypoxia in senile dementia and other biotrophies. Brain 1976;99:459–496.
5. Perry EK, Gibson PH, Blessed G, Perry RH, Tomlinson BE. Neurotransmitter enzyme abnormalities in senile dementia. J Neurol Sci 1977;34:247–265.
6. Whitehouse PJ, Price DL, Struble RG, Clark AW, Coyle JT, DeLong MR. Alzheimer's disease and senile dementia: loss of neurones in the basal forebrain. Science 1982;215:1237–1238.
7. Fibiger HC. Cholinergic mechanisms in learning, memory and dementia: a review of recent evidence. Trends Neurosci 1991;14:220–223.
8. Dunnett SB, Everitt BJ, Robbins TW. The basal forebrain-cortical cholinergic system: interpreting the functional consequences of excitotoxic lesions. Trends Neurosci 1991;14:494–501.
9. Rossor M, Iversen LL. Non-cholinergic neurotransmitter abnormalities in Alzheimer's disease. Br Med Bull 1986;42:70–74.
10. Mann DMA. Pyramidal nerve cell loss in Alzheimer's disease. Neurodegeneration 1996;5:423–427.
11. Braak H, Braak E. Neuropathological staging of Alzheimer-related changes. Acta Neuropathol 1991;82:239–259.
12. Perry EK, Tomlinson BE, Blessed G, Bergmann K, Gibson PH, Perry RH. Correlation of cholinergic abnormalities with senile plaques and mental test scores in senile dementia. BMJ 1978;2:1457–1459.
13. Bierer LM, Haroutunian V, Gabriel S, et al. Neurochemical correlates of dementia severity in Alzheimer's disease: relative importance of the cholinergic deficits. J Neurochem 1995;64:749–760.
14. Bierer LM, Hof PR, Purohit DP, et al. Neocortical neurofibrillary tangles correlate with dementia severity in Alzheimer's disease. Arch Neurol 1995;52:81–88.
15. Terry RD, Masliah E, Salmon DP, et al. Physical basis of cognitive alterations in Alzheimer's disease: synapse loss is the major correlate of cognitive impairment. Ann Neurol 1991;30:572–580.
16. DeKosky ST, Scheff SW. Synapse loss in frontal cortex biopsies in Alzheimer's disease: correlation with cognitive severity. Ann Neurol 1990;27:457–464.

17. Kopelman MD. Multiple memory deficits in Alzheimer-type dementia: implications for pharmacotherapy. Psychol Med 1985;15:527–541.
18. Medin DL, O'Neil P, Smeltz E, Davis RT. Age differences in retention of concurrent discrimination problems in monkeys. J Gerontol 1973;28:63–67.
19. Bachevalier J, Landis LS, Walker LC, et al. Aged monkeys exhibit behavioral deficits indicative of widespread cerebral dysfunction. Neurobiol Aging 1991;12:99–111.
20. Bartus RT, Fleming D, Johnson H. Aging in the rhesus monkey: debilitating effects on short-term memory. J Gerontol 1978;33:858–971.
21. Bartus RT. On neurodegenerative diseases, models, and treatment strategies: lessons learned and lessons forgotten a generation following the cholinergic hypothesis. Exp Neurol 2000;163:495–529.
22. Beach TG, Potter PE, Kuo YM, et al. Cholinergic deafferentation of the rabbit cortex: a new model of A beta deposition. Neurosci Lett 2000;283:9–12.
23. Beach TG, Kuo YM, Schwab C, Walker DG, Roher AE. Reduction of cortical amyloid beta levels in guinea pig brain after systemic administration of physostigmine. Neurosci Lett 2001;310:21–24.
24. Ridley RM, Warner KA, Maclean CJ, Gaffan D, Baker HF. Visual agnosia and Klüver-Bucy syndrome in marmosets (*Callithrix jacchus*) following ablation of the inferotemporal cortex, with additional mnemonic effects of immunotoxic lesions of cholinergic projections to medial temporal areas. Brain Res 2001;898:136–151.
25. Ridley RM, Timothy CJ, Maclean CJ, Baker HF. Conditional learning and memory impairments following neurotoxic lesion of the CA1 field of the hippocampus. Neuroscience 1995;67:263–275.
26. Ridley RM, Thornley HD, Baker HF, Fine A. Cholinergic neural transplants into hippocampus restore learning ability in monkeys with fornix transections. Exp Brain Res 1991;83:533–538.
27. Ridley RM, Baker HF. Mental representation in human and monkey neuropsychology. In: Milner AD, ed. *Comparative Neuropsychology*. Oxford, UK: Oxford University Press; 1998:245–270.
28. Ridley RM, Baker HF. A critical evaluation of monkey models of amnesia and dementia. Brain Res Rev 1991;16:15–37.
29. Mesulam MM, Mufson EJ, Levey AI, Wainer BH. Cholinergic innervation of cortex by the basal forebrain: cytochemistry and cortical connections of the septal area, diagonal band nuclei, nucleus basalis (substantia innominata) and hypothalamus in the rhesus monkey. J Comp Neurol 1983;214:170–197.
30. Mesulam MM, Mufson EJ, Levey AI, Wainer BH. Atlas of cholinergic neurons in the forebrain and upper brainstem of the macaque based on monoclonal choline acetyltransferase immunohistochemistry and acetylcholinesterase histochemistry. Neuroscience 1984;3:669–686.
31. Everitt BJ, Sirkia TE, Roberts AC, Jones GH, Robbins TW. Distribution and some projections of cholinergic neurones in the brain of the common marmoset. J Comp Neurol 1988;271:533–558.

32. Mesulam MM, Mufson EJ. Neural inputs into the nucleus basalis of the substantia innominata (Ch4) in the rhesus monkey. Brain 1984;107:253–274.
33. Mesulam MM. The systems-level organization of cholinergic innervation in the human cerebral cortex and its alterations in Alzheimer's disease. Prog Brain Res 1996;109:285–297.
34. Jones BE, Cuello AC. Afferents to the basal forebrain cholinergic cell area from pontomesencephalic—catecholamine, serotonin, and acetylcholine—neurons. Neuroscience 1989;31:37–61.
35. Zaborszky L, Cullinan WE, Luine VN. Catecholaminergic–cholinergic interactions in the basal forebrain. Prog Brain Res 1993;98:31–49.
36. Wiley RG, Oeltmann TN, Lappi DA. Immunolesioning: selective destruction of neurons using immunotoxin to rat NGF receptor. Brain Res 1991;562:149–153.
37. Hefti F, Hartikka J, Salvaterra P, Weinen WJ, Mash D. Localization of nerve growth factor receptors on cholinergic neurons of the human basal forebrain. Neurosci Lett 1986;69:275–281.
38. Mufson EJ, Bothwell M, Hersh LB, Kordower J. Nerve growth factor receptor profiles in the normal, aged human basal forebrain: colocalization with cholinergic neurons. J Comp Neurol 1989;285:196–217.
39. Kordower JH, Bartus RT, Bothwell M, Schatteman G, Gash D. Nerve growth factor receptor immunoreactivity in the non-human primate (*Cebus apella*): distribution, morphology and colocalization with cholinergic enzyme. J Comp Neurol 1988;277:465–486.
40. Maclean CJ, Baker HF, Fine A, Ridley RM. The distribution of p75 neurotrophin receptor-immunoreactive cells in the forebrain of the common marmoset (*Callithrix jacchus*). Brain Res Bull 1997;43:197–208.
41. Smith C, Farrah T, Goodwin R. The TNF receptor superfamily of cellular and viral proteins: activation, costimulation, and death. Cell 1994;76:959–962.
42. Ebendal T. Function and evolution in the NGF family and its receptors. J Neurosci Res 1992;32:461–470.
43. Mrzljak L, Levey AI, Belcher S, Goldman-Rakic PS. Localization of the m2 muscarinic acetylcholine receptor protein and mRNA in cortical neurons of the normal and the cholinergically deafferented rhesus monkey. J Comp Neurol 1998;390:112–132.
44. Easton A, Ridley RM, Baker HF, Gaffan D. Unilateral lesions of the cholinergic basal forebrain and fornix in one hemisphere and inferotemporal cortex in the opposite hemisphere produce severe learning impairments in rhesus monkeys. Cerebral Cortex 2002;12:729–736.
45. Bartus RT. Physostigmine and recent memory: effects in young and aged non-human primates. Science 1979;206:1087–1089.
46. Bartus RT, Dean RL, Fleming DL. Aging in the rhesus monkey: effects on visual discrimination learning and reversal learning. J Gerontol 1979;34:209–219.
47. Ridley RM, Bowes PM, Baker HF, Crow TJ. An involvement of acetylcholine in object discrimination learning and memory in the marmoset. Neuropsychologia 1984;22:253–263.

48. Bartus RT, Johnson HR. Short term memory in the rhesus monkey: disruption from the anticholinergic scopolamine. Pharmacol Biochem Behav 1976;5:39–46.

49. Penetar DM, McDonough J-HJ. Effects of cholinergic drugs on delayed match-to-sample performance of rhesus monkeys. Pharmacol Biochem Behav 1983;19:963–967.

50. Ridley RM, Baker HF, Drewett B, Johnson JA. Effects of ibotenic acid lesions of the basal forebrain on serial reversal learning in marmosets. Psychopharmacology 1985;86:438–443.

51. Ridley RM, Murray TK, Johnson JA, Baker HF. Learning impairment following lesion of the basal nucleus of Meynert in the marmoset: modification by cholinergic drugs. Brain Res 1986;376:108–116.

52. Aigner TG, Mitchell SJ, Aggleton JP, et al. Effects of scopolamine and physostigmine on recognition memory in monkeys with ibotenic-acid lesions of the nucleus basalis of Meynert. Psychopharmacology 1987;92:292–300.

53. Voytko ML, Olton DS, Richardson RT, Gorman IK, Tobin JT, Price DL. Basal forebrain lesions in monkeys disrupt attention but not learning and memory. J Neurosci 1994;14:167–186.

54. Sunderland T, Tariot PN, Cohen RM, Weingartner H, Mueller EA, Murphy DL. Anticholinergic sensitivity in patients with dementia of the Alzheimer-type and age-matched controls. Arch Gen Psychiatry 1987;44:418–426.

55. Flicker C, Ferris SH, Serby M. Hypersensitivity to scopolamine in the elderly. Psychopharmacology (Berl) 1992;107:437–441.

56. Voytko ML. Impairments in acquisition and reversals of two-choice discriminations by aged rhesus monkeys. Neurobiol Aging 1999;20:617–627.

57. Harder JA, Baker HF, Ridley RM. The role of the central cholinergic projections in cognition: Implications of the effects of scopolamine on discrimination learning by monkeys. Brain Res Bull 1998;45:319–326.

58. Irle E, Markowitsch HJ. Basal forebrain-lesioned monkeys are severely impaired in tasks of association and recognition memory. Ann Neurol 1987;22:735–743.

59. Ridley RM, Samson NA, Baker HF, Johnson JA. Visuospatial learning impairment following lesion of the cholinergic projection to the hippocampus. Brain Res 1988;456:71–87.

60. Ridley RM, Aitken DM, Baker HF. Learning about rules but not about reward is impaired following lesions of the cholinergic projection to the hippocampus. Brain Res 1989;502:306–318.

61. Ridley RM, Pugh P, Maclean CJ, Baker HF. Severe learning impairment caused by combined immunotoxic lesion of the cholinergic projections to the cortex and hippocampus in monkeys. Brain Res 1999;836:120–138.

62. Maclean CJ, Gaffan D, Baker HF, Ridley RM. Visual discrimination learning impairments produced by combined transections of the anterior temporal stem, amygdala and fornix in marmoset monkeys. Brain Res 2001;888:34–50.

63. Ridley RM, Barefoot HC, Maclean CJ, Pugh P, Baker HF. Different effects on learning ability following injection of the cholinergic immunotoxin ME20.4 IgG-saporin into the diagonal band of Broca, basal nucleus of Meynert, or both in monkeys. Behav Neurosci 1999;113:303–315.

64. Ridley RM, Hardy A, Maclean CJ, Baker HF. Non-spatial acquisition and retention deficits following small excitotoxic lesions within the hippocampus in monkeys. Neuroscience 2001;107:239–248.
65. Murray TK, Ridley RM. The effect of excitotoxic hippocampal lesions on simple and conditional discrimination learning in the rat. Behav Brain Res 1999;99:103–113.
66. Fine A, Hoyle C, Maclean CJ, LeVatte TL, Baker HF, Ridley RM. Learning impairments following injection of a selective cholinergic immunotoxin, ME20.4 IgG-saporin, into the basal nucleus of Meynert in monkeys. Neuroscience 1997;81:331–343.
67. Cowey A, Gross CG. Effects of foveal prestriate and inferotemporal lesions on visual discrimination by rhesus monkeys. Exp Brain Res 1970;11:128–144.
68. Gaffan EA, Harrison S, Gaffan D. Single and concurrent discrimination learning by monkeys after lesions of inferotemporal cortex. Q J Exp Psychol 1986;38B:31–52.
69. Gaffan D, Harrison S, Gaffan EA. Visual identification following inferotemporal ablation in the monkey. Q J Exp Psychol 1986;38B:5–30.
70. Suzuki WA, Amaral DG. Perirhinal and parahippocampal cortices of the macaque monkey: cortical afferents. J Comp Neurol 1994;350:497–533.
71. Suzuki WA, Amaral DG. Topographic organization of the reciprocal connections between the monkey entorhinal cortex and the perirhinal and parahippocampal cortices. J Neurosci 1994;14:1856–1877.
72. Suzuki WA, Amaral DG. Cortical inputs to the CA1 field of the monkey hippocampus originate from the perirhinal and parahippocampal cortex but not from area TE. Neurosci Lett 1990;115:43–48.
73. Witter MP, Amaral DG. Entorhinal cortex of the monkey: V. Projections to the dentate gyrus, hippocampus, and subicular complex. J Comp Neurol 1991;307:437–459.
74. Barefoot HC, Maclean CJ, Baker HF, Ridley RM. Unilateral hippocampal and inferotemporal cortex lesions in opposite hemispheres impair learning of single-pair visual discriminations as well as visuovisual conditional tasks in monkeys. Behav Brain Res 2003;141:51–62.
75. Gaffan D, Parker A, Easton A. Dense amnesia in the monkey after transection of fornix, amygdala and anterior temporal stem. Neuropsychologia 2001;39:51–70.
76. Moss M, Mahut H, Zola-Morgan SM. Concurrent discrimination learning in monkeys after hippocampal, entorhinal or fornix lesions. J Neurosci 1981;1:227–240.
77. Teng E, Stefanacci L, Squire LR, Zola SM. Contrasting effects on discrimination learning after hippocampal lesions and conjoint hippocampal-caudate lesions in monkeys. J Neurosci 2000;20:3853–3863.
78. Barefoot HC, Baker HF, Ridley RM. Synergistic effects of unilateral immunolesions of the cholinergic projections from the basal forebrain and contralateral ablations of the inferotemporal cortex and hippocampus in monkeys. Neuroscience 2000;98:243–251.

79. Barefoot HC, Baker HF, Ridley RM. Crossed unilateral lesions of temporal lobe structures and cholinergic cell bodies impair visual conditional and object discrimination learning in monkeys. Eur J Neurosci 2002;15:507–516.
80. Stephan H, Baron G, Schwerdtfeger WK. *The Brain of the Common Marmoset* (Callithrix jacchus); *a Stereotaxic Atlas.* Berlin: Springer; 1980.
81. Gaffan D, Parker A. Interaction of perirhinal cortex with the fornix-fimbria: memory for objects and "object-in-place" memory. J Neurosci 1996;16:5864–5869.
82. Gaffan D, Easton A, Parker A. Interaction of inferior temporal cortex with frontal cortex and basal forebrain: double dissociation in strategy implementation and associative learning. J Neurosci 2002;22:7288–7296.
83. Francis PT, Cross AJ, Bowen DM. Neurotransmitters and neuropeptides. In: Terry RD, Katzman R, Bick KL, eds. *Alzheimer Disease.* New York: Raven Press Ltd.; 1994:247–261.
84. Francis PT, Pangaloss MN, Bowen DM. Animal and drug modelling for Alzheimer synaptic pathology. Prog Neurobiol 1992;39:517–545.
85. Ottersen OP. Excitatory amino acid neurotransmitters: anatomical systems. In: Meldrum B, ed. *Excitatory Amino Acid Antagonists.* Oxford, UK: Blackwell Scientific; 1991:14–38.
86. Chessell IP, Pearson RC, Heath PR, Bown DM, Francis PT. Selective loss of cholinergic receptors following unilateral intracortical injection of volkensin. Exp Neurol 1997;147:183–191.
87. Alonso JR, U HS, Amaral DG. Cholinergic innervation of the primate hippocampal formation: II. Effects of fimbria/fornix transection. J Comp Neurol 1996;375:527–551.
88. Kitt CA, Mitchell SJ, DeLong MR, Wainer BH, Price DL. Fibre pathways of basal forebrain cholinergic neurons in monkeys. Brain Res 1987;406:192–206.
89. Ogura H, Aigner TG. MK-801 impairs recognition memory in rhesus monkeys: comparison with cholinergic drugs. J Pharmacol Exp Ther 1993;266:60–64.
90. Matsuoka N, Aigner TG. Cholinergic–glutamatergic interactions in visual recognition memory of rhesus monkeys. Neuroreport 1996;7:565–568.
91. Harder JA, Aboobaker A, Hodgetts T, Ridley RM. Learning impairments induced by glutamate blockade using dizocilpine (MK801) in monkeys. Br J Pharmacol 1998;125:1013–1018.
92. Dijk SN, Francis PT, Stratmann GC, Bowen DM. NMDA-induced glutamate and aspartate release from rat cortical pyramidal neurones: evidence for modulation by a 5-HT1A antagonist. Br J Pharmacol 1995;115:1169–1174.
93. Harder JA, Ridley RM. The $5HT_{1A}$ antagonist, WAY100635, alleviates cognitive impairments induced by dizocilpine (MK801) in monkeys. Neuropharmacology 2000;39:547–552.
94. Harder JA, Maclean CJ, Alder JT, Francis PT, Ridley RM. The $5HT_{1A}$ antagonist, WAY100635, ameliorates the cognitive impairment induced by fornix transection in the marmoset. Psychopharmacology 1996;127:245–254.

95. Gaffan D. Scene-specific memory for objects: a model of episodic impairment in monkeys with fornix transection. J Cogn Neurosci 1994;6:305–320.

96. Hood KL, Postle BR, Corkin S. An evaluation of the concurrent discrimination task as a measure of habit learning: performance of amnesic subjects. Neuropsychologia 1999;37:1375–1386.

97. Aggleton JP, Nicol RM, Huston AE, Fairbairn AF. The performance of amnesic subjects on tests of experimental amnesia in animals: delayed matching-to-sample and concurrent learning. Neuropsychologia 1988;26:265–272.

98. Squire LR, Zola-Morgan SM, Chen KS. Human amnesia and animal model of amnesia: performance of amnesic patients on tests designed for the monkey. Behav Neurosci 1988;102:210–221.

99. Gaffan D, Gaffan EA. Amnesia in man following transection of the fornix. A review. Brain 1991;114:2611–2618.

100. Rempel-Clower NL, Zola SM, Squire LR, Amaral DG. Three cases of enduring memory impairment after bilateral damage limited to the hippocampal formation. J Neurosci 1996;16:5233–5255.

101. Mishkin M, Malamut B, Bachevalier J. Memories and habits: two neural systems. In: Lynch G, McGough JL, Weinberger NM, eds. *Neurobiology of Learning and Memory*. New York: Guilford Press; 1984:65–77.

102. Corkin S. Acquisition of motor skill after bilateral medial temporal-lobe excision. Neuropsychologia 1968;6:225–264.

103. Hodges JR, Patterson K, Oxbury S, Funnell E. Semantic dementia: progressive fluent aphasia with temporal lobe atrophy. Brain 1992;115:1783–1806.

104. O'Keefe J, Nadel L. *The Hippocampus as a Cognitive Map*. Oxford, UK: Oxford University Press; 1978.

105. Hirsh R. The hippocampus and contextual retrieval of information from memory: a theory. Behav Biol 1974;12:421–444.

106. Sutherland RJ, Rudy JW. Configural association theory: the role of the hippocampal formation in learning, memory, and amnesia. Psychobiology 1989;17:129–144.

107. Hirsh R. The hippocampus, conditional operations and cognition. Physiol Psychol 1986;8:175–182.

108. Buckley MJ, Booth MCA, Rolls ET, Gaffan D. Selective perceptual impairments after perirhinal cortex ablation. J Neurosci 2001;21:9824–9836.

109. Bussey TJ, Saksida LM, Murray EA. Perirhinal cortex resolves feature ambiguity in complex visual discriminations. Eur J Neurosci 2002;15:365–374.

110. Ridley RM, Baker HF, Harder JA, Pearson C. Effects of lesions of different parts of the septo-hippocampal system in primates on learning and retention of information acquired before or after surgery. Brain Res Bull 1996;40:21–32.

111. McCormick DA. Cellular mechanisms of cholinergic control of neocortical and thalamic neuronal excitability. In: Steriade M, Biesold D, eds. *Brain Cholinergic Systems*. Oxford, UK: Oxford University Press; 1990:236–264.

112. Metherate R, Tremblay N, Dykes RW. The effects of acetylcholine on response properties of cat somatosensory cortical neurons. J Neurophysiol 1988;59:1231–1252.

113. Sato H, Hata V, Hagihara K, Tsumoto T. Effects of cholinergic depletion on neuron activities in the cat visual cortex. J Neurophysiol 1987;58:781–794.
114. Wilson FAW, Rolls ET. Neuronal responses related to reinforcement in the primate basal forebrain. Brain Res 1990;509:213–231.
115. Wilson FAW, Rolls ET. Neuronal responses related to novelty and familiarity of visual stimuli in the substantia innominata, diagonal band of Broca and periventricular region of the primate basal forebrain. Exp Brain Res 1990;80:104–120.
116. Burton MJ, Rolls ET, Mora F. Effects of hunger on the responses of neurons in the lateral hypothalamus to the sight and taste of food. Exp Neurol 1976;51:668–677.
117. Mora F, Rolls ET, Burton MJ. Modulation during learning of the responses of neurons in the lateral hypothalamus to the sight of food. Exp Neurol 1976;53:508–519.
118. Richardson RT, DeLong MR. A reappraisal of the functions of the nucleus basalis of Meynert. Trends Neurosci 1988;11:264–267.
119. Tanaka Y, Sakurai M, Hayashi S. Effect of scopolamine and HP029, a cholinesterase inhibitor, on long-term potentiation in hippocampal slices of guinea pig. Neurosci Lett 1989;98:179–183.
120. Fell J, Klaver P, Lehnertz K, et al. Human memory formation is accompanied by rhinal-hippocampal coupling and decoupling. Nature Neurosci 2001;4:1259–1264.
121. Mesulam MM. Large-scale neurocognitive networks and distributed processing for attention, language, and memory. Ann Neurol 1990;28:597–613.
122. Gorry JD. Studies on the comparative anatomy of the ganglion basale of Meynert. Acta Anat 1963;55:51–104.
123. Mesulam MM, Volicer L, Marquis JK, Mufson EJ, Green RC. Systematic regional differences in the cholinergic innervation of the primate cerebral cortex: distribution of enzyme activities and some behavioral implications. Ann Neurol 1986;19:144–151.
124. Mesulam MM, Geula C. Acetylcholinesterase-rich pyramidal neurons in the human neocortex and hippocampus: absence at birth, development during the life span, and dissolution in Alzheimer's disease. Ann Neurol 1988;24:765–773.
125. Mesulam MM. Cholinergic pathways and the ascending reticular activating system of the human brain. Ann NY Acad Sci 1995;757:169–179.
126. Easton A, Gaffan D. Comparison of perirhinal cortex ablation and crossed unilateral lesions of the medial forebrain bundle from the inferior temporal cortex in the rhesus monkey: effects on learning and retrieval. Behav Neurosci 2000;114:1041–1057.
127. Easton A, Gaffan D. Crossed unilateral lesions of the medial forebrain bundle and either inferior temporal or frontal cortex impair object-reward association learning in rhesus monkeys. Neuropsychologia 1902;39:71–82.
128. Easton A, Parker A, Gaffan D. Crossed unilateral lesions of medial forebrain bundle and either inferior temporal or frontal cortex im111111pair object recognition memory in Rhesus monkeys. Behav Brain Res 2001;121:1–10.

129. Perry E, Walker M, Grace J, Perry R. Acetylcholine in mind: a neurotransmitter correlate of consciousness? Trends Neurosci 1999;22:273–280.

7

Cortical Cholinergic Deafferentation Induces Aβ Deposition

Toward a Physiological Animal Model of Alzheimer's Disease

Thomas G. Beach, D. G. Walker, P. E. Potter, L. I. Sue, S. Scott, K. J. Layne, A. J. Newell, P. K. Rauschkolb, M. E. Poston, S. D. Webster, R. A. Durham, M. R. Emmerling, K. Sawada, W. G. Honer, A. Fisher, and A. E. Roher

INTRODUCTION

There are 4 million Americans with Alzheimer's disease (AD), and the cost of the disease to the United States is estimated at $100 billion annually (Alzheimer's Association). Finding a cure or prevention for AD is therefore an important goal. To do this, however, the cause(s) of AD must first be determined.

Research has established that brain accumulation and histological deposition of a single peptide known as Aβ is a critical event in AD. Many investigators believe that Aβ deposition leads to all of the other relevant pathological changes in the disease, including neurofibrillary tangle formation, loss of synapses, neuronal death, and dementia *(1–3)*. Preventing this accumulation may prevent AD. In simple genetic forms of AD, accumulation of Aβ is caused by inherited gene mutations that result in increased Aβ production *(4)*. Only a very small subset of AD occurs this way, however. In the common, "sporadic" form of AD, the reason for Aβ accumulation is not known.

If Aβ deposition can be considered the essence of AD, then the disease in fact transcends human genetics because Aβ deposition is an aging change

From: *Molecular Neurosurgery With Targeted Toxins*
Edited by: R. G. Wiley and D. A. Lappi © Humana Press Inc., Totowa, NJ

common to many mammalian species *(5–11)*. The prevalence of AD increases exponentially with age *(12)*, and the histopathology of AD affects all humans who approach the maximum human lifespan *(13,14)*. The initial pathogenic event of AD therefore must lie within the physiological process of aging.

We have developed an animal model of AD that is initiated by a physiological aging change *(15,16)*. In primates, cholinergic afferents to the cerebral cortex are depleted during aging, probably because of the loss or physiological inadequacy of the parent cell bodies in the basal forebrain *(17–30)*. Evidence from human postmortem studies, as well as cell culture and animal experiments, has linked cholinergic neurotransmission to Aβ metabolism and deposition. In aging human cerebral cortex, cholinergic deafferentation begins around ages 40–50 yr *(20,25)* and is shortly followed by biochemically detectable elevations of cortical Aβ (31) and Aβ deposition *(32)*. In aging, nondemented humans, there is a statistical association between the depletion of cortical cholinergic markers and measures of Aβ accumulation *(27,33,34)*.

In vitro studies have shown that m1 and m3 muscarinic receptor activation leads to changes in the cleavage pattern of Aβ's amyloid precursor protein (βAPP) that favor decreased production of Aβ (processing changes that result in more Aβ formation are termed *amyloidogenic*; changes that favor secretory APP [sAPPα], a different cleavage product, are termed *nonamyloidogenic*) *(35–50)*. This effect has been confirmed in vivo in animals *(51–53)* and humans *(54,55)*. Conversely, decreased activation of muscarinic receptors, whether through lesions of cholinergic afferents *(56–63)* or pharmacological blockade *(64)*, leads to increased expression of βAPP or evidence of increased amyloidogenic cleavage. We therefore hypothesized that cortical cholinergic deafferentation would cause increased cortical Aβ production and deposition.

Cortical cholinergic deafferentation, accomplished through lesioning of the nucleus basalis of Meynert (NBM) has long been employed as an animal model of AD. Following the discovery of the cortical cholinergic deficit in AD, many investigators suggested that this could be the initial critical pathogenic event in the disease. Some predicted that degenerating cholinergic fibers might participate in plaque formation *(65–67)*. Two groups even reported the development of Aβ deposition in rats with NBM lesions *(68,69)*, but this was not replicated by others, and these findings were later disputed *(70)*. One group reported that NBM lesions increased amyloidogenic processing of βAPP *(62,63)*, but they did not measure Aβ directly. Our approach differs from these previous efforts in a number of ways.

We used rabbits as our experimental animal rather than rats, which were employed by most earlier studies. Rodent Aβ differs from the human peptide by three different amino acids, and there is some evidence that this difference leads to decreased amyloidogenic processing of βAPP *(71–73)*. It is possible therefore that the rodent Aβ sequence may make rodents resistant to Aβ overproduction and deposition. Because the rabbit and human Aβ peptide are identical *(74,75)*, this possibility is avoided. The first models of cholinergic deafferentation *(76–78)* used lesioning methods that were relatively nonspecific in terms of the cell types affected *(79)*. We used an immunotoxin that is much more selective *(63,80–86)*. Finally, previous attempts to link amyloidogenic metabolism and cholinergic deafferentation used surrogate markers for Aβ induction, such as full-length βAPP and sAPPα *(56–63)*. This approach is inadequate. Increased Aβ production can arise from altered processing of βAPP in the absence of concentration changes of the parent molecule; secretion of sAPPα does not always have a reciprocal relationship with secretion of Aβ *(87–90)*. We therefore measured Aβ directly using sensitive enzyme-linked immunosorbent assay (ELISA) methods.

We showed that lesions of the rabbit NBM resulted in cortical Aβ deposition *(15,16)*. Lesioned animals had as much as an eightfold increase in cortical Aβ concentration. The Aβ deposits were primarily vascular, with occasional perivascular plaques. We think it likely, based on molecular mechanisms worked out in cell culture studies *(35–50)*, that cholinergic deafferentation leads to increased Aβ production and secretion by deafferented cortical neurons. The increased extracellular fluid concentrations of Aβ lead to precipitation of Aβ onto the vascular basal lamina because of physicochemical affinities between Aβ and extracellular matrix molecules of the basal lamina *(91,92)*. The dependence of lesion-induced Aβ deposition on cholinergic processes has been demonstrated by its reduction with cholinergic therapy and by showing that lesioning of the noradrenergic locus coeruleus (LC) does not cause Aβ deposition.

The relevance of our animal model for AD depends on the place of the cholinergic deficit within the AD pathogenetic cascade. In AD, the cholinergic deficit is accentuated relative to normal aging, so that AD patients, especially those toward the younger age ranges, have statistically lower concentrations of cholinergic markers relative to age-matched controls. Controversy exists as to whether the cholinergic deficit in AD is an early or a later stage in the disease. Multiple studies were consistent with an early cholinergic deficit *(24,93–102)*, but some work has contradicted this, suggesting that it is a late change in the disease *(103–106)*. It has also been suggested that the cholinergic deficit is merely a secondary change, a retrograde degeneration occurring after cortical degeneration *(107)*.

We feel that the studies advocating a late-stage occurrence are flawed in that they used clinical staging of AD and mixed true, histopathological stages of the disease. These studies also ignored earlier investigators, who had found that the continuing loss of cortical cholinergic markers with age eventually resulted in AD-like cholinergic deficits in age-matched controls *(17,18,21,22,25,26)*. Therefore, it will always be difficult in the oldest old to distinguish between AD and controls on the basis of cholinergic markers. We consider that, because the cortical cholinergic deficit in normal aging humans precedes and is statistically linked to age-related Aβ deposition *(20,25,27,31,33,34)*, that it must precede clinical AD. Nucleus basalis neuronal cell bodies are also affected at the preclinical stage because neurofibrillary tangles are universally present in the NBM of nondemented elderly humans (79/80 cases aged 67 yr and older) *(108;109)*, in many cases in the complete absence of neocortical plaques or tangles.

Finally, we have causally linked cholinergic deafferentation to Aβ deposition in our animal model; other animal models have shown that neither cortical neuronal destruction *(110)* nor massive Aβ deposition *(111–116)* resulted in a quantitatively significant retrograde cortical cholinergic deficit. The aggregate data strongly indicate that the cholinergic NBM begins to degenerate early in the aging process, leading to cortical cholinergic deafferentation, Aβ deposition, and AD.

Our animal model of AD is still incomplete, however, because animals surviving 6 mo show much less Aβ deposition than what is seen in AD, and the deposits are confined largely to the vasculature. Examination of longer survival periods has been complicated by the regeneration of cholinergic afferents. Repetitive NBM lesions sustained cholinergic deafferentation but Aβ deposition did not increase beyond what was seen at 6 mo.

SUMMARY OF EXPERIMENTS UNDERTAKEN TO DATE

Time-Course of Aβ Deposition After Cortical Cholinergic Deafferentation

Methods

Twelve-week-old (2–2.5 kg) female New Zealand white rabbits received unilateral intracerebroventricular (icv) stereotaxic injections of either 12 μL (32.4 mg) of an immunotoxin conjugate (Advanced Targeting Systems, San Diego, CA) dissolved in sterile saline or 12 μL of sterile saline alone. The conjugate is composed of saporin, a ribosomal toxin, conjugated to mono-clonal antibody ME20.4, which is specific for the p75 neurotrophin receptor (p75^{NTR}; low-affinity nerve growth factor receptor) that is expressed selectively on cholinergic NBM neurons *(86)*. The optimum dose of conjugate was determined by pilot experiments. Higher doses of conjugate, whether delivered by unilateral or bilateral injections, caused increased toxicity (anorexia, lethargy, diarrhea, abnormal posturing, convulsions, death) without an appreciable increase in lesion extent. Coordinates for the injection, relative to bregma, were: anteroposterior axis [AP] = 0, lateral axis [L] = 2.2, depth axis [D] = 7.5 (mm).

After survival periods of 3 wk, 5 wk, 3 mo, 6 mo, and 1 yr, the animals were euthanized, and the brains were removed and cut into 0.4-cm coronal slices. One or two slices containing frontal cortex and hippocampus were fixed in 4% paraformaldehyde for immunohistochemical studies; the remaining slices were fresh-frozen on slabs of dry ice. Immunoperoxidase histochemistry was performed on free-floating sections as previously described *(117)*. Cortical cholinergic fibers were visualized using an enhanced acetylcholinesterase (AChE) enzyme histochemical method *(118)*; cholinergic NBM neuronal cell bodies were demonstrated using the same ME20.4 p75^{NTR} antibody used for immunotoxin construction.

Tissue localization of Aβ was performed using several antibodies, including 10D5 (amino acids 1–16; Elan Pharmaceuticals, South San Francisco, CA), 4G8 (amino acids 17–24, Signet Laboratories, Dedham, MA), 6E10 (amino acids 1–16, Signet Laboratories), 3D6 (N-terminal specific for Aβ, Elan Pharmaceuticals), 21F12 (end specific for Aβ42, Elan Pharmaceuticals), and 5C3 (end specific for Aβ40, Calbiochem, La Jolla, CA). For colocalization experiments, we used monoclonal antibody 10C9 to heparan sulfate proteoglycan (IISPG; Biogenesis, Brentwood, NH). Control sections were treated by omitting the primary antibody and (for 10D5 stained sections) by preabsorbing the primary antibody with 100 µg/mL synthetic Aβ 1-40 (California Peptides, Napa, CA) for 2 h prior to use. Thioflavine S staining was used to assess for the presence of β-pleated sheet amyloid and the Campbell–Switzer silver stain *(119)* was used to demonstrate argyrophilic diffuse and compact amyloid deposits.

Quantification of histological Aβ deposition and of cholinergic fiber depletion was performed by counting the intersections of positively stained blood vessels or fibers with the lines on an ocular grid. The grid position was successively moved through the cortical column, and a mean value was determined per column for each animal. This method was described in earlier publications *(67,120,121)*.

Confocal scanning laser fluorescence microscopy was performed on sections stained immunohistochemically for Aβ and HSPG as described above except for the substitution of fluorescent signal development in place of the immunoperoxidase method. Sections were first reacted for HSPG with the 10C9 antibody and then for Aβ with the 10D5 antibody. Signal development was achieved with fluorochrome-linked secondary antibodies (Molecular Probes, Eugene, OR). These were goat antirat immunoglobulin G (IgG) conjugated to Alexa 488 for HSPG and sheep antimouse IgG conjugated to Alexa 568 for Aβ. Control sections were treated identically except for omission of one of the two primary antibodies (antibody to HSPG omitted on one control section, antibody to Aβ omitted on the other control section). Sections were viewed on an Olympus confocal microscope at appropriate excitation wavelengths.

For electron microscopy, sections were initially processed identically as for Aβ immunohistochemistry with the 10D5 antibody except for omission of nickel ammonium sulfate intensification of the 3,3'-diaminobenzidine reaction product. Following immunostaining, sections were sequentially postfixed for 1 h at 4°C in 1% glutaraldehyde and 1% osmium tetroxide, both made up in 0.1M sodium cacodylate buffer, pH 7.4. Following dehydration in a graded ethanol series and propylene oxide, the sections were infiltrated in Polybed 812 resin (Polysciences Inc., Warrington, PA) and polymerized at 65°C. Ultrathin sections were cut at 100 nm and examined without heavy metal staining.

Biochemical analyses of fresh-frozen brain tissue (dorsolateral frontal cerebral cortex ipsilateral to the injection site for all groups, with contralateral cortex and ipsilateral hippocampus also measured in some groups) included choline acetyltransferase (ChAT) enzyme assay *(122)*, ELISA quantification of Aβ, and Western blot quantification of sAPPα and full-length βAPP.

Levels of Aβ (N-40) and Aβ (N-42) were assayed in cerebral cortex by ELISA methods after tissue homogenization. Three different extraction techniques were employed. For the 5-wk and 6-mo survival groups, the first step consisted of homogenization in 0.5M Tris-HCl buffer, pH 7.5, with protease inhibitors (2.0 μg/mL each of pepstatin A, antipain, leupeptin, and aprotinin) and 5mM EDTA (ethylenediaminetetraacetic acid), followed by centrifugation at 100,000g for 1 h. The pellet from this first centrifugation was then resuspended and sonicated in either 90% formic acid (for the 5-wk survival group) *(123)* or 2% diethylamine (DEA) *(89)* (for the 6-mo survival group), following which the supernatant from a subsequent centrifugation step was analyzed. For the 6-mo survival group, a third extraction was performed on the pellet from this step, using 90% formic acid. For the 3-wk and 1-yr survival groups, a one-step extraction in guanidine hydrochloride was employed *(124)*. The supernatants from all of these extractions were analyzed by ELISA.

The ELISA methods also differed between studies. For the 5-wk survival group, the capture antibody was 6E10 (for total Aβ). For the 6-mo survival group, the C-terminal-specific antibodies *(125,126)* R163 (Aβ40) and R165 (Aβ42) were used for antigen capture. Signal development employed europium-conjugated 4G8 for the 5-wk survival group, with streptavidin-HRP-conjugated 4G8 for the 6-mo survival group. Standard curves were constructed using synthetic Aβ1–40 and Aβ1–42 (California Peptides). A commercially obtained ELISA (Biosource International, Camarillo, CA) for Aβ40 and 42 was used for the 3 wk and 1 yr survival groups. This uses an N-terminal-specific Aβ antibody for capture, end-specific Aβ40 and Aβ42 antibodies in a second step, and HRP-conjugated antirabbit IgG as a third step. Standards for Aβ40 and Aβ42 are supplied. We have verified the accuracy of the Biosource ELISA by running both quantitative Western blots and ELISA analyses on samples of rabbit cerebrospinal fluid (CSF). There is a strong correlation ($r = 0.82$, $p = 0.0003$) between the arithmetic mean of Aβ40 and Aβ42 concentrations as measured by ELISA and the intensity of the approx 4-kDa band on Western blots, probed with the 6E10 antibody.

Cortical concentrations of full-length APP and sAPPα were determined for the 6-mo survival group using Western blots. Tissue was homogenized in Tris-HCl buffer with protease inhibitors (as described in the ELISA methods) and centrifuged at $100,000g$ for 1 h. The supernatant was collected, and the pellet was solubilized in sodium dodecyl sulfate (SDS). Samples of the supernatant and solubilized pellet were separated on 10–20% Tris-Glycine polyacrylamide gradient gels (Invitrogen, Carlsbad, CA), transferred to membranes (Invitrogen), and reacted with the 22C11 antibody, which recognizes the N-terminal portion of βAPP (Roche Biochemicals, Indianapolis, IN). Bound antibody was detected with peroxidase-labeled antimouse IgG, followed by incubation with chemiluminescent substrate (Pierce Biotechnology, Rockford, IL). The location and intensity of bands were assessed using a ChemiImager 4000 blot imaging system (Alpha Innotech, San Leandro, CA).

Results

The efficacy of the NBM lesion has been demonstrated by ChAT assay, AChE histochemistry, and immunohistochemistry for p75[NTR]. Cortical ChAT activity ipsilateral to the toxin injection site was significantly reduced ($p < 0.01$) in all lesioned groups with respect to their control groups. Lesioned animals had ChAT activity that ranged from 31% of control (6-mo survival group), to 50% of control (5-wk survival group), to 64% of control

(3-wk survival group). The variability was likely caused by differences in the efficacy of the initial lesion rather than evolution of the lesion over time. The immunotoxin conjugate appeared to lose potency with prolonged storage, even at –80°C. Contralateral to the injection site, the reduction was less marked, to 68% of control values (compared to 31% of control on ipsilateral side; measured for 6-mo survival group only). The hippocampus was assayed at one time-point only (5-wk survival; ipsilateral to injection) and showed a reduction to 49.5% of control values.

AChE enzyme histochemistry revealed very marked depletion of cortical cholinergic fibers in immunotoxin-injected animals (Fig. 1A,B). Depletion of cholinergic fibers was perceptibly more marked on the ipsilateral side and was restricted to medial and dorsolateral cerebral cortex; the ventro-lateral cerebral cortex did not show apparent fiber depletion. The subiculum and hippocampus were severely depleted of cholinergic fibers. Quantification of cholinergic fiber density was performed in areas of maximum depletion (medial frontal cortex and CA1 of hippocampus) in the 3-wk survival animals. Cholinergic fibers were depleted to 17% of control in the medial frontal cortex and 24.6% of control in area CA1 (Fig. 2G,J). Histochemical staining for AChE (Fig. 1D,E) and immunohistochemical staining for p75^{NTR} (not shown) demonstrated a marked depletion of cholinergic NBM neuronal cell bodies in all lesioned animals.

Immunohistochemistry for Aβ with all antibodies revealed frequent positively stained blood vessels throughout the cerebri of immunotoxin-treated animals (Figs. 1C, 2C). The greatest number of vessels were located in the cerebral cortex, but occasional positive vessels were present in diencephalic areas, including the thalamus and basal ganglia. Within the cerebral cortex, the superficial layers had the greatest vessel densities. Blood vessels of all sizes were stained, from large arterioles to capillaries; large arterioles were most frequently involved. Staining was localized to the blood vessel walls (Fig. 1F); there was no staining of the vessel luminal contents and no staining of red blood cells.

The 5C3 antibody, specific for Aβ40, gave similar results as antibody 21F12, specific for Aβ42, indicating that both forms of Aβ were present in the vascular deposits. Staining with the 3D6 antibody, specific for the N-terminus of Aβ, was also of similar quality and density, indicating that the complete Aβ peptide was deposited. Intracellular Aβ staining was not present in any brain region.

In all immunotoxin-treated animals, the neuropil around occasional blood vessels was also stained (Figs. 1C,I, 2C), resembling the perivascular diffuse plaques sometimes seen in human AD cases. No staining of any type was observed in any control animal or in control sections.

Neither the vascular nor the perivascular deposits were stained with thioflavine S, indicating that the deposited Aβ was in a diffuse, nonamyloid form. The vascular deposits, however, were stained with the Campbell–Switzer method for amyloid (not shown). Quantification of the density of Aβ-immunoreactive blood vessels showed that histological Aβ deposition tended to increase between 3-wk and 3-mo survival, but did not increase appreciably between 3 and 6 mo (Fig. 3A).

Electron microscopic examination revealed that the immunohistochemical reaction product marking Aβ was localized to the basal lamina covering arteriolar smooth muscle, pericyctes and endothelial cells (Fig. 1G,H). The reaction product consisted of granular material; no amyloid fibrils were present. Images obtained using scanning confocal fluorescent laser microscopy were also consistent with a basal lamina localization for Aβ because the immunofluorescent staining pattern for Aβ matched that of HSPG (Fig. 1J–C), an integral component of the vascular basal lamina *(15)*.

Assays of dorsolateral cerebral cortex for Aβ using ELISA methods showed statistically significant increases ($p < 0.05$) in both Aβ40 and Aβ42 in lesioned animals relative to controls (Fig. 3B; Table 1) in the 3-wk, 5-wk, and 6-mo survival groups (no measurements were done of the 3-mo survival group). These increases ranged between 1.4-fold and 2-fold for the 3- and 5-wk survival groups; the lesioned animals that survived 6 mo had 2.5-fold and 8-fold elevations of Aβ40 and Aβ42, respectively (Fig. 3B). In the 6-mo survival group, Aβ42 was increased disproportionately compared to Aβ40. Mean concentrations of Aβ ranged between 2.5 and 26 pmol/g of tissue in lesioned animals (Table 1).

These data were derived from the formic acid-extracted fraction for the 5-wk survival group, from the DEA-extracted fraction for the 6-mo survival group, and from the guanidine-extracted fraction for the 3-wk survival group. Extraction with Tris-HCl buffer alone (6-mo group) did not yield measurable amounts of Aβ. There was some variability in concentration of Aβ possibly because of the differing extraction and detection methods used. This was demonstrated by the values obtained for control animals in the different experiments (Table 1). Concentrations of cortical Aβ ranged from 1 to 7 pmol/g tissue in control animals, with the highest values present in the 6-mo survival group.

Western blots of Tris-HCl buffer cortical extracts from the 6-mo survival group were probed with the 22C11 antibody, which recognizes the N-termi-

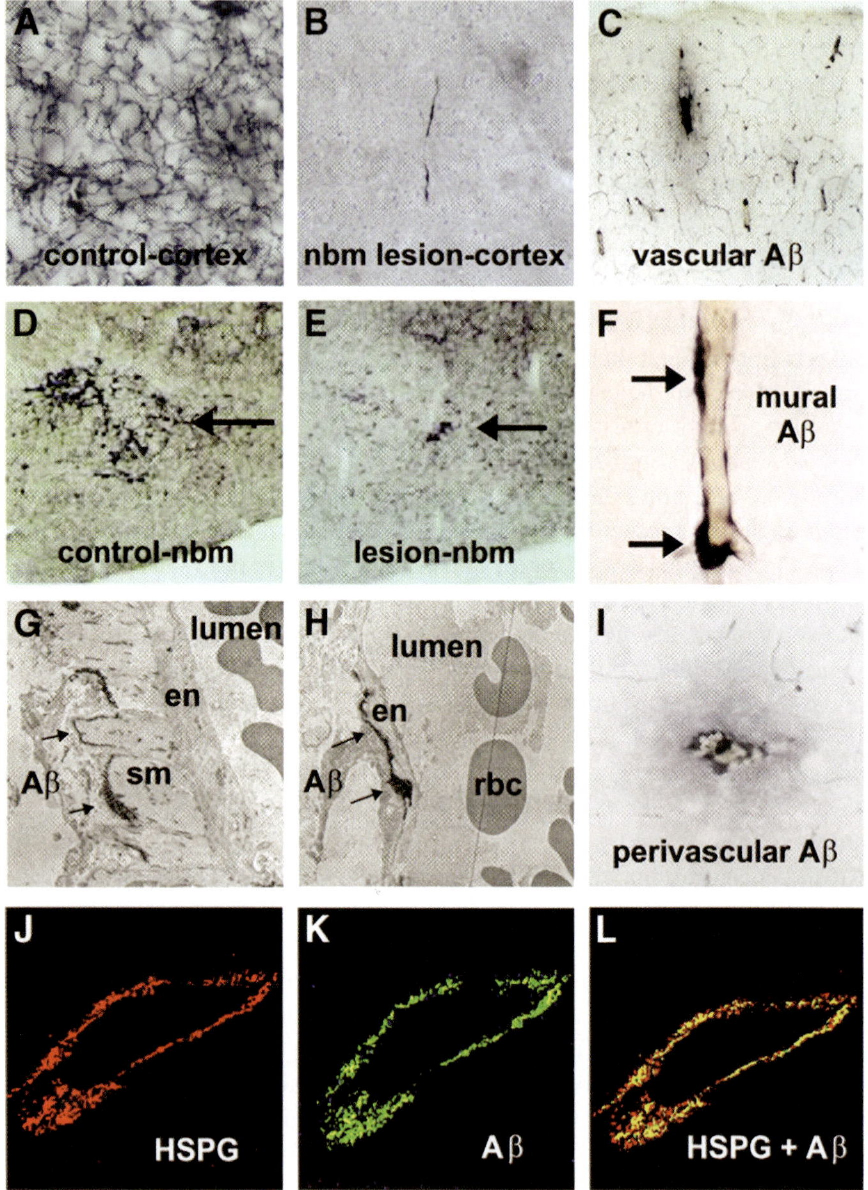

Fig. 1. Comparison of nucleus basilis of Meynert (NBM)-lesioned and control animals. All panels are from the 6-mo survival group. Lesioned animals showed a profound reduction of (**B**) acetylcholinesterase -reactive cortical cholinergic fibers and (**E**) NBM neurons compared to (**A**) and (**D**) controls. Lesioned animals display frequent cortical blood vessels that are immunoreactive for (**C**) Aβ. Deposits of Aβ

nal portion of β-APP. As full-length βAPP is entirely contained within cell membranes; secretory βAPP (mainly sAPPα) is mainly found in extracellular fluid, and blots of the supernatant give a band representing predominantly sAPPα (Fig. 4A); blots of the pelleted membrane fraction further solubilized with SDS give a band representing full-length βAPP (Fig. 4B). Quantification of these bands found that there was no significant difference between lesioned and control animals.

Histological examination of the 1-yr survival group with the Tago AChE method showed that lesioned animals had regenerated profuse fiber networks in the cerebral cortex and hippocampus (Fig. 2G,H,J,K). There were no apparent differences, in terms of cortical cholinergic fiber density, between control animals and animals that had received NBM lesions. Cortical ChAT assays confirmed that there was no significant difference between the two groups (Fig. 3C). Immunohistochemical analysis for Aβ deposition revealed sparse positively stained blood vessels in one lesioned animal and rare vessels in another (not shown). Three additional lesioned animals had no Aβ immunoreactivity. ELISA results showed no significant differences in levels of Aβ40 or Aβ42 between lesioned and control animals (Fig. 3C).

Discussion

These results demonstrate that cortical cholinergic deafferentation leads to Aβ deposition in the cerebral vasculature and perivascular neuropil of rabbits. Control animals did not have such deposition, and previous studies have failed to demonstrate any form of Aβ deposition in normal aged rabbits *(127)*. The immunohistochemistry results show that deposited Aβ consists of all portions of the molecule, including the N-terminus and the 40 and 42 amino acid C-termini.

Previous studies of animals with NBM lesions reported increases *(56,57,60,62)* or decreases *(128,129)* in the expression of cortical full-length βAPP. We found that full-length βAPP was not increased or decreased in the cortex of lesioned animals. This suggests that the increased Aβ was not caused by simple upregulation of the precursor protein but rather was prob-

---

Fig. 1. *(continued from opposite page)* are found in (**F**) blood vessel walls and (**I**) perivascular neuropil. Electron microscopic observation demonstrates that Aβ deposits (black granular material) are found on the abluminal surface of (**G**) smooth muscle cells and (**H**) endothelium, consistent with the location of the basal lamina. Confocal fluorescent microscopy confirmed this, as immunofluorescence for Aβ colocalizes with that for (**J–L**) heparan sulfate proteoglycan (HSPG), which is a known component of the vascular basal lamina.

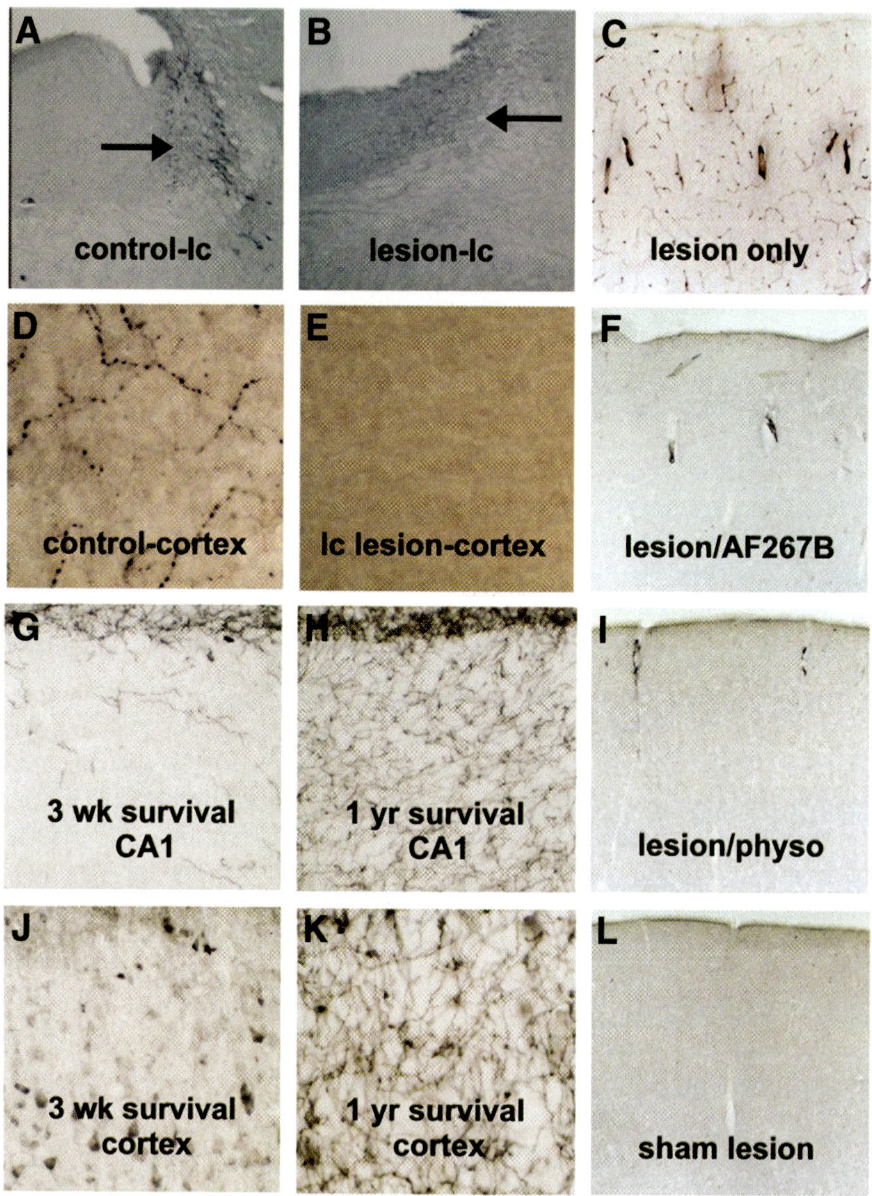

Fig. 2. Immunotoxin lesion of the locus coeruleus (LC) was effective in ablating both dopamine-β-hydroxylase-immunoreactive noradrenergic neuronal perikarya (arrow in **B**) and (**E**) cortical nerve fibers; compare with (**A**) and (**D**) control animals. LC lesion did not, however, cause Aβ deposition (not shown), suggesting that nucleus basilis of Meynert (NBM)-lesion-induced Aβ deposition is not a nonspe-

ably derived from increased amyloidogenic processing. Increased amyloidogenic processing of βAPP in cell culture studies usually leads to reciprocal changes in Aβ and sAPPα, but unlike two previous groups *(62,63)*, we found no change in the concentration of sAPPα in cortical extracts from lesioned animals. It has previously been noted that a reciprocal relationship between Aβ and sAPPα does not always exist in either cell culture *(87)* or animal studies *(88–90)*.

The NBM lesion results in increasingly predominant accumulation of Aβ42 with increasing survival times. This phenomenon has also been reported for βAPP transgenic mice *(124,130)* and may be caused by the increased tendency of Aβ42 to form aggregates *(131,132)*. This form of Aβ is also thought to be the initially deposited form of Aβ in human aging, Down syndrome, and AD *(133–135)*. Early-onset forms of familial AD are caused by gene alterations that result in increased Aβ42 production *(4)*.

It is remarkable that histological Aβ deposition can begin with as little as a 1.5-fold increase in cortical Aβ concentration and can begin as early as 3 wk after such an increase. It has previously been thought that the threshold concentration for Aβ deposition was about 14 pmol/g *(136)*, and the earliest reported appearance of Aβ deposition in transgenic βAPP mice has been at 13 wk *(130)*. In comparison, we observed Aβ after only 3 wk and at a total (40 + 42) Aβ concentration of 4.9 pmol/g.

The sensitivity of our immunohistochemical protocol may partially account for these differing time and concentration thresholds for demonstrating Aβ deposition. We used free-floating, fixed, and cryoprotected frozen sections, in which there is less antigen masking than occurs with paraffin-embedded tissue. Antigen retrieval with formic acid is not required with our tissue sections but is necessary for paraffin-embedded tissue. The relatively low threshold for Aβ deposition that we have found may have significance for AD therapy or prevention as this could mean that lowering Aβ concentrations by as little as 50% may be sufficient to prevent the formation of histological deposits.

Fig. 2. *(continued from opposite page)* cific cortical response to deafferentation. The cholinergic dependence of Aβ deposition was further illustrated by the marked reduction of Aβ deposition in NBM-lesioned animals (**C, F, I, L**) treated with cholinergic agents. One yr after NBM lesion, (**K**) cortical and (**H**) hippocampal (CA1) cortical fiber networks had completely regenerated, illustrated by comparison with (**J**) cortical and (**G**) hippocampal CA1 sections from animals surviving for 3 wk after NBM lesion.

A Cortical Aβ Deposition: Time Course Post-Lesion
mean and SEM
no Aβ deposition in controls
Aβ Deposits Relative Density
7.5
5.0
2.5
0.0
3 wk
5 wk
3 mo
6 mo
Post-Lesion Survival

B Cortical Aβ Concentration: Time Course Post-Lesion
* p < .05
Aβ40
Aβ42
Aβ, percent of control
800
700
600
500
400
300
200
100
Aβ40+42
3 wks
5 wks
6 mos
Post-Lesion Survival

C Cortical Aβ And ChAT 1 Year Post-Lesion
Aβ40
Aβ42
ChAT
mean and SD
ChAT activity pg/mg protein/min
1.00
0.75
0.50
0.25
0.00
Aβ, pmol/g
10.0
7.5
5.0
2.5
0.0
control
lesioned

D Muscarinic Agonist Effect on CSF Aβ40 & 42
mean and SEM
* p < .05   ** p < .01
AF267B
AF150S
AF102B
control
Aβ, ng/ml
7.5
5.0
2.5
0.0
*
*
**
*
**
Aβ40
Aβ42

E Muscarinic Agonist Effect on Cortical Aβ42
mean and SD
* p = .02 vs control
Aβ, pmol/g
3
2
1
0
Control
AF102B
AF150S
AF267B

F Physostigmine Effect on Cortical Aβ40 & 42
Control
physostigmine
mean and SD
p = .002
*
Aβ, pmol/g
3
2
1
0
Aβ40
Aβ42

G Effect of Cholinergic Therapy on Lesion-Induced Cortical Aβ Deposition
Aβ Deposits Relative Density
3
2
1
0
mean and SEM
* p < .01
*
*
AF267B
physo
no therapy

H Effect of Cholinergic Therapy on Lesion-Induced Cortical Aβ Concentration
mean and SEM
Sham-lesioned = 100%
Aβ40
Aβ42
p < .05
*
Aβ, Percent of Sham-Lesioned
300
200
100
0
lesion/physo
lesion/AF267B
lesion only

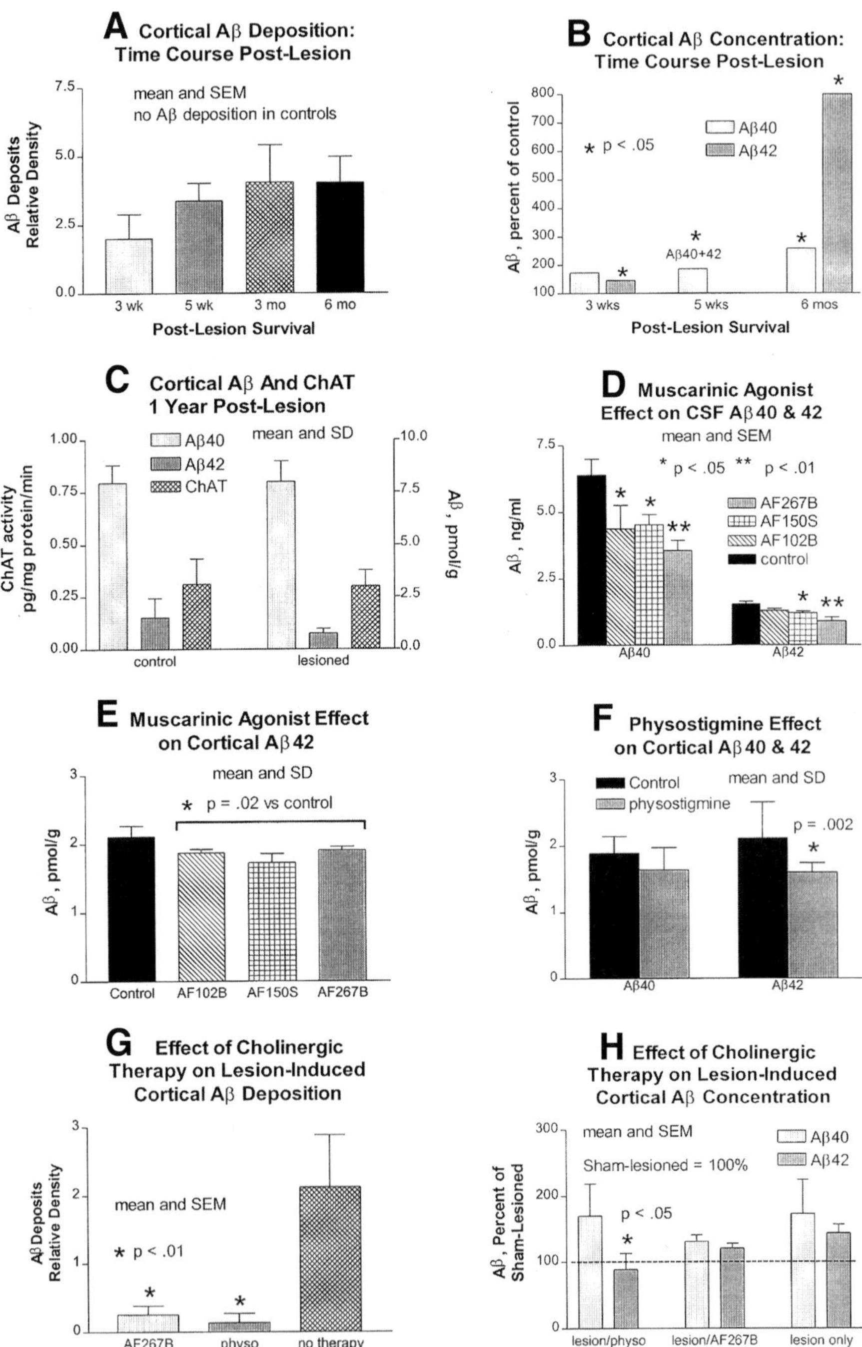

Fig. 3

Vascular Aβ deposition is very common in AD, occurring in 80% or more of cases *(137)*, but is usually less noticeable than the neuropil deposits (plaques). In contrast, in our animal model, vascular deposition is the most prominent feature, with only sparse neuropil deposits. The reason for this is not known. The predominantly vascular location of the Aβ deposits may be caused by the propensity of Aβ to adhere to the vascular basal lamina *(91,92)*. We suggest that cholinergic deafferentation leads to increased release of Aβ by deafferented neurons, and this Aβ diffuses through the extracellular space, eventually coating the basal laminae of nearby blood vessels. In support of this, two lines of βAPP transgenic mice developed prominent vascular Aβ deposits even though their promoters direct exclusively neuronal expression *(138–141)*.

One year after NBM lesioning, all animals had completely regenerated their cortical cholinergic fiber networks. This was most probably accomplished as a result of sprouting from fibers that survived the initial lesion. The immunotoxin lesion did not completely ablate cortical fibers. Even in the most severely affected dorsomedial cortical regions, there were always scattered fibers present, especially in the deeper cortical layers. Similarly, appreciable numbers of p75^{NTR}-immunoreactive neuronal cell bodies survived the immunotoxin lesion. It is likely that surviving cortical cholinergic fibers undergo a massive sprouting response and repopulate the cortex. Several groups have previously documented a similar regenerative response in rats with NBM lesions *(142–146)*; others have not seen this *(147–151)*. Reconciliation of these differing results may come from reports that recovery of cholinergic markers occurs in rats with unilateral lesions, but not in rats with bilateral lesions *(143,152)*. We have repeated the 1-yr survival experiment using repetitive, bilateral immunotoxin injections; this maintained cho-

---

Fig. 3. *(continued from opposite page)* Cortical Aβ **(A)** histological deposition and **(B)** tissue concentrations increased with increasing survival times after nucleus basilis of Meynert (NBM) lesions. **(C)** At 1 yr postlesion, both cortical choline acetyltransferase levels and Aβ concentrations had returned to normal after regeneration of cortical cholinergic afferents. Muscarinic agonist therapy in normal animals reduced Aβ in **(D)** CSF and **(E)** cortex; physostigmine treatment reduced **(F)** cortical but not cerebrospinal fluid (not shown) Aβ levels. Cholinergic therapy markedly reduced **(G)** histological Aβ deposition and **(H)** Aβ concentrations in animals with NBM lesions. In these experiments, the dose of the muscarinic agonists was 2 mg/kg given twice daily by subcutaneous injection. Physostigmine was administered at 3 mg/kg/d by continuous infusion using osmotic pumps.

Table 1
Cortical Aβ Concentrations (pmol/g) and Postlesion Survival Time

Group	Aβ40	Aβ42	Aβ40 + Aβ42
3-wk controls	0.87 (0.16)	1.60 (0.16)	2.47 (0.42)
3-wk lesioned	1.50 (1.09)[a]	2.31 (0.30)	3.86 (1.79)[a]
5-wk controls			1.35 (0.32)
5-wk lesioned			2.50 (0.52)[a]
6-mo controls	5.09 (0.64)	1.58 (1.15)	6.67 (1.20)
6-mo lesioned	13.14 (6.32)[a]	12.65 (9.72)[a]	25.80 (16.0)[b]

[a]$p < 0.05$ in comparison with control group.

[b]$p < 0.01$ in comparison with control group.

Standard deviations are given in parentheses. Statistical analyses used Fisher least significant difference for Aβ40 and Aβ42 in 3-wk group (because of multiple comparisons with drug treatment groups); total Aβ values (Aβ40 + Aβ42) were compared using the Wilcoxon rank sum test. For the 5-wk group and for Aβ40 and Aβ42 in the 6-mo group, unpaired, two-tailed t-tests were used. The Wilcoxon rank sum test was used for total Aβ (Aβ40 + Aβ42) in the 6-mo group.

linergic deafferentation, but did not increase cortical Aβ deposition over that seen at the 6-mo survival period.

In our model, the reestablishment of cortical cholinergic afferents is accompanied by a subsidence of cortical Aβ concentrations to control levels and a loss of cortical Aβ deposits. This is another demonstration of the link between cholinergic neurotransmission and the regulation of cortical Aβ levels. Cessation of cholinergic neurotransmission leads to increased Aβ concentrations; resumption of cholinergic neurotransmission restores Aβ concentrations to normal. This result also illustrates that Aβ deposition, at least in its early stages, is a dynamic equilibrium between production and clearance; deposits are removed if production is curtailed.

The failure to produce significant numbers of neuropil plaques, β-pleated sheet amyloid, and τ- or silver-stained neurofibrillary changes (*see* the next section) are shortcomings of our model with respect to AD. Most βAPP transgenic mice produce thioflavine S-positive Aβ deposition only after 6- to 12-mo survival, and changes in τ require additional time (*124,138,153,154*). Alternatively, cholinergic deafferentation may not be sufficient to produce massive neuropil deposition of Aβ; additional, additive physiological aging changes may be required.

Aβ DEPOSITION IS DEPENDENT ON CHOLINERGIC MECHANISMS

It could be argued that the Aβ deposition induced by cortical cholinergic deafferentation is caused by some kind of nonspecific injury response mechanism or by a general reaction to deafferentation. There is circumstantial evidence that Aβ production and deposition may occur in response to trauma in humans *(155–160)*. In βAPP transgenic mice, however, brain trauma was associated with decreased Aβ deposition *(161)*. Our hypothesis is that Aβ deposition in our model is a result of decreased cholinergic neurotransmission. We therefore designed two experiments to test this.

In the first experiment, rabbits were subjected to a lesion of the LC, which, like the NBM, supplies the cerebral cortex with a subcortically originating, neurotransmitter-specific input. Like the NBM, the LC is subject to neurofibrillary degeneration and neuron loss in AD. The LC presynaptic terminals, however, release noradrenaline rather than acetylcholine. If Aβ deposition is a general response to deafferentation, then it should occur after LC lesion, as well as after NBM lesion. If Aβ deposition is specifically caused by decreased cholinergic neurotransmission, then it should not occur after LC lesion.

The second experiment was based on the expectation that, if Aβ deposition subsequent to NBM lesion is caused by loss of cholinergic neurotransmission, then treatment of lesioned animals with cholinergic agents should prevent or reduce such deposition. Preliminary work indicated that both muscarinic m1-selective agonists and an AChE inhibitor lower CSF or cortical Aβ concentrations in normal animals. Subsequently, rabbits with NBM lesions were treated, immediately after immunotoxin injection, with a muscarinic agonist or an AChE inhibitor.

Methods

LC noradrenergic neuronal lesions were performed on female New Zealand white rabbits (2–2.5 kg) similarly to NBM lesions by intracerebroventricular (icv) injection of a specific immunotoxin. The immunotoxin, like that used for the NBM lesion (Advanced Targeting Systems), is composed of a monoclonal antibody bound to the ribosomal toxin saporin. The monoclonal antibody MAB394 used for the LC lesion specifically recognizes dopamine β-hydroxylase, which is expressed selectively on noradrenergic neurons of the LC. The immunotoxin has previously been shown to lesion the LC effectively in rats, with marked depletions of both noradrenergic neuronal cell bodies in the LC and noradrenergic fibers in the cerebral cortex *(162)*. The dose of immunotoxin given, 10 μg in 12 μL, was determined optimal in a pilot experiment. Three other groups of rabbits were subjected to alternative treatments. One group received NBM lesions as described previously. Another group received both NBM and LC lesions; a third group received icv saline injections. The animals were euthanized 3 mo after lesioning. For the cholinergic therapy study, three muscarinic agonists, an AChE inhibitor (physostigmine), and nicotine were first administered to

A Cortical Synaptic Antigen
Density: 3 Months Post-Lesion
mean and SD
Control group = 100%
Percent of Control
150
125
100
75
50
25
0
SP11 SP33 LP27 SP6 SP18 SP12 EP10
Antibodies

B Cortical Synaptic Antigen
Density: 6 Months Post-Lesion
mean and SD, * p < .05
Control group = 100%
Percent of Control
150
125
100
75
50
25
0
EP10 SP15 SP12 SP18 SP11 SP6
Antibodies

C Cortical Synaptic Antigen
Density: 1 Year Post-Lesion
* p < .05
mean and SD
Control group = 100%
Percent of Control
150
100
50
0
SP15 SP12 SP6 SP10 SP18 SP33 LP27
Antibodies

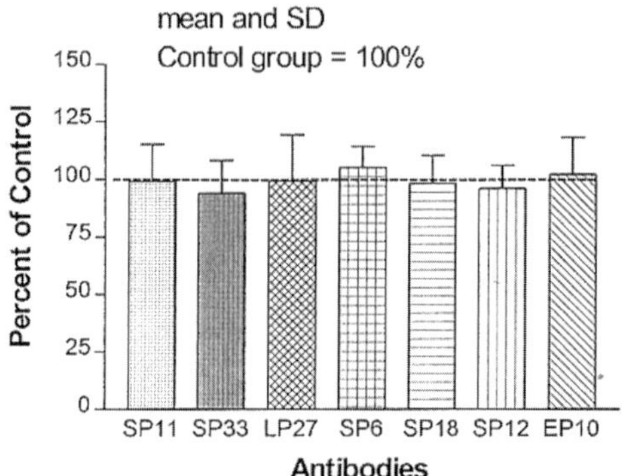

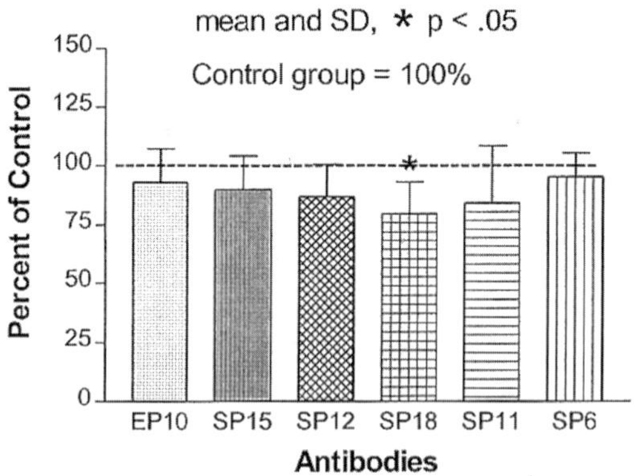

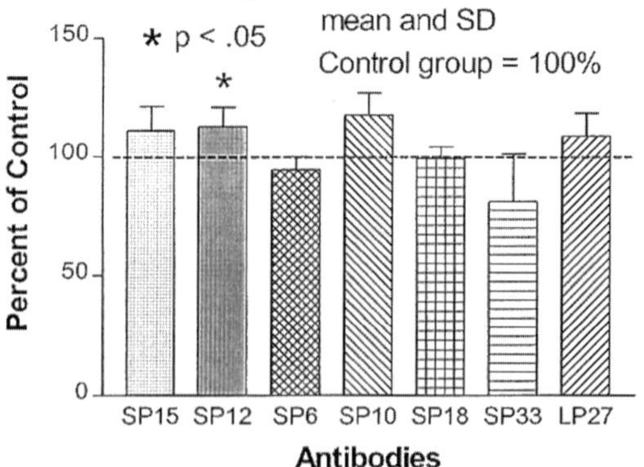

Fig. 4

normal rabbits to determine the effects of these cholinergic agents on CSF and cortical Aβ levels. The effects were contrasted with those of a noncholinergic compound, noradrenaline. Three m1-selective muscarinic agonists from the AF series were tested: AF102B, AF150(S), and AF267B *(163)*. Rabbits received twice-daily subcutaneous injections (total of 2 mg/ kg/d). Physostigmine was administered by subcutaneous osmotic pump (model 2ML4, Durect Corp., Cupertino, CA) at a dose of 3 mg/kg/d; nicotine was administered by twice-daily subcutaneous injections at a dose of 2.4 mg/ kg/d. The noradrenaline dose and route were 7.0 mg/kg/d by subcutaneous osmotic pumps (model 2ML1, Durect Corp.), which exceeds the dose previously reported to have physiological central nervous system effects in rabbits (164). For each drug treatment, a control group received sham therapy with vehicle. All animals were euthanized after 5 d of treatment.

Following the studies on normal animals, the effect of cholinergic therapy on lesioned animals was determined. Three groups of New Zealand white rabbits (female, 2–2.5 kg) were subjected to unilateral intracerebroventricular injection of the NBM immunotoxin as described previously. One group also received twice-daily subcutaneous injections of AF267B (2 mg/kg/d); a second group received physostigmine at a rate of 3 mg/kg/d by subcutaneous osmotic pump (model 2ML4, Durect Corp.). The third group received twice-daily subcutaneous injections of saline. A fourth group received saline intracerebroventricular injection (sham NBM lesion) and twice-daily subcutaneous injections of saline. The animals were euthanized 3 wk after surgery.

Fig. 4. *(continued from opposite page)* Synaptic antigen enzyme-linked immunosorbent assay (ELISA) analysis showed **(A)** no changes in any of the synaptic antigens at 3 mo postlesion relative to control (dotted line). **(B)** At 6 mo postlesion, all antigens were decreased relative to control animals. The decrease seen with antibody SP18 (asterisk), against the synaptic protein septin, was significant relative to controls ($p < 0.05$, unpaired, uncorrected, two-tailed *t*-test). The aggregate result, with all six antigens decreased in lesioned animals, was also significant ($p = 0.014$, one sample goodness-of-fit test). **(C)** One year after nucleus basalis of Meynert lesion, on regeneration of cortical cholinergic afferents, some antigens were decreased, and some were increased; the increase seen with the SP12 antibody (asterisk), which recognizes the synaptic protein SNAP-25, was significant (uncorrected, unpaired, two-tailed *t*-test). For these experiments, frozen cortical tissue was subjected to multiple ELISA for the following: VAMP/synexin, complexin I, complexin II, syntaxin, CDCrel, SNAP-25 and synaptophysin.

Tissue from all experimental groups was processed as described earlier. The efficacy of the LC lesion was determined using immunohistochemical staining for dopamine β-hydroxylase.

Results

In the experiment comparing LC and NBM lesion effect on Aβ deposition, observation of histologically demonstrated cholinergic (not shown) and noradrenergic (Fig. 2A,B,D,E) neuronal cell bodies and cortical nerve fibers confirmed that there was an effective lesion of both types of cortical afferents. The cholinergic lesion was qualitatively similar to that seen at the 3-wk, 5-wk, and 6-mo survival points. Noradrenergic fiber density was quantified in dorsolateral frontal cortex; fiber density in lesioned animals was reduced to 3.2% of controls ($p < 0.05$, unpaired, two-tailed t-test).

Only animals with NBM lesions developed histological Aβ deposition. As previously described, this consisted of frequent Aβ-immunoreactive cortical blood vessels with occasional perivascular diffuse Aβ deposits. There was no positive immunoreaction in sections from animals that received either the LC lesion alone or control saline injection. The group that received both LC and NBM lesions did not have perceptibly increased Aβ deposition in comparison with animals that received NBM lesion alone.

Studies with normal animals indicated that all of the cholinergic agents lowered central nervous system levels of Aβ in normal animals; noradrenaline did not. The three muscarinic agonists significantly reduced CSF levels of Aβ40, and two of the three agents significantly reduced CSF Aβ42 (Fig. 3D, analysis of variance with *post hoc* compensated pairwise significance testing using Fisher least significant difference [LSD]). For Aβ40, the CSF concentrations were lowered to 55.5, 68.5, and 70.7% of control values for AF267B, AF102B, and AF150S, respectively; for Aβ42, animals had CSF concentrations that were 59.2, 83.6, and 77.8%, respectively, of control animals. Concentrations of CSF sAPPα were not significantly affected by drug treatment (Fig. 4C). All three agonists also lowered cortical Aβ, although this reached the significance level only for Aβ42 and only when the data for all three agents were combined and compared to control (Fig. 3E, Wilcoxon rank sum test). Physostigmine and nicotine did not significantly lower CSF Aβ, but both decreased cortical Aβ. Physostigmine lowered Aβ40 and Aβ42 to 86 and 70% of control levels, respectively (Fig. 3F; latter comparison significant using an unpaired, two-tailed t-test), and nicotine decreased Aβ40 and Aβ42 to 78.3 and 76.9%, respectively (not shown; latter comparison significant with unpaired, one-tailed t-test; combined data for Aβ40 and Aβ42 were significant vs control at $p = 0.005$ using Wilcoxon rank sum test). Noradrenaline did not significantly alter either CSF or cortical Aβ, and there was no appreciable trend discernible (data not shown).

The lesion-and-treatment study showed that both AF267B and physostigmine reduced histological deposition (Figs. 2C,F,I,L and 3G) and biochemical levels (Fig. 3H) of Aβ. Histological Aβ deposition was reduced to 6.4 and 12% of the lesioned, untreated group for physostigmine and AF267B, respectively. Analysis of variance found that the treatment groups differed significantly, and both AF267B- and physostigmine-treated groups differed significantly from the lesioned, untreated group (Fisher's LSD).

Cortical Aβ42 concentrations were reduced by physostigmine treatment to 61.8% of that in lesioned, untreated animals; Aβ42 levels in physostigmine-treated animals were even slightly lower than those of sham-lesioned animals (Fig. 3H). Treatment with AF267B reduced Aβ42 levels to 83.4% of those of the lesioned, untreated group. The treatment groups were significantly different on analysis of variance, and *post hoc* pairwise comparisons found that physostigmine-treated animals differed significantly from lesioned, untreated animals (Fisher's LSD). For Aβ40, only AF267B-treated animals had reduced concentrations (to 85.9%) as compared to lesioned, untreated animals.

Discussion

The results of these two sets of experiments demonstrated that Aβ deposition induced by cortical cholinergic deafferentation is caused by decreased cholinergic neurotransmission and is not a nonspecific effect of cortical deafferentation. Destruction of the LC, which supplies the cortex with noradrenergic fibers, did not induce Aβ deposition. Treatment of normal animals with cholinergic agents, including muscarinic agonists, physostigmine, and nicotine, all reduced biochemical levels of Aβ, and treatment with a muscarinic agonist and physostigmine reduced both biochemical levels and deposition of Aβ in NBM-lesioned animals.

Cholinergic therapy has also been used with mixed results in an attempt to decrease or prevent Aβ deposition in βAPP transgenic mice. Metrifonate, an AChE inhibitor, failed to reduce Aβ deposition or concentrations in doubly transgenic (Tg2575/PS1-A246E) mice *(165)*; nicotine treatment resulted in an 80% decrease in plaque load and 50–60% reductions in cortical Aβ concentrations in the same mice *(166)*. These differing results could be because of compensatory mechanisms that reduce the effects of AChE inhibitors over time because it has been reported that tacrine administration to humans causes a significant drop in plasma Aβ after 2 wk of treatment, but this effect is no longer present after 6 wk of treatment *(167)*. In contrast to this, however, patients with AD had sustained inhibition of serum AChE after 12 mo of treatment with rivastigmine *(168)*, and rats treated for 5 wk with metrifonate had persistent brain inhibition of the enzyme *(169)*. Another study found that metrifonate causes increased release of sAPPα from SH-SY5Y cells, but only transiently because the effect is lost after 24 h in spite of preserved inhibition of AChE *(170)*. One investigator suggested that different AChE inhibitors may differ in their actions on βAPP metabolism *(171)*.

It was remarkable in our model that Aβ deposition could be prevented by less than a twofold decrease in tissue concentrations of the peptide. The concentration of Aβ in NBM-lesioned, physostigmine-treated animals was only reduced to about 62% of that in lesioned, untreated animals, but this almost eliminated histological Aβ deposition. At least in its beginning stages, it appears that Aβ deposition may be readily reversed by pharmacological agents that reduce Aβ production.

EFFECTS OF THE NBM LESION AND Aβ DEPOSITION ON SYNAPTIC ANTIGEN DENSITY AND OTHER MARKERS OF NEUROPIL STATUS

Although lesioning the NBM effectively models Aβ deposition, are other aspects of AD pathology produced by the lesion? In human AD, Aβ deposition has been proposed as the central pathogenic event, leading to neurofibrillary tangle formation, synaptic loss, astrocytic and microglial activation and proliferation, neuronal death, and cognitive impairment *(2)*. Several βAPP transgenic mouse models of AD support this progression as they begin with Aβ deposition and are followed by abnormal τ formation in neurites *(138,172–174)*, reduction in the densities of synaptic antigens *(174–176)*, neuronal loss *(139,177)*, and deficits in learning and memory *(154,178,179)*. These changes, however, have generally been much less marked than what is observed in AD *(180–182)*.

In this section, we describe efforts we have made to evaluate our model for its effects on "downstream" events in AD, including astrocytic and microglial proliferation, induction of abnormal tau protein or neurofibrillary tangles, and synaptic antigen density.

Methods

Assessment of glial response was done using the Griffonia lectin method for microglia *(183)* and glial fibrillary acidic protein immunohistochemistry for astrocytes (glial fibrillary acidic protein antibody obtained from Dako). To detect neurofibrillary changes, sections were stained with the Gallyas silver method *(119)* and with immunohistochemistry for abnormally phosphorylated τ protein using the PHF-1 and AT8 antibodies.

Synaptic antigen density was determined in cerebral cortex from the 3-mo, 6-mo, and 1-yr survival groups. Multiple synaptic antigens were assayed using ELISA methods as described in earlier publications *(184,185)*. Monoclonal antibodies and synaptic antigens assayed included SP15 and EP10 (synaptophysin), SP12 (SNAP-25), SP6 (syntaxin), SP11 (VAMP/synaptobrevin), SP18 (septin), LP27 (complexin I), and SP33 (complexin II).

Results

Staining for microglia and astrocytes revealed no evidence of a significant glial response in the cerebral cortex. Blinded microscopic sorting of sections from lesioned and control animals from 3-mo, 6-mo, and 1-yr time-points did not consistently distinguish one group from the other. There was no histological evidence of neurofibrillary or tau protein changes in animals from the 3-mo, 6-mo, or 1-yr time-points.

Synaptic ELISAs done at the 3-mo survival time-point included animals with lesions of the LC, as well as animals with lesions of both the LC and the NBM. Rabbits with NBM lesions did not show significant changes compared to control animals in any of the synaptic antigens tested (Fig. 4A). Two of the antigens showed increases, averaging 9.5%; five showed small decreases, averaging 2.6%. In comparison, rabbits with lesions of the LC showed a trend toward decreased antigen density, with decreases in six antigens, averaging 9.8%, and a 1% increase in one antigen (results not shown). Rabbits with both LC and NBM lesions showed decreases in three, averaging 8%; increases in three, averaging 10%; and no change in one. One antigen, complexin I (antibody SP33), showed a significant 18% decrease in this double-lesioned group ($p < 0.05$, uncorrected, unpaired, two-tailed *t*-test).

At the 6-mo survival time-point, all six synaptic antibodies tested showed decreased density relative to control animals (Fig. 4B). The decreases ranged from 4.6 to 20.2%, with a mean decrease of 11.7%. The greatest decrease, and the only significant pairwise change from control, was for the synaptic antigen septin (antibody SP18) ($p < 0.05$, uncorrected, unpaired, two-tailed *t*-test). The aggregate result, with all six antibodies showing decreased intensity and none increased intensity, was statistically significant ($p = 0.014$, one sample goodness-of-fit test).

Synaptic antigen ELISAs at the 1-yr survival time-point (Fig. 4C) showed increases for four antigens (average increase 12.4%) and decreases for three (average 8.4%). The 12% increase seen with the SP12 antibody (SNAP-25) was significant ($p = 0.017$, uncorrected, unpaired, two-tailed *t*-test).

Discussion

There was no evidence of a glial response to the lesion in our model. It is possible, however, that quantitative methods might disclose a small proliferative or hypertrophic response. We have recently detected a microglial response in cerebral cortex of lesioned animals using an antibody that recognizes activated microglial in rabbits (RAM11). We are now preparing a manuscript describing these results.

There was also no evidence of argyrophilic neurofibrillary changes or of abnormal phosphorylation of τ. Again, this possibility has not been fully excluded as it is possible that other antibodies could detect τ phosphorylation at other sites than that recognized by the AT8 antibody.

The aggregate results of the synaptic ELISAs suggested that there was no synaptic loss at 3 mo postlesion but significant loss, averaging about 12%, at 6 months postlesion. At 1 yr postlesion, net synaptic antigen density was similar to control animals. Synaptic loss at 6 mo could be caused by the deafferentation caused by immunotoxin injection, increased Aβ concentrations, or both. Because appreciable synaptic loss was not present in NBM-lesioned animals at 3 mo but was present at 6 mo, this suggests that prolonged exposure to increased Aβ concentrations was the cause. The number of synaptic terminals lost because of the initial immunotoxin lesion would not be expected to change between the 3-mo survival point and the 6-mo survival point; Aβ concentrations increased (for Aβ42) from about 2.8-fold over control to 8-fold over control during this interval. Cholinergic deafferentation alone was not likely to account for the observed 12% average decrease in synaptic antigen density because cholinergic nerve terminals are estimated to account for only about 6–7% of total cortical terminals *(186)*. At the 1-yr time-point, regeneration of cholinergic afferents and return of Aβ concentrations to normal levels are the probable reasons for the reestablishment of normal synaptic density. There is even some suggestion of an overshoot in this regenerative response. The LC lesion was associated with a nonsignificant trend toward decreased synaptic antigen density.

Synaptic loss in our model may be compared with that reported in βAPP transgenic mice. One group found no loss of synaptic antigens or messenger ribonucleic acid in 18-mo-old βAPP transgenic mice *(187,188)*; others have shown significant loss of synaptic markers: about 15% from 7 mo onward *(189)*, 10–15% loss at 2–4 mo, with 20–30% loss at 21–28 mo *(175)*. There was electron microscopic evidence of degenerating synaptic boutons from 14.5 mo *(190)*.

SUMMARY

Transgenic βAPP mice are valid and useful models of AD because they effectively recreate Aβ deposition, which is widely regarded as the central pathogenic event in the disease. Transgenic mice do not, however, replicate the initial pathogenic event of the most common form of AD. The majority of AD is not caused by any of the gene mutations employed to create these mice. As cortical Aβ deposition is a common, if not universal, occurrence in many mammalian species, its cause is likely to lie within the physiological process of aging. We created an animal model of Aβ deposition by inducing cortical cholinergic deafferentation, a well-known aging change, in the brains of young rabbits. Lesioning the cholinergic NBM resulted in cortical cholinergic deafferentation and cortical Aβ deposition. The Aβ deposits were primarily vascular, with occasional perivascular plaques. The specificity of this change for cholinergic processes was demonstrated by (1) the reduction of lesion-induced Aβ deposition by cholinergic therapy with AF267B, an m1-selective muscarinic agonist, and physostigmine, an acetylcholinesterase inhibitor; and (2) by showing that cortical noradrenergic deafferentation did not cause Aβ deposition. Significant decreases in cortical synaptic antigen density were evident at 6 mo postlesion. Age-related degeneration of the NBM in humans may be a major contributor to Aβ deposition in normal aging and AD.

ACKNOWLEDGMENTS

This work was supported by grants to T. G. B. from the Alzheimer's Association and the National Institute on Aging/National Institute of Neurological Disorders and Stroke.

REFERENCES

1. Neve RL, Robakis NK. Alzheimer's disease: a re-examination of the amyloid hypothesis. Trends Neurosci 1998;21:15–19.
2. Hardy J, Selkoe DJ. The amyloid hypothesis of Alzheimer's disease: progress and problems on the road to therapeutics. Science 2002;297:353–356.
3. Sommer B. Alzheimer's disease and the amyloid cascade hypothesis: 10 years on. Curr Opin Pharmacol 2002;2:87–92.
4. Younkin SG. The role of A beta 42 in Alzheimer's disease. J Physiol Paris 1998;92:289–292.
5. Cummings BJ, Satou T, Head E, et al. Diffuse plaques contain C-terminal A beta 42 and not A beta 40: evidence from cats and dogs. Neurobiol Aging 1996;17:653–659.

6. Geula C, Nagykery N, Wu CK. Amyloid-beta deposits in the cerebral cortex of the aged common marmoset (*Callithrix jacchus*): incidence and chemical composition. Acta Neuropathol (Berl) 2002;103:48–58.

7. Maclean CJ, Baker HF, Ridley RM, Mori H. Naturally occurring and experimentally induced beta-amyloid deposits in the brains of marmosets (*Callithrix jacchus*). J Neural Transm 2000;107:799–814.

8. Head E, McCleary R, Hahn FF, Milgram NW, Cotman CW. Region-specific age at onset of beta-amyloid in dogs. Neurobiol Aging 2000;21:89–96.

9. Selkoe DJ, Bell DS, Podlisny MB, Price DL, Cork LC. Conservation of brain amyloid proteins in aged mammals and humans with Alzheimer's disease. Science 1987;235:873–877.

10. Price DL, Martin LJ, Sisodia SS, et al. Aged non-human primates: an animal model of age-associated neurodegenerative disease. Brain Pathol 1991;1:287–296.

11. Gearing M, Rebeck GW, Hyman BT, Tigges J, Mirra SS. Neuropathology and apolipoprotein E profile of aged chimpanzees: implications for Alzheimer disease. Proc Natl Acad Sci USA 1994;91:9382–9386.

12. McDowell I. Alzheimer's disease: insights from epidemiology. Aging (Milano) 2001;13:143–162.

13. Delaere P, He Y, Fayet G, Duyckaerts C, Hauw JJ. Beta A4 deposits are constant in the brain of the oldest old: an immunocytochemical study of 20 French centenarians. Neurobiol Aging 1993;14:191–194.

14. Bouras C, Hof PR, Giannakopoulos P, Michel JP, Morrison JH. Regional distribution of neurofibrillary tangles and senile plaques in the cerebral cortex of elderly patients: a quantitative evaluation of a 1-year autopsy population from a geriatric hospital. Cereb Cortex 1994;4:138–150.

15. Beach TG, Potter PE, Kuo YM, et al. Cholinergic deafferentation of the rabbit cortex: a new animal model of Aβ deposition. Neurosci Lett 2000;283:9–12.

16. Roher AE, Kuo YM, Potter PE, et al. Cortical cholinergic denervation elicits vascular A beta deposition. Ann NY Acad Sci 2000;903:366–373.

17. Mann DM, Yates PO, Marcyniuk B. Monoaminergic neurotransmitter systems in presenile Alzheimer's disease and in senile dementia of Alzheimer type. Clin Neuropathol 1984;3:199–205.

18. Mann DM, Yates PO, Marcyniuk B. Changes in nerve cells of the nucleus basalis of Meynert in Alzheimer's disease and their relationship to ageing and to the accumulation of lipofuscin pigment. Mech Ageing Dev 1984;25:189–204.

19. Mann DM, Yates PO, Marcyniuk B. Alzheimer's presenile dementia, senile dementia of Alzheimer type and Down's syndrome in middle age form an age related continuum of pathological changes. Neuropathol Appl Neurobiol 1984;10:185–207.

20. McGeer PL, McGeer EG, Suzuki J, Dolman CE, Nagai T. Aging, Alzheimer's disease, and the cholinergic system of the basal forebrain. Neurology 1984;34:741–745.

21. Mountjoy CQ, Rossor MN, Iversen LL, Roth M. Correlation of cortical cholinergic and GABA deficits with quantitative neuropathological findings in senile dementia. Brain 1984;107(pt 2):507–518.

22. Rossor MN, Iversen LL, Johnson AJ, Mountjoy CQ, Roth M. Cholinergic deficit in frontal cerebral cortex in Alzheimer's disease is age dependent. Lancet 1981;2:1422.

23. Lowes-Hummel P, Gertz HJ, Ferszt R, Cervos-Navarro J. The basal nucleus of Meynert revised: the nerve cell number decreases with age. Arch Gerontol Geriatr 1989;8:21–27.

24. Perry EK, Blessed G, Tomlinson BE, et al. Neurochemical activities in human temporal lobe related to aging and Alzheimer-type changes. Neurobiol Aging 1981;2:251–256.

25. Perry EK, Johnson M, Kerwin JM, et al. Convergent cholinergic activities in aging and Alzheimer's disease, Neurobiol Aging 1992;13:393–400.

26. Bird TD, Stranahan S, Sumi SM, Raskind M. Alzheimer's disease: choline acetyltransferase activity in brain tissue from clinical and pathological subgroups. Ann Neurol 1983;14:284–293.

27. Beach TG, Honer WG, and Hughes LH, Cholinergic fibre loss associated with diffuse plaques in the non-demented elderly: the preclinical stage of Alzheimer's disease? Acta Neuropathol (Berl) 1997;93:146–153.

28. Wenk GL, Pierce DJ, Struble RG, Price DL, Cork LC. Age-related changes in multiple neurotransmitter systems in the monkey brain. Neurobiol Aging 1989;10:11–19.

29. Beal MF, Walker LC, Storey E, Segar L, Price DL, Cork LC. Neurotransmitters in neocortex of aged rhesus monkeys. Neurobiol Aging 1991;12:407–412.

30. Smith DE, Roberts J, Gage FH, Tuszynski MH. Age-associated neuronal atrophy occurs in the primate brain and is reversible by growth factor gene therapy. Proc Natl Acad Sci USA 1999;96:10,893–10,898.

31. Funato H, Yoshimura M, Kusui K, et al. Quantitation of amyloid beta-protein (A beta) in the cortex during aging and in Alzheimer's disease. Am J Pathol 1998;152:1633–1640.

32. Davies L, Wolska B, Hilbich C, et al. A4 amyloid protein deposition and the diagnosis of Alzheimer's disease: prevalence in aged brains determined by immunocytochemistry compared with conventional neuropathologic techniques. Neurology 1988;38:1688–1693.

33. Beach TG, Kuo YM, Spiegel K, et al. The cholinergic deficit coincides with Aβ deposition at the earliest histopathologic stages of Alzheimer disease. J Neuropathol Exp Neurol 2000;59:308–313.

34. Katzman R, Terry R, DeTeresa R, et al. Clinical, pathological, and neurochemical changes in dementia: a subgroup with preserved mental status and numerous neocortical plaques. Ann Neurol 1988;23:138–144.

35. Buxbaum JD, Oishi M, Chen HI, et al. Cholinergic agonists and interleukin 1 regulate processing and secretion of the Alzheimer beta/A4 amyloid protein precursor. Proc Natl Acad Sci USA 1992;89:10,075–10,078.

36. Nitsch RM, Slack BE, Wurtman RJ, Growdon JH. Release of Alzheimer amyloid precursor derivatives stimulated by activation of muscarinic acetylcholine receptors. Science 1992;258:304–307.

37. Bymaster FP, Wong DT, Mitch CH, et al. Neurochemical effects of the M1 muscarinic agonist xanomeline (LY246708/NNC11-0232). J Pharmacol Exp Ther 1994;269:282–289.

38. Bymaster FP, Carter PA, Peters SC, et al. Xanomeline compared to other muscarinic agents on stimulation of phosphoinositide hydrolysis in vivo and other cholinomimetic effects. Brain Res 1998;795:179–190.

39. Nitsch RM, Growdon JH. Role of neurotransmission in the regulation of amyloid beta-protein precursor processing. Biochem Pharmacol 1994;47:1275–1284.

40. Nitsch RM. From acetylcholine to amyloid: neurotransmitters and the pathology of Alzheimer's disease. Neurodegeneration 1996;5:477–482.

41. Nitsch RM, Wurtman RJ, Growdon JH. Regulation of APP processing. Potential for the therapeutical reduction of brain amyloid burden. Ann NY Acad Sci 1996;777:175–182.

42. Haring R, Gurwitz D, Barg J, et al. Amyloid precursor protein secretion via muscarinic receptors: reduced desensitization using the M1-selective agonist AF102B. Biochem Biophys Res Commun 1994;203:652–658.

43. Haring R, Gurwitz D, Barg J, et al. NGF promotes amyloid precursor protein secretion via muscarinic receptor activation. Biochem Biophys Res Commun 1995;213:15–23.

44. Eckols K, Bymaster FP, Mitch CH, Shannon HE, Ward JS, DeLapp NW. The muscarinic M1 agonist xanomeline increases soluble amyloid precursor protein release from Chinese hamster ovary-m1 cells. Life Sci 1995;57:1183–1190.

45. Wolf BA, Wertkin AM, Jolly YC, et al. Muscarinic regulation of Alzheimer's disease amyloid precursor protein secretion and amyloid beta-protein production in human neuronal NT2N cells. J Biol Chem 1995;270:4916–4922.

46. Hung AY, Haass C, Nitsch RM, et al. Activation of protein kinase C inhibits cellular production of the amyloid beta-protein. J Biol Chem 1993;268:22,959–22,962.

47. Pittel Z, Heldman E, Barg J, Haring R, Fisher A. Muscarinic control of amyloid precursor protein secretion in rat cerebral cortex and cerebellum. Brain Res 1996;742:299–304.

48. Muller D, Wiegmann H, Langer U, Moltzen-Lenz S, Nitsch RM. Lu 25-109, a combined m1 agonist and m2 antagonist, modulates regulated processing of the amyloid precursor protein of Alzheimer's disease. J Neural Transm 1998;105:1029–1043.

49. Muller DM, Mendla K, Farber SA, Nitsch RM. Muscarinic M1 receptor agonists increase the secretion of the amyloid precursor protein ectodomain. Life Sci 1997;60:985–991.

50. Farber SA, Nitsch RM, Schulz JG, Wurtman RJ. Regulated secretion of beta-amyloid precursor protein in rat brain. J Neurosci 1995;15:7442–7451.

51. Beach TG, Kuo Y, Schwab C, Walker DG, Roher AE. Reduction of cortical amyloid beta levels in guinea pig brain after systemic administration of physostigmine. Neurosci Lett 2001;310:21–24.

52. Beach TG, Walker DG, Potter PE, Sue LI, Fisher A. Reduction of cerebrospinal fluid amyloid beta after systemic administration of M1 muscarinic agonists. Brain Res 2001;905:220–223.

53. Lin L, Georgievska B, Mattsson A, Isacson O. Cognitive changes and modified processing of amyloid precursor protein in the cortical and hippocampal system after cholinergic synapse loss and muscarinic receptor activation. Proc Natl Acad Sci USA 1999;96:12,108–12,113.

54. Hock C, Maddalena A, Heuser I, et al. Treatment with the selective muscarinic agonist talsaclidine decreases cerebrospinal fluid levels of total amyloid beta-peptide in patients with Alzheimer's disease. Ann NY Acad Sci 2000;920:285–291.

55. Nitsch RM, Deng M, Tennis M, Schoenfeld D, Growdon JH. The selective muscarinic M1 agonist AF102B decreases levels of total Abeta in cerebrospinal fluid of patients with Alzheimer's disease. Ann Neurol 2000;48:913–918.

56. Wallace W, Ahlers ST, Gotlib J, et al. Amyloid precursor protein in the cerebral cortex is rapidly and persistently induced by loss of subcortical innervation. Proc Natl Acad Sci USA 1993;90:8712–8716.

57. Wallace WC, Bragin V, Robakis NK, et al. Increased biosynthesis of Alzheimer amyloid precursor protein in the cerebral cortex of rats with lesions of the nucleus basalis of Meynert. Brain Res Mol Brain Res 1991;10:173–178.

58. Wallace WC, Lieberburg I, Schenk D, Vigo-Pelfrey C, Davis KL, Haroutunian V. Chronic elevation of secreted amyloid precursor protein in subcortically lesioned rats, and its exacerbation in aged rats. J Neurosci 1995;15:4896–4905.

59. Beeson JG, Shelton ER, Chan HW, Gage FH. Age and damage induced changes in amyloid protein precursor immunohistochemistry in the rat brain. J Comp Neurol 1994;342:69–77.

60. Leanza G. Chronic elevation of amyloid precursor protein expression in the neocortex and hippocampus of rats with selective cholinergic lesions. Neurosci Lett 1998;257:53–56.

61. Lin L, LeBlanc CJ, Deacon TW, Isacson O. Chronic cognitive deficits and amyloid precursor protein elevation after selective immunotoxin lesions of the basal forebrain cholinergic system. Neuroreport 1998;9:547–552.

62. Rossner S, Ueberham U, Yu J, et al. In vivo regulation of amyloid precursor protein secretion in rat neocortex by cholinergic activity. Eur J Neurosci 1997;9:2125–2134.

63. Geula C, Zhan SS. Altered processing of amyloid precursor protein following specific cholinergic denervation of rat cortex. Soc Neurosci Abstr 1997;23:820.

64. Beach TG, Walker DG, Cynader MS, Hughes LH. Increased beta-amyloid precursor protein mRNA in the rat cerebral cortex and hippocampus after chronic systemic atropine treatment. Neurosci Lett 1996;210:13–16.

65. Struble RG, Cork LC, Whitehouse PJ, Price DL. Cholinergic innervation in neuritic plaques. Science 1982;216:413–415.

66. Arendt T, Bigl V, Tennstedt A, Arendt A. Neuronal loss in different parts of the nucleus basalis is related to neuritic plaque formation in cortical target areas in Alzheimer's disease. Neuroscience 1985;14:1–14.

67. Beach TG, McGeer EG. Senile plaques, amyloid beta-protein, and acetylcholinesterase fibres: laminar distributions in Alzheimer's disease striate cortex. Acta Neuropathol (Berl) 1992;83:292–299.

68. Arendash GW, Millard WJ, Dunn AJ, Meyer EM. Long-term neuropathological and neurochemical effects of nucleus basalis lesions in the rat. Science 1987;238:952–956.

69. Fuentes C, Roch G, Konig N. Light and electron microscopical observations in the nucleus basalis of Meynert and in hippocampus of the rat after injection of a cholinotoxin: degeneration and reorganization. Z Mikrosk Anat Forsch 1987;101:451–460.

70. Thal LJ, Mandel RJ, Terry RD, Buzsaki G, Gage FH. Nucleus basalis lesions fail to induce senile plaques in the rat. Exp Neurol 1990;108:88–90.

71. DeStrooper B, Simons M, Multhaup G, Van Leuven F, Beyreuther K, Dotti CG. Production of intracellular amyloid-containing fragments in hippocampal neurons expressing human amyloid precursor protein and protection against amyloidogenesis by subtle amino acid substitutions in the rodent sequence. EMBO J 1995;14:4932–4938.

72. Otvos L Jr, Szendrei GI, Lee VM, Mantsch HH. Human and rodent Alzheimer beta-amyloid peptides acquire distinct conformations in membrane-mimicking solvents. Eur J Biochem 1993;211:249–257.

73. Reaume AG, Howland DS, Trusko SP, et al. Enhanced amyloidogenic processing of the beta-amyloid precursor protein in gene-targeted mice bearing the Swedish familial Alzheimer's disease mutations and a "humanized" Abeta sequence. J Biol Chem 1996;271:23,380–23,388.

74. Davidson JS, West RL, Kotikalapudi P, Maroun LE. Sequence and methylation in the beta/A4 region of the rabbit amyloid precursor protein gene. Biochem Biophys Res Commun 1992;188:905–911.

75. Johnstone EM, Chaney MO, Norris FH, Pascual R, Little SP. Conservation of the sequence of the Alzheimer's disease amyloid peptide in dog, polar bear and five other mammals by cross-species polymerase chain reaction analysis. Brain Res Mol Brain Res 1991;10:299–305.

76. Johnston MV, McKinney M, Coyle JT. Evidence for a cholinergic projection to neocortex from neurons in basal forebrain. Proc Natl Acad Sci USA 1979;76:5392–5396.

77. Mantione CR, Fisher A, Hanin I. The AF64a-treated mouse: possible model for central cholinergic hypofunction. Science 1981;213:579–580.

78. Muir JL, Page KJ, Sirinathsinghji DJ, Robbins TW, Everitt BJ. Excitotoxic lesions of basal forebrain cholinergic neurons: effects on learning, memory and attention. Behav Brain Res 1993;57:123–131.

79. Lindefors N, Boatell ML, Mahy N, Persson H. Widespread neuronal degeneration after ibotenic acid lesioning of cholinergic neurons in the nucleus basalis revealed by in situ hybridization. Neurosci Lett 1992;135:262–264.

80. Book AA, Wiley RG, Schweitzer JB. Specificity of 192 IgG-saporin for NGF receptor-positive cholinergic basal forebrain neurons in the rat. Brain Res 1992;590:350–355.

81. Book AA, Wiley RG, Schweitzer JB. 192 IgG-saporin: I. Specific lethality for cholinergic neurons in the basal forebrain of the rat. J. Neuropathol Exp Neurol 1994;53:95–102.

82. Heckers S, Ohtake T, Wiley RG, Lappi DA, Geula C, Mesulam MM. Complete and selective cholinergic denervation of rat neocortex and hippocampus but not amygdala by an immunotoxin against the p75 NGF receptor. J Neurosci 1994;14:1271–1289.

83. Walsh TJ, Kelly RM, Dougherty KD, Stackman RW, Wiley RG, Kutscher CL. Behavioral and neurobiological alterations induced by the immunotoxin 192-IgG-saporin: cholinergic and non-cholinergic effects following icv injection. Brain Res 1995;702:233–245.

84. Wenk GL, Stoehr JD, Quintana G, Mobley S, Wiley RG. Behavioral, biochemical, histological, and electrophysiological effects of 192 IgG-saporin injections into the basal forebrain of rats. J Neurosci 1994;14:5986–5995.

85. Wiley RG, Oeltmann TN, Lappi DA. Immunolesioning: selective destruction of neurons using immunotoxin to rat NGF receptor. Brain Res 1991;562:149–153.

86. Fine A, Hoyle C, Maclean CJ, Levatte TL, Baker HF, Ridley RM. Learning impairments following injection of a selective cholinergic immunotoxin, ME20.4 IgG-saporin, into the basal nucleus of Meynert in monkeys. Neuroscience 1997;81:331–343.

87. Fuller SJ, Storey E, Li QX, Smith AI, Beyreuther K, Masters CL. Intracellular production of beta A4 amyloid of Alzheimer's disease: modulation by phosphoramidon and lack of coupling to the secretion of the amyloid precursor protein. Biochemistry 1995;34:8091–8098.

88. Petanceska SS, Nagy V, Frail D, Gandy S. Ovariectomy and 17beta-estradiol modulate the levels of Alzheimer's amyloid beta peptides in brain. Exp Gerontol 2000;35:1317–1325.

89. Savage MJ, Trusko SP, Howland DS, et al. Turnover of amyloid beta-protein in mouse brain and acute reduction of its level by phorbol ester. J Neurosci 1998;18:1743–1752.

90. Vincent B, Smith JD. Effect of estradiol on neuronal Swedish-mutated beta-amyloid precursor protein metabolism: reversal by astrocytic cells. Biochem Biophys Res Commun 2000;271:82–85.

91. Weller RO, Massey A, Newman TA, Hutchings M, Kuo YM, Roher AE. Cerebral amyloid angiopathy: amyloid beta accumulates in putative interstitial fluid drainage pathways in Alzheimer's disease. Am J Pathol 1998;153:725–733.

92. Weller RO, Massey A, Kuo YM, Roher AE. Cerebral amyloid angiopathy: accumulation of A beta in interstitial fluid drainage pathways in Alzheimer's disease. Ann NY Acad Sci 2000;903:110–117.

93. Bowen DM, Benton JS, Spillane JA, Smith CC, Allen SJ. Choline acetyltransferase activity and histopathology of frontal neocortex from biopsies of demented patients. J Neurol Sci 1982;57:191–202.

94. Bowen DM, Allen SJ, Benton JS, et al. Biochemical assessment of serotonergic and cholinergic dysfunction and cerebral atrophy in Alzheimer's disease. J Neurochem 1983;41:266–272.

95. Francis PT, Palmer AM, Sims NR, et al. Neurochemical studies of early-onset Alzheimer's disease. Possible influence on treatment. N Engl J Med 1985;313:7–11.

96. Francis PT, Webster MT, Chessell IP, et al. Neurotransmitters and second messengers in aging and Alzheimer's disease. Ann NY Acad Sci 1993;695:19–26.

97. Lowe SL, Francis PT, Procter AW, Palmer AM, Davison AN, Bowen DM. Gamma-aminobutyric acid concentration in brain tissue at two stages of Alzheimer's disease. Brain 1988;111:785–799.

98. Perry EK, Perry RH. A review of neuropathological and neurochemical correlates of Alzheimer's disease. Dan Med Bull 1985;32(suppl 32):27–34.

99. Palmer AM, Gershon S. Is the neuronal basis of Alzheimer's disease cholinergic or glutamatergic? FASEB J 1990;4:2745–2752.

100. Palmer AM. Neurochemical studies of Alzheimer's disease. Neurodegeneration 1996;5:381–391.

101. Procter AW, Lowe SL, Palmer AM, et al. Topographical distribution of neurochemical changes in Alzheimer's disease. J Neurol Sci 1988;84:125–140.

102. Procter AW. Neurochemical correlates of dementia. Neurodegeneration 1996;5:403–407.

103. Davis KL, Mohs RC, Marin D, et al. Cholinergic markers in elderly patients with early signs of Alzheimer disease. JAMA 1999;281:1401–1406.

104. DeKosky ST, Ikonomovic MD, Styren SD, et al. Upregulation of choline acetyltransferase activity in hippocampus and frontal cortex of elderly subjects with mild cognitive impairment. Ann Neurol 2002;51:145–155.

105. Gilmor ML, Erickson JD, Varoqui H, et al. Preservation of nucleus basalis neurons containing choline acetyltransferase and the vesicular acetylcholine transporter in the elderly with mild cognitive impairment and early Alzheimer's disease. J Comp Neurol 1999;411:693–704.

106. Tiraboschi P, Hansen LA, Alford M, Masliah E, Thal LJ, Corey-Bloom J. The decline in synapses and cholinergic activity is asynchronous in Alzheimer's disease. Neurology 2000;55:1278–1283.

107. Pearson RC, Powell TP. Anterograde vs retrograde degeneration of the nucleus basalis medialis in Alzheimer's disease. J Neural Transm 1987;24:139–146.

108. Beach TG, Sue LI, Scott S, Sparks DL. Neurofibrillary tangles are constant in aging human nucleus basalis. Alzheimer's Rep 1998;1:375–380.

109. Sassin I, Schultz C, Thal DR, et al. Evolution of Alzheimer's disease-related cytoskeletal changes in the basal nucleus of Meynert. Acta Neuropathol (Berl) 2000;100:259–269.

110. Minger SL, and Davies P. Persistent innervation of the rat neocortex by basal forebrain cholinergic neurons despite the massive reduction of cortical target neurons. I. Morphometric analysis. Exp Neurol 1992;117:124–138.

111. Gau JT, Steinhilb ML, Kao TC, et al. Stable beta-secretase activity and presynaptic cholinergic markers during progressive central nervous system amyloidogenesis in Tg2576 mice. Am J Pathol 2002;160:731–738.

112. Jaffar S, Counts SE, Ma SY, et al. Neuropathology of mice carrying mutant APP(swe) and/or PS1(M146L) transgenes: alterations in the p75(NTR) cholinergic basal forebrain septohippocampal pathway. Exp Neurol 2001;170:227–243.

113. Bronfman FC, Moechars D, Van Leuven F. Acetylcholinesterase-positive fiber deafferentation and cell shrinkage in the septohippocampal pathway of aged amyloid precursor protein London mutant transgenic mice. Neurobiol Dis 2000;7:152–168.

114. Hernandez D, Sugaya K, Qu T, McGowan E, Duff K, McKinney M. Survival and plasticity of basal forebrain cholinergic systems in mice transgenic for presenilin-1 and amyloid precursor protein mutant genes. Neuroreport 2001;12:1377–1384.

115. Wong TP, Debeir T, Duff K, Cuello AC. Reorganization of cholinergic terminals in the cerebral cortex and hippocampus in transgenic mice carrying mutated presenilin-1 and amyloid precursor protein transgenes. J Neurosci 1999;19:2706–2716.

116. Boncristiano S, Calhoun ME, Kelly PH, et al. Cholinergic changes in the APP23 transgenic mouse model of cerebral amyloidosis. J Neurosci 2002;22:3234–3243.

117. Beach TG, Tago H, Nagai T, Kimura H, McGeer PL, McGeer EG. Perfusion-fixation of the human brain for immunohistochemistry: comparison with immersion-fixation. J Neurosci Methods 1987;19:183–192.

118. Tago H, Kimura H, Maeda T. Visualization of detailed acetylcholinesterase fiber and neuron staining in rat brain by a sensitive histochemical procedure. J Histochem Cytochem 1986;34:1431–1438.

119. Braak H, Braak E. Demonstration of amyloid deposits and neurofibrillary changes in whole brain sections. Brain Pathol 1991;1:213–216.

120. Beach TG, McGeer EG. Cholinergic fiber loss occurs in the absence of synaptophysin depletion in Alzheimer's disease primary visual cortex. Neurosci Lett 1992;142:253–256.

121. Geula C, Mesulam MM. Cortical cholinergic fibers in aging and Alzheimer's disease: a morphometric study. Neuroscience 1989;33:469–481.

122. Fonnum F. Radiochemical micro assays for the determination of choline acetyltransferase and acetylcholinesterase activities. Biochem J 1969;115:465–472.
123. Kuo YM, Crawford F, Mullan M, et al. Elevated A beta and apolipoprotein E in A betaPP transgenic mice and its relationship to amyloid accumulation in Alzheimer's disease. Mol Med 2000;6:430–439.
124. Johnson-Wood K, Lee M, Motter R, et al. Amyloid precursor protein processing and A β42 deposition in a transgenic mouse model of Alzheimer disease. Proc Natl Acad Sci USA 1997;94:1550–1555.
125. Mehta PD, Dalton AJ, Mehta SP, Kim KS, Sersen EA, Wisniewski HM. Increased plasma amyloid beta protein 1-42 levels in Down syndrome. Neurosci Lett 1998;241:13–16.
126. Mehta PD, Pirttila T, Mehta SP, Sersen EA, Aisen PS, Wisniewski HM. Plasma and cerebrospinal fluid levels of amyloid beta proteins 1-40 and 1-42 in Alzheimer disease. Arch Neurol 2000;57:100–105.
127. Woodruff-Pak DS, Trojanowski JQ. The older rabbit as an animal model: implications for Alzheimer's disease. Neurobiol Aging 1996;17:283–290.
128. Ramirez MJ, Heslop KE, Francis PT, Rattray M. Expression of amyloid precursor protein, tau and presenilin RNAs in rat hippocampus following deafferentation lesions. Brain Res 2001;907:222–232.
129. Apelt J, Schliebs R, Beck M, Rossner S, Bigl V. Expression of amyloid precursor protein mRNA isoforms in rat brain is differentially regulated during postnatal maturation and by cholinergic activity. Int J Dev Neurosci 1997;15:95–112.
130. Borchelt DR, Ratovitski T, van Lare J, et al. Accelerated amyloid deposition in the brains of transgenic mice coexpressing mutant presenilin 1 and amyloid precursor proteins. Neuron 1997;19:939–945.
131. Hilbich C, Kisters-Woike B, Reed J, Masters CL, Beyreuther K. Aggregation and secondary structure of synthetic amyloid beta A4 peptides of Alzheimer's disease. J Mol Biol 1991;218:149–163.
132. Jarrett JT, Berger EP, Lansbury PTJ. The carboxy terminus of the beta amyloid protein is critical for the seeding of amyloid formation: implications for the pathogenesis of Alzheimer's disease. Biochemistry 1993;32:4693–4697.
133. Lemere CA, Blusztajn JK, Yamaguchi H, Wisniewski T, Saido TC, Selkoe DJ. Sequence of deposition of heterogeneous amyloid beta-peptides and APO E in Down syndrome: implications for initial events in amyloid plaque formation. Neurobiol Dis 1996;3:16–32.
134. Iwatsubo T, Odaka A, Suzuki N, Mizusawa H, Nukina N, Ihara Y. Visualization of A beta 42(43) and A beta 40 in senile plaques with end- specific A beta monoclonals: evidence that an initially deposited species is A beta 42(43). Neuron 1994;13:45–53.
135. Iwatsubo T, Mann DM, Odaka A, Suzuki N, Ihara Y. Amyloid beta protein (A beta) deposition: A beta 42(43) precedes A beta 40 in Down syndrome. Ann Neurol 1995;37:294–299.
136. Duff K. Alzheimer transgenic mouse models come of age. Trends Neurosci 1997;20:279–280.

137. Revesz T, Holton JL, Lashley T, et al. Sporadic and familial cerebral amyloid angiopathies. Brain Pathol 2002;12:343–357.

138. Sturchler-Pierrat C, Abramowski D, Duke M, et al. Two amyloid precursor protein transgenic mouse models with Alzheimer disease-like pathology. Proc Natl Acad Sci USA 1997;94:13,287–13,292.

139. Sturchler-Pierrat C, Staufenbiel M. Pathogenic mechanisms of Alzheimer's disease analyzed in the APP23 transgenic mouse model. Ann NY Acad Sci 2000;920:134–139.

140. Van Dorpe J, Smeijers L, Dewachter I, et al. Prominent cerebral amyloid angiopathy in transgenic mice overexpressing the London mutant of human APP in neurons. Am J Pathol 2000;157:1283–1298.

141. Burgermeister P, Calhoun ME, Winkler DT, Jucker M. Mechanisms of cerebrovascular amyloid deposition. Lessons from mouse models. Ann NY Acad Sci 2000;903:307–316.

142. Hohmann GF, Wenk GL, Lowenstein P, Brown ME, Coyle JT. Age-related recurrence of basal forebrain lesion-induced cholinergic deficits. Neurosci Lett 1987;82:253–259.

143. Casamenti F, Di Patre PL, Bartolini L, Pepeu G. Unilateral and bilateral nucleus basalis lesions: differences in neurochemical and behavioural recovery. Neuroscience 1988;24:209–215.

144. Nakamura S, Kawamoto Y, Nakano S, Akiguchi I, Kimura J. p35nck5a and cyclin-dependent kinase 5 colocalize in Lewy bodies of brains with Parkinson's disease. Acta Neuropathol (Berl) 1997;94:153–157.

145. Cossette P, Umbriaco D, Zamar N, Hamel E, Descarries L. Recovery of choline acetyltransferase activity without sprouting of the residual acetylcholine innervation in adult rat cerebral cortex after lesion of the nucleus basalis. Brain Res 1993;630:195–206.

146. Zhang Z-J, Lappi DA, Wrenn CC, Milner TA, Wiley RG. Selective lesion of the cholinergic basal forebrain causes a loss of cortical neuropeptide Y and somatostatin neurons. Brain Res 1998; 800:198–206.

147. Bartus RT, Flicker C, Dean RL, Pontecorvo M, Figueiredo JC, Fisher SK. Selective memory loss following nucleus basalis lesions: long term behavioral recovery despite persistent cholinergic deficiencies. Pharmacol Biochem Behav 1985;23:125–135.

148. Bartus RT, Pontecorvo MJ, Flicker C, Dean RL, Figueiredo JC. Behavioral recovery following bilateral lesions of the nucleus basalis does not occur spontaneously. Pharmacol Biochem Behav 1986;24:1287–1292.

149. Ojima H, Sakurai T, Yamasaki T. Changes in choline acetyltransferase immunoreactivity and the number of immunoreactive fibers remaining after lesions to the magnocellular basal nucleus of rats. Neurosci Lett 1988;95:31–36.

150. Gomeza J, Aragon C, Gimenez C. High-affinity transport of choline and amino acid neurotransmitters in synaptosomes from brain regions after lesioning the nucleus basalis magnocellularis of young and aged rats. Neurochem Res 1992;17:345–350.

151. Connor DJ, Thal LJ, Mandel RJ, Langlais PJ, Masliah E. Independent effects of age and nucleus basalis magnocellularis lesion: maze learning, cortical neurochemistry, and morphometry. Behav Neurosci 1992;106:776–788.

152. Nakamura S, Ishihara T. Task-dependent memory loss and recovery following unilateral nucleus basalis lesion: behavioral and neurochemical correlation. Behav Brain Res 1990;39:113–122.
153. Games D, Adams D, Alessandrini R, et al. Alzheimer-type neuropathology in transgenic mice overexpressing V717F beta-amyloid precursor protein. Nature 1995;373:523–527.
154. Hsiao K, Chapman P, Nilsen S, et al. Correlative memory deficits, Abeta elevation, and amyloid plaques in transgenic mice. Science 1996;274:99–102.
155. Roberts GW, Allsop D, Bruton C. The occult aftermath of boxing. J Neurol Neurosurg Psychiatry 1990;53:373–378.
156. Roberts GW, Gentleman SM, Lynch A, Murray L, Landon M, Graham DI. Beta amyloid protein deposition in the brain after severe head injury: implications for the pathogenesis of Alzheimer's disease. J Neurol Neurosurg Psychiatry 1994;57:419–425.
157. Gentleman SM, Greenberg BD, Savage MJ, et al. A beta 42 is the predominant form of amyloid beta-protein in the brains of short-term survivors of head injury. Neuroreport 1997;8:1519–1522.
158. Graham DI, Gentleman SM, Lynch A, Roberts GW. Distribution of beta-amyloid protein in the brain following severe head injury. Neuropathol Appl Neurobiol 1995;21:27–34.
159. Emmerling MR, Morganti-Kossmann MC, Kossmann T, et al. Traumatic brain injury elevates the Alzheimer's amyloid peptide A beta 42 in human CSF. A possible role for nerve cell injury. Ann NY Acad Sci 2000;903:118–122.
160. Raby CA, Morganti-Kossmann MC, Kossmann T, et al. Traumatic brain injury increases beta-amyloid peptide 1-42 in cerebrospinal fluid. J Neurochem 1998;71:2505–2509.
161. Nakagawa Y, Reed L, Nakamura M, et al. Brain trauma in aged transgenic mice induces regression of established abeta deposits. Exp Neurol 2000;163:244–252.
162. Wrenn CC, Picklo MJ, Lappi DA, Robertson D, Wiley RG. Central noradrenergic lesioning using anti-DBH-saporin: anatomical findings. Brain Res 1996;740:175–184.
163. Fisher A. Therapeutic strategies in Alzheimer's disease: M1 muscarinic agonists. Jpn J Pharmacol 2000;84:101–112.
164. Czepita D. Influence of alpha and beta-adrenergic stimulators and blockers on the electroretinogram and visually evoked potentials of the rabbit. Biomed Biochim Acta 1990;49:509–513.
165. Liu L, Ikonen S, Heikkinen T, Tapiola T, van Groen T, Tanila H. The effects of long-term treatment with metrifonate, a cholinesterase inhibitor, on cholinergic activity, amyloid pathology, and cognitive function in APP and PS1 doubly transgenic mice. Exp Neurol 2002;173:196–204.
166. Nordberg A, Hellstrom-Lindahl E, Lee M, et al. Chronic nicotine treatment reduces beta-amyloidosis in the brain of a mouse model of Alzheimer's disease (APPsw). J Neurochem 2002;81:655–658.

167. Basun H, Nilsberth C, Eckman C, Lannfelt L, Younkin S. Plasma Levels of Abeta42 and Abeta40 in Alzheimer patients during treatment with the acetylcholinesterase inhibitor tacrine. Dement Geriatr Cogn Disord 2002;14:156–160.

168. Darreh-Shori T, Almkvist O, Guan ZZ, et al. Sustained cholinesterase inhibition in AD patients receiving rivastigmine for 12 months. Neurology 2002;59:563–572.

169. Rakonczay Z, Papp H. Effects of chronic metrifonate treatment on cholinergic enzymes and the blood-brain barrier. Neurochem Int 2001;39:19–24.

170. Racchi M, Sironi M, Caprera A, Konig G, Govoni S. Short- and long-term effect of acetylcholinesterase inhibition on the expression and metabolism of the amyloid precursor protein. Mol Psychiatry 2001;6:520–528.

171. Lahiri DK, Farlow MR, Hintz N, Utsuki T, Greig NH. Cholinesterase inhibitors, beta-amyloid precursor protein and amyloid beta-peptides in Alzheimer's disease. Acta Neurol Scand 2000;176:60–67.

172. Tomidokoro Y, Ishiguro K, Harigaya Y, et al. Abeta amyloidosis induces the initial stage of tau accumulation in APP(Sw) mice. Neurosci Lett 2001;299:169–172.

173. Tomidokoro Y, Harigaya Y, Matsubara E, et al. Brain Abeta amyloidosis in APPsw mice induces accumulation of presenilin-1 and tau. J Pathol 2001;194:500–506.

174. Masliah E, Sisk A, Mallory M, Games D. Neurofibrillary pathology in transgenic mice overexpressing V717F beta-amyloid precursor protein. J Neuropathol Exp Neurol 2001;60:357–368.

175. Mucke L, Masliah E, Yu GQ, et al. High-level neuronal expression of abeta 1-42 in wild-type human amyloid protein precursor transgenic mice: synaptotoxicity without plaque formation. J Neurosci 2000;20:4050–4058.

176. Rockenstein E, Mallory M, Mante M, Sisk A, Masliaha E. Early formation of mature amyloid-beta protein deposits in a mutant APP transgenic model depends on levels of Aβ(1-42). J Neurosci Res 2001;66:573–582.

177. Bondolfi L, Calhoun M, Ermini F, et al. Amyloid-associated neuron loss and gliogenesis in the neocortex of amyloid precursor protein transgenic mice. J Neurosci 2002;22:515–522.

178. Moran PM, Higgins LS, Cordell B, Moser PC. Age-related learning deficits in transgenic mice expressing the 751-amino acid isoform of human beta-amyloid precursor protein. Proc Natl Acad Sci USA 1995;92:5341–5345.

179. Holcomb L, Gordon MN, McGowan E, et al. Accelerated Alzheimer-type phenotype in transgenic mice carrying both mutant amyloid precursor protein and presenilin 1 transgenes. Nat Med 1998;4:97–100.

180. Dewachter I, Van Dorpe J, Spittaels K, et al. Modeling Alzheimer's disease in transgenic mice: effect of age and of presenilin1 on amyloid biochemistry and pathology in APP/London mice. Exp Gerontol 2000;35:831–841.

181. Xu G, Gonzales V, Borchelt DR. Abeta deposition does not cause the aggregation of endogenous tau in transgenic mice. Alzheimer Dis Assoc Disord 2002;16:196–201.

182. Richardson JA, Burns DK. Mouse models of Alzheimer's disease: a quest for plaques and tangles. ILAR J 2002;43:89–99.

183. Streit WJ. An improved staining method for rat microglial cells using the lectin from *Griffonia simplicifolia* (GSA I-B4). J Histochem Cytochem 1990;38:1683–1686.

184. Honer WG, Dickson DW, Gleeson J, Davies P. Regional synaptic pathology in Alzheimer's disease. Neurobiol Aging 1992;13:375–382.

185. Honer WG, Falkai P, Young C, et al. Cingulate cortex synaptic terminal proteins and neural cell adhesion molecule in schizophrenia. Neuroscience 1997;78:99–110.

186. Richardson PJ. Quantitation of cholinergic synaptosomes from guinea pig brain. J Neurochem 1981;37:258–260.

187. Irizarry MC, Soriano F, McNamara M, et al. Abeta deposition is associated with neuropil changes, but not with overt neuronal loss in the human amyloid precursor protein V717F (PDAPP) transgenic mouse. J Neurosci 1997;17:7053–7059.

188. Irizarry MC, McNamara M, Fedorchak K, Hsiao K, Hyman BT. APPSw transgenic mice develop age-related A beta deposits and neuropil abnormalities, but no neuronal loss in CA1. J Neuropathol Exp Neurol 1997;56:965–973.

189. Mucke L, Yu GQ, McConlogue L, et al. Astroglial expression of human alpha(1)-antichymotrypsin enhances Alzheimer-like pathology in amyloid protein precursor transgenic mice. Am J Pathol 2000;157:2003–2010.

190. Oster-Granite ML, McPhie DL, Greenan J, Neve RL. Age-dependent neuronal and synaptic degeneration in mice transgenic for the C terminus of the amyloid precursor protein. J Neurosci 1996;16:6732–6741.

8

Chemical Dissection of Brain Glucoregulatory Circuitry

Sue Ritter, Thu T. Dinh, Kishor Bugarith, and Dawna M. Salter

INTRODUCTION

Glucose is the essential substrate for brain energy metabolism *(1)*. Although glycogen, the major storage form of glucose, contributes dynamically to brain energy metabolism, it is present in very limited quantities *(2)*. Thus, the brain requires continuous delivery of glucose by the blood. Clearly, then, the control of blood glucose is of fundamental importance for brain metabolism. Work in our laboratory has focused on the neural organization of controls that maintain blood glucose concentrations. The immunotoxin, antidopamine β-hydroxylase (anti-DβH) conjugated to saporin (anti-DβH-sap) *(3–7)*, has been an invaluable tool for establishing the importance of hindbrain catecholamine neurons for coordinated arousal of critical behavioral, autonomic, and neuroendocrine responses to glucose deficit. The goal of this review is to describe our use of anti-DβH-sap in demonstrating the essential roles of hindbrain catecholamine neurons in glucoregulation.

To date, we have concentrated primarily on three key responses to a glucose deficit (glucoprivation). These are increased adrenal medullary catecholamine secretion, increased corticosterone secretion, and stimulation of food intake. These responses can be readily elicited by hypoglycemic doses of insulin or by central or systemic administration of nonmetabolizable glucose analog, such as 2-deoxy-D-glucose (2DG) or 5-thio-D-glucose (5TG) *(8–12)*, which competitively inhibit intracellular utilization of glucose *(13,14)*. Adrenal medullary catecholamine secretion increases hepatic and muscle glycogenolysis, decreases insulin secretion, and increases lipolysis.

From: *Molecular Neurosurgery With Targeted Toxins*
Edited by: R. G. Wiley and D. A. Lappi © Humana Press Inc., Totowa, NJ

These responses almost immediately elevate blood glucose while reducing its uptake by peripheral tissues. Corticosterone promotes gluconeogenesis by several mechanisms and directs peripheral metabolism away from glucose and toward utilization of fat. Finally, glucoprivic stimulation of food intake elevates blood glucose directly on absorption of ingested carbohydrates and provides calories for replenishment of depleted energy stores.

Control of Glucoregulatory Responses by Hindbrain Glucoreceptor Cells

The first and most definitive attempts to localize glucoreceptor cells involved in systemic glucoregulation focused on those controlling feeding and adrenal medullary responses. Early cannula-mapping studies showed that glucoprivic feeding could be elicited by injection of 2DG into the forebrain ventricles but not by localized glucoprivation of a variety of forebrain tissue sites *(15,16)*. Later studies using chronically maintained decerebrate rats showed that neural circuits sufficient to detect glucoprivation and stimulate hyperglycemic and feeding responses are present within the midbrain or hindbrain *(17,18)*. Also pivotal were experiments showing that acute obstruction of the mesencephalic aqueduct completely blocked feeding and hyperglycemic responses to lateral ventricular, but not to fourth ventricular, 5TG injection *(19),* demonstrating that glucoreceptors controlling feeding and hyperglycemic responses most likely are restricted to the hindbrain.

In more recent cannula-mapping studies, we have been able to localize glucoreceptors controlling feeding and hyperglycemic responses to distinct areas of the ventrolateral and dorsomedial hindbrain (Fig. 1) *(20).* We have also found that corticosterone secretion and glucagon secretion can be elicited by localized glucoprivation of these same hindbrain sites but not by localized glucoprivation of the hypothalamus (unpublished data).

Although the phenotype of hindbrain glucoreceptor cells and the transduction mechanism by which they monitor glucose availability are not yet known, the cannulation maps indicating their localization within specific hindbrain regions has allowed us to make substantial progress in defining the circuitry through which they evoke glucoregulatory responses.

The Neural Circuitry for Glucoregulatory Responses Includes Hypothalamic and Spinal Sites

Although receptor cells that elicit glucoprivic feeding and corticosterone secretion are not located in the hypothalamus, there is abundant evidence that the hypothalamus contains circuitry important for these responses. Glucoprivic feeding is impaired by acute administration of neuropeptide Y (NPY) antibodies into the paraventricular nucleus of the hypothalamus

(PVH) *(21)* or hypothalamic delivery of catecholamine receptor antagonists *(22,23)*. Moreover, the messenger ribonucleic acids (mRNAs) for the potent orexigenic peptides, NPY and agouti gene-related protein (AGRP) are increased in the ARC by systemic glucoprivation *(24–26)*. In the case of corticosterone secretion, the PVH is essential for the response. Corticotrophin-releasing hormone (CRH), the major secretagogue for adrenocorticotropic hormone (ACTH), is synthesized in the PVH. Finally, the glucoprivic control of adrenal medullary secretion is dependent on activation of adrenal medullary preganglionic neurons in the intermediolateral column of the spinal cord. Although several brain sites appear to be involved in control of adrenal medullary secretion *(27–29)*, there is relatively little evidence to suggest which sites are involved specifically in the glucoprivic control of secretion. However, the presence of a hyperglycemic response in decerebrate rats given systemic 2DG *(18)* and in aqueduct-occluded rats given fourth ventricular 5TG injections *(19)* indicated that pathways controlling this response descend from hindbrain directly into the spinal cord.

Early Evidence Suggests Involvement of Hindbrain Norepinephrine and Epinephrine Neurons in Glucoregulatory Responses

A variety of evidence accumulating over the last three decades suggests the involvement of hindbrain norepinephrine (NE) or epinephrine (E) neurons in glucoprivic responses.

Glucoprivation increases turnover of catecholamines in the hypothalamus and elsewhere *(30,31)*. Pharmacological studies have shown that central adrenergic receptor blockade *(22,23)*, electrolytic or 6-hydroxydopamine lesions of ascending catecholamine fibers *(32,33)*, and knife cuts transecting the ascending catecholamine fibers all impair glucoprivic feeding *(34,35)*. Catecholamine neurons also constitute an important afferent input for CRH neurons in the medial parvicellular part of the PVH and are capable of increasing both CRH gene expression and ACTH release by direct innervation of CRH neurons or indirectly through glutamatergic interneurons *(36–40)*.

Finally, a number of pharmacological studies have revealed important interactions between the activity of central catecholamine neurons and blood glucose concentration *(41–45)*. In our work, we noted that Fos, the protein product of the c-*fos* gene expressed in response to neuronal activation *(46)*, is preferentially induced by systemic glucoprivation in specific subgroups of catecholamine neurons concentrated within the glucoreceptive zones identified in our cannula mapping studies *(20)*. These catecholamine neurons innervate the intermediolateral column of the spinal cord, as well as hypothalamic sites crucial for control of food intake and corticosterone secretion *(47–50)*.

Food Intake
Hyperglycemia
sp5
Gr
Cu
Sp5C
A2
Sol
sol
AP
12
ROb
A1
12n
A1
RPa
LRt
py
Mean = -0.1 g
Mean = 2.8 g
Mean = 3.3 mg/dl
Mean = 63.2 mg/dl
sol
Sol
C2
ECu
Sp5
C2
10
12
RVL/CVL
PMn
Gi
C1/A1
LRt
12n
RPa
py
Mean = 0.2 g
Mean = 2.9 g
Mean = 5.4 mg/dl
Mean = 61.4 mg/dl

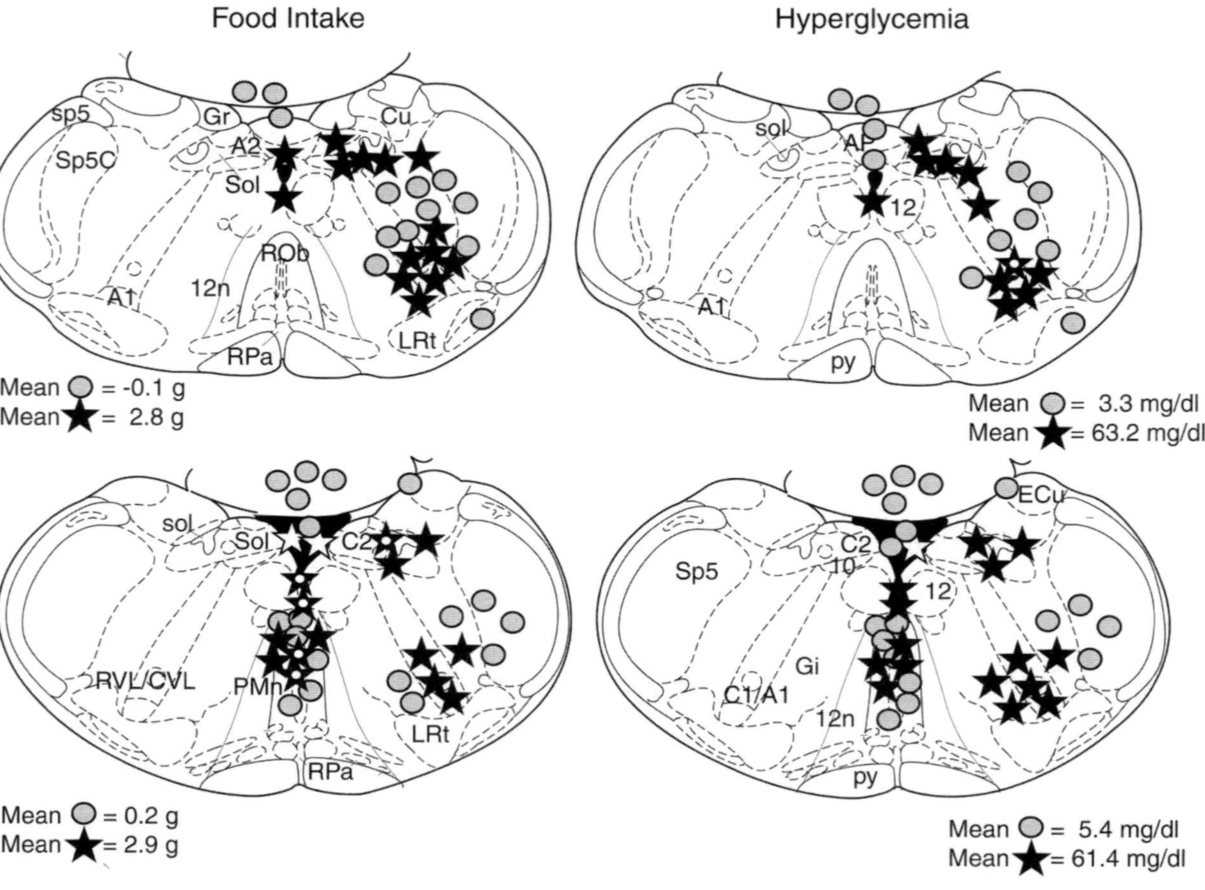

Fig. 1

Despite evidence for their involvement in feeding, corticosterone secretion, and adrenal medullary secretion, it has not been possible with presently available techniques to determine the relative importance of hindbrain catecholamine neurons in glucoprivic responses or to specify the particular cell groups involved. This difficulty is attributable to the previous lack of highly selective lesioning agents. Until recently, 6-hydroxydopamine was the most selective of the catecholamine lesioning agents used to investigate these questions, but the selectivity of even this toxin is limited *(51)*. If 6-hydroxydopamine is administered into the ascending catecholaminergic axonal bundles, catecholamine projections with very different destinations may be simultaneously lesioned. In addition, noncatecholaminergic ascending and descending fibers intermingled with the catecholamine neurons may be destroyed *(52,53)*.

Especially troublesome is the possibility that some of these damaged projections may participate in functions of global importance for behavior, such as motivation or arousal, and that their destruction might cause generalized disruption of appetitive responses. Dopamine neurons of vital importance for motivation and motor function may be damaged by injections of 6-hydroxydopamine into the ventral ascending catecholamine bundle at mesencephalic or lateral hypothalamic levels, causing severe neurological deficits *(54)*.

Another consideration is that 6-hydroxydopamine is also variable in its effect on different parts of the catecholamine neuron and on different catecholamine phenotypes *(51,55)*. Furthermore, administration of 6-hydroxydopamine into terminal areas is likely to leave the associated catecholamine cell bodies intact, adding the possibility of axonal sprouting and recovery of function to complicate the interpretation of the results.

Fig. 1. Diagrams of coronal sections through two levels of the medulla oblongata showing location of cannula tips positive (stars) and negative (circles) for elicitation of feeding (left side) and hyperglycemic (right side) responses to localized glucoprivation induced by the glycolytic inhibitor, 5-thio-D-glucose (5TG) (200 nL). The criterion for positivty was 1.5 g of feeding or 25 mg/dL rise in blood glucose above the respective responses to control injection. Stars containing white dots were the most positive sites, defined as 4 g of feeding and 100 mg/dL above control responses. Positive sites were found only the hindbrain and were not found in the hypothalamus. Subsequent cannulation studies have identified a similar distribution of sites where glucagon and corticosterone secretion can be elicited by localized injection of 5TG. Results indicate that glucoreceptor cells controlling these particular responses to glucose deficit are present in and apparently restricted to the hindbrain. Adapted from ref. *20*, Fig. 2.

Injection of 6-hydroxydopamine directly into the hindbrain cell groups has not generally been a useful approach because the cell bodies are dispersed throughout large extents of hindbrain and overlap critical homeostatic control sites. Moreover, catecholamine cell bodies projecting to distinctly different anatomical sites, and presumably therefore possessing distinctly different functions, are intermingled in some areas, such that even a selective lesioning agent applied to such areas would produce a complex lesion. Pharmacological treatments provide the other major alternative for studies of catecholamine neuron function, but pharmacological treatments may be nonselective if administered systemically and may be unsuitable for chronic central administration.

USE OF ANTI-DβH-SAP TO ESTABLISH THE PIVOTAL ROLES OF DISTINCT BRAIN E AND NE NEURON POPULATIONS IN BEHAVIORAL, AUTONOMIC, AND NEUROENDOCRINE GLUCOREGULATORY RESPONSES

Early reports describing the effects of anti-DβH-sap immunolesions suggested that this technique might overcome some of the major obstacles noted in the previous section that have severely limited our ability to progress in our research. Of foremost importance for our applications was the fact that anti-DβH-sap could be taken up selectively by DβH-containing terminals and retrogradely transported to the cell body, where its ribosomal toxicity destroyed the entire neuron *(56)*. The potential for retrograde transport from a discrete injection site was extremely important for us because of the intermingling within the hindbrain of NE and E cell bodies with very different projection patterns and functions and because of the widespread distribution within the hindbrain of cell bodies with projections to any single location, such as the medial hypothalamus. Thus, by exploiting the ability of anti-DβH-sap to be transported retrogradely, we were able to increase further the selectivity of this lesioning agent to include only those cells that innervate the injection site.

Also important for us was the potential for accurate assessment of the effectiveness of the anti-DβH-sap lesion in each individual animal, which we have done primarily by quantification of NE and E cell bodies innervating the anti-DβH-sap injection site and evaluation of the terminal loss at the injection site and related sites. The ability to assess the extent and effectiveness of the anti-DβH-sap lesion accurately using such measures is in fact crucial because anti-DβH-sap lesions are so selective for NE and E neurons that the microinjection site frequently cannot be localized by signs of tissue damage typically used to localize conventional lesions (*see* the section on assessment of lesion specificity).

Anti-DβH-Sap Destroys Only NE and E Neurons That Innervate the Injection Site

Individual NE/E neurons do not send collateral projections to both the spinal cord and the PVH. Rather, innervation of these two sites arises from separate cell populations *(47,49,50,57,58)*. Therefore, we were able to show that injections of anti-DβH-sap into the spinal cord or PVH, the two anti-DβH-sap injection sites we have studied most extensively, produced distinct and clearly definable lesions *(59)* (Fig. 2).

PVH injections virtually eliminate DβH-immunoreactive (-ir) terminals in the PVH and surrounding medial hypothalamic structures, as well as the associated hindbrain cell bodies. PVH anti-DβH-sap injections profoundly reduce cell numbers in cell groups A1 and C1, which supply the major innervation to the PVH and medial hypothalamus. Only the most rostral portion of C1 and the most caudal part of A1 are spared. Cell numbers are also substantially reduced in cell groups A2, A6, C2, and C3. In the last groups, some, but not all, cells project to the PVH, so the loss is not as complete as in the A1/C1 region. In groups A5 and A7, subcoeruleus, and the rostral pole of C1, NE, and E neurons project to the spinal cord but not to the hypothalamus. Cells in these locations were not affected by the PVH anti-DβH-sap injection but were virtually eliminated by intraspinal injection of anti-DβH-sap at T2–T4. Schreihofer and Guyenet also found that intraspinal anti-DβH-sap lesions produced a selective loss of spinally projecting NE and E neurons *(60)*. Thus, PVH and spinal cord microinjections of anti-DβH-sap selectively lesion the NE/E neurons that innervate each injection site.

Loss of NE and E terminals in the medial hypothalamus and spinal cord after anti-DβH-sap injections into the PVH or at T2–T4 are consistent with the pattern of cell loss described. Terminals were profoundly reduced in the medial hypothalamus (including the PVH, ARC, and median eminence) and in the paraventricular nucleus of the thalamus, but were only minimally reduced in the supraoptic nucleus and other more lateral regions (Fig. 3) after PVH anti-DβH-sap injection. After intraspinal injection of anti-DβH-sap, but not SAP (unconjugated saporin control solution, Advanced Targeting Systems), terminals were severely reduced throughout the intermediolateral column below the injection site (Fig. 4).

Despite the extensive loss of NE and E terminals in the anti-DβH-sap-injected rats, virtually no nonspecific damage associated specifically with anti-DβH-sap was observed in our experiments. However, some spinal cord damage may be produced by the injection procedure itself (*see* the Methodological and Technical Issues) *(59,61)*. An especially important aspect of these anti-DβH-sap lesions is that they do not compromise the health and

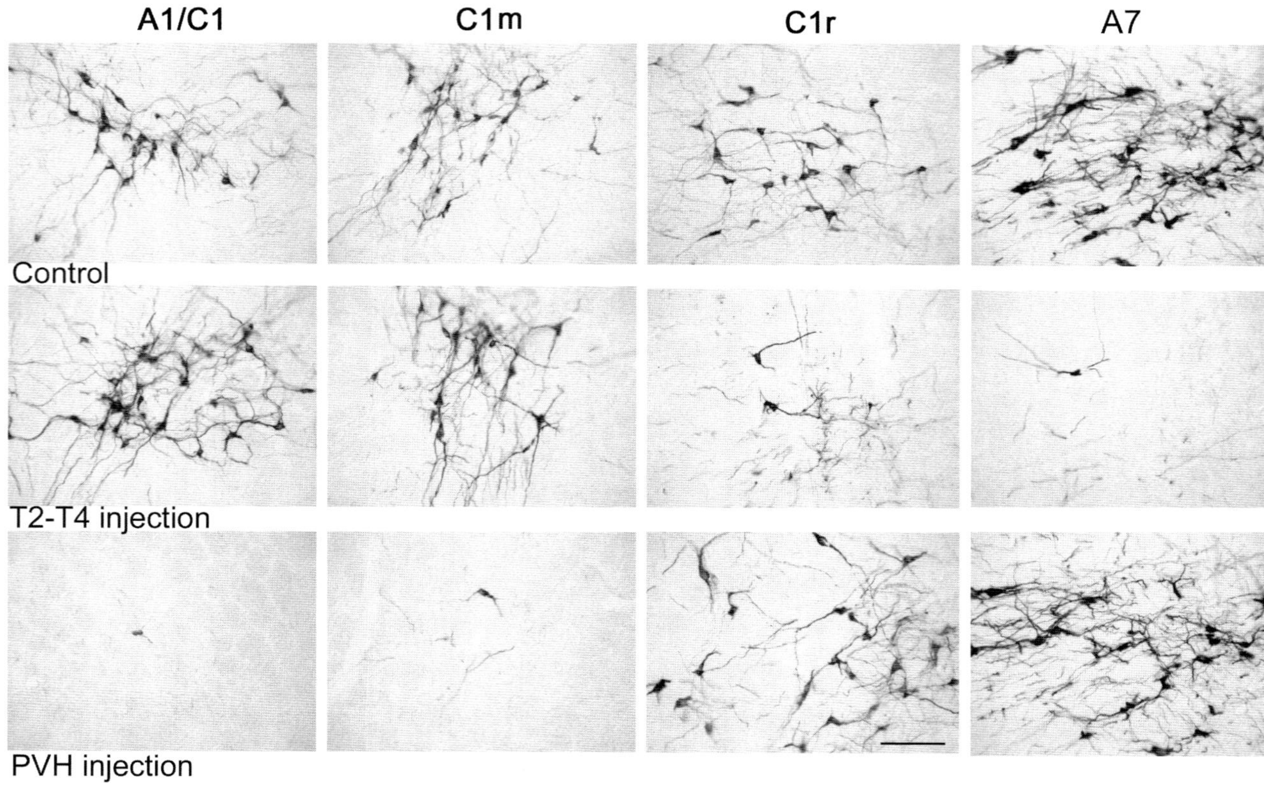

Fig. 2

behavioral competence of the rats, unlike other methods of lesioning these neurons. Therefore, rats can be tested extensively and over long periods of time.

Anti-DβH-Sap Lesions Selectively Impair Glucoprivic Feeding

Because of the vast literature demonstrating important influences of central catecholamine systems on food intake, PVH anti-DβH-sap rats were tested in a number of feeding paradigms *(59)*. Our most important finding was that the anti-DβH-sap-injected rats did not increase their food intake in response to systemic 2DG-induced glucoprivation or to insulin-induced hypoglycemia (Fig. 5). The impairment of food intake was specific for the glucoprivic condition. Daily food intake under basal conditions was not altered. In addition, anti-DβH-sap-injected rats increased their food intake in a manner identical to controls in response to overnight food deprivation and in response to a different metabolic challenge, mercaptoacetate (MA)-induced blockade of fatty acid oxidation *(62,63)*. Furthermore, the adrenal medullary hyperglycemic response to 2DG-induced glucoprivation remained intact (Fig. 6), indicating that this response is not mediated by the same NE or E neurons responsible for the feeding response.

We completed an additional study in which PVH anti-DβH-sap rats were trained to drink milk delivered directly into the mouth through a chronic intraoral fistula *(64)*. This experiment was done to examine the effect of anti-DβH-sap on the consummatory phase of the glucoprivic feeding response, that is, chewing and swallowing food once it is in the mouth. When food is delivered directly into the mouth, animals can accept and swallow the food or allow it to drip out of their mouths, but an appetitive response (i.e., food-seeking behavior) is not required. Previous work showed that de-

---

Fig. 2. Coronal sections of rat hindbrain showing effects of control injections (top row), intraspinal (middle row), and paraventricular nucleus of the hypothalamus (PVH) (bottom row) injections of anti-dopamine β hydroxylase-saporin (DβH-sap) on tyrosine hydroxylase immunoreactivity in anatomically equivalent areas representing hindbrain norepinephrine and epinephrine cell groups (designated A and C groups, respectively). Columns (left to right) show anatomically equivalent sections at the level of A1/C1 overlap, midlevel C1 (C1m), rostral C1 (C1r), and A7. In A1/C1 and C1m, cells project heavily to the PVH and were destroyed by PVH anti-DβH-sap, but not by intraspinal anti-DβH-sap injections. In C1r and A7, cells project spinally, but not to the PVH, and were destroyed by intraspinal DSAP injections, but not by PVH anti-DβH-sap injections. Scale bar = 200 μ*M*. Adapted from ref. *59*, Figs. 2 and 4.

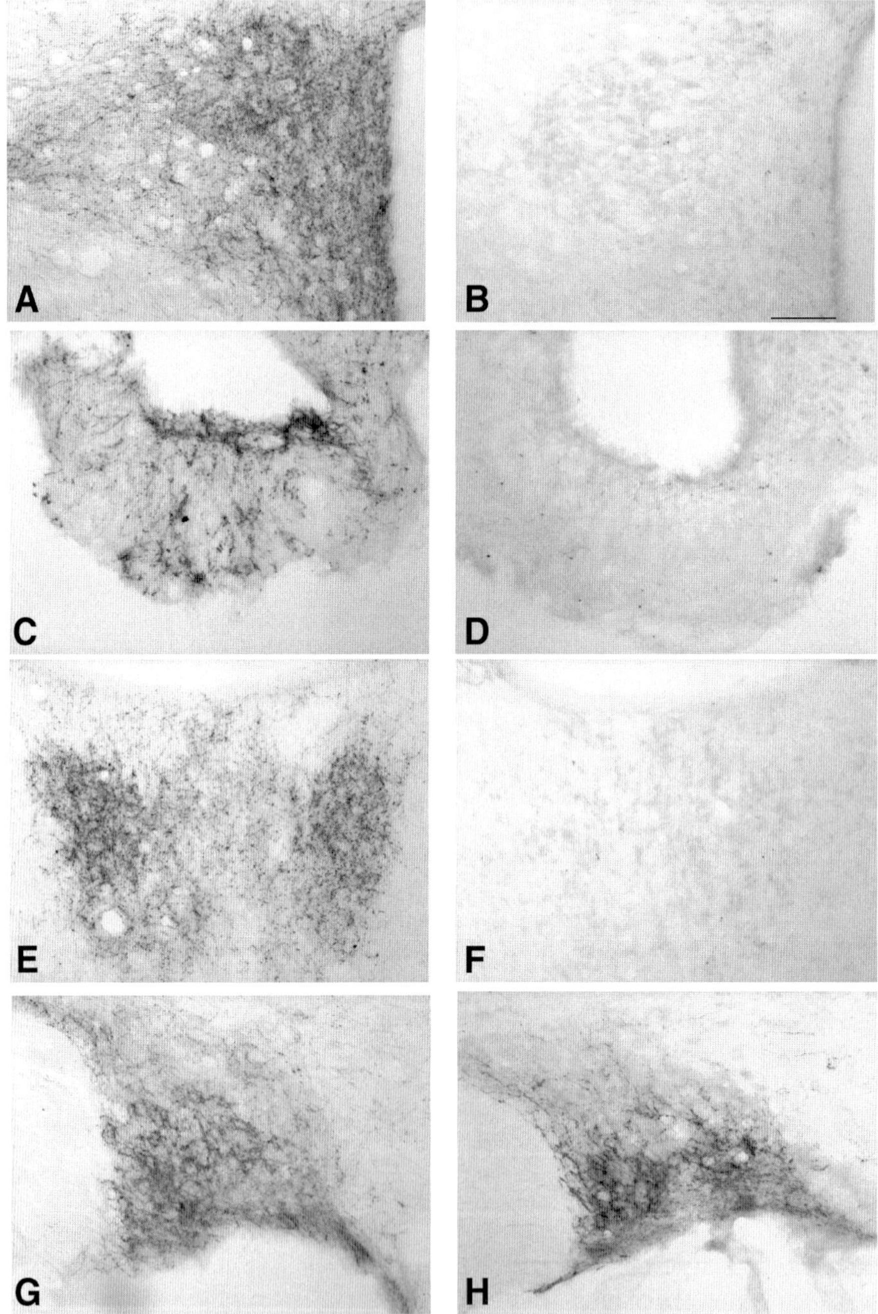

Fig. 3

cerebrate rats in which all of the connections between hindbrain and forebrain were severed continued to increase their food intake in response to glucoprivation when food was delivered intraorally *(17)*. These data indicated that circuitry for consummatory responding and the sensory receptors for detecting the glucose deficit are located in the hindbrain. Therefore, it was important to determine whether the anti-DβH-sap injection, like decerebration, had disabled or disengaged the more complex motivational and appetitive mechanisms of the ingestive response to glucoprivation without impairing the presumably simpler hindbrain circuitry underlying the consummatory response. However, we found that PVH anti-DβH-sap rats did not increase milk intake in response to either insulin-induced hypoglycemia or 2DG, even when food was placed directly into their mouth (Fig. 7). MA-induced blockade of fatty acid oxidation and food deprivation stimulated intraoral feeding significantly in both SAP and anti-DβH-sap rats, and responses did not differ between groups, suggesting that anti-DβH-sap did not destroy the circuitry for consummatory responding, but only the mechanism for activating this circuitry specifically by glucoprivation.

The fact that the consummatory response to glucoprivation was preserved after the complete decerebration, but impaired by the more selective anti-DβH-sap lesion, although at first puzzling, provides clues to the neural organization of this ingestive response. Although decerebration eliminates the forebrain terminals of NE and E neurons, it leaves their cell bodies and hindbrain projections intact. In contrast, PVH anti-DβH-sap destroys the entire catecholamine neuron. Therefore, NE or E neurons with projections to the PVH anti-DβH-sap injection site must also engage the circuitry responsible for stimulation of the consummatory component of the glucoprivic feeding response. The fact that the consummatory response to

---

Fig. 3. Photomicrographs showing dopamine β-hydroxylase (DβH) immunoreactivity (black particulate) in anatomically comparable levels of the medial hypothalamus from a rat injected bilaterally into the paraventricular nucleus of the hypothalamus (PVH) with 200 nL solution containing unconjugated saporin (SAP) control (left column) or anti-DβH-saporin (right column). Levels shown are PVH (**A,B**), median eminence (**C,D**), paraventricular nucleus of the thalamus (**E,F**), and supraoptic nucleus (**G,H**). Anti-DβH-sap eliminated DβH-immunoreactive terminals in medial periventricular structures of the hypothalamus and in the paraventricular nucleus of the thalamus, but not in more lateral sites, such as the supraoptic nucleus. This pattern of denervation depicted in B,D, and F may be due in part to diffusion of the anti-DβH-sap from the injection site and in part to extensive collateralization of the axons of cell bodies innervating these medial structures.

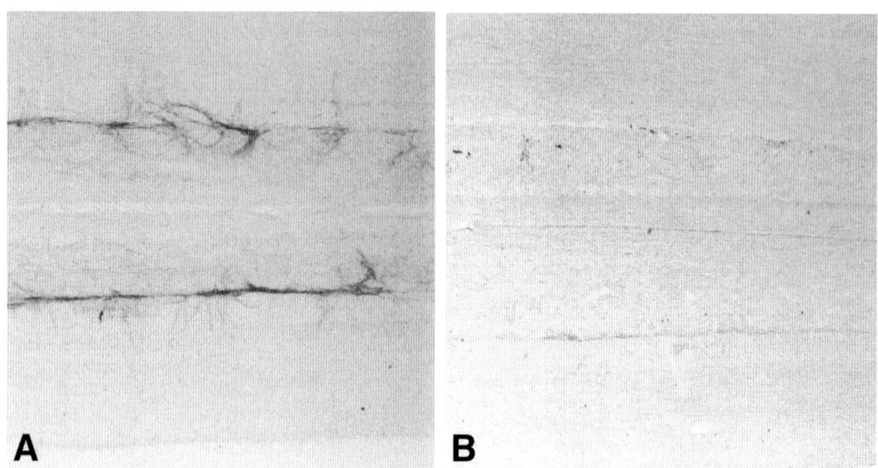

Fig. 4. Horizontal sections through the intermediolateral column of thoracic spinal cord from rats injected previously at T2-T4 with unconjugated saporin control solution (**A**) or anti-dopamine β hydroxylase (DβH)-saporin. (**B**) Injection of anti-DβH-sap, but not saporin, severely reduced or eliminated DβH-immunoreactive terminals in the spinal cord below the injection site.

glucoprivation persists in decerebrate rats indicates that hindbrain collaterals of PVH-projecting neurons, not their PVH or other forebrain terminals, must stimulate this response. Hindbrain catecholamine neurons therefore appear to be involved in multilevel processing of behavioral responses to glucoprivic stimulation, incorporating appetitive and consummatory phases of ingestion into the behavioral response by activation of circuits distributed along the neuroaxis.

Results from PVH anti-DβH-sap-injected rats have also shed light on another question regarding the neural circuitry for glucoprivic feeding. That question has to do with the involvement of the PVH in the feeding response. Because of the historical focus on the PVH as a critical site for control of feeding behavior, the finding by several investigators *(65,66)* that glucoprivic feeding is not abolished by electrolytic lesion of the PVH has puzzled us. The fact that PVH anti-DβH-sap injections abolish glucoprivic feeding, but electrolytic lesions do not, strongly suggests that catecholamine terminals outside the PVH are most critical for the feeding response. Catecholamine innervation of other hypothalamic or extrahypothalamic sites by these same neurons may be involved. Our PVH anti-DβH-sap injections substantially reduced DβH-ir terminals throughout the medial hypo-

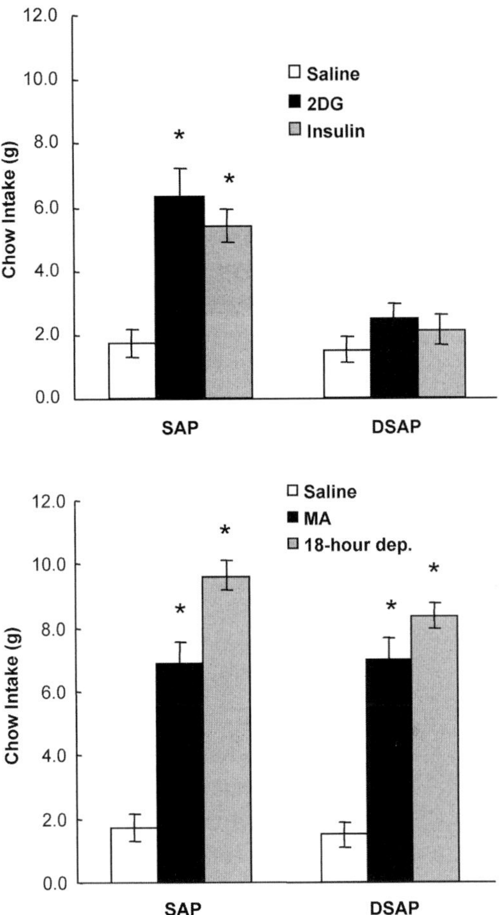

Fig. 5. Intake of pelleted rat chow (4-h tests) by rats injected bilaterally with unconjugated saporin (SAP) control solution or anti-dopamine hydroxylase (DβH)-saporin (DSAP) in the paraventricular nucleus of the hypothalamus. The top panel shows responses to glucoprivation induced by 2-deoxy-D-glucose (200 mg/kg) or a hypoglycemic dose of insulin (1.5 U/kg) and to saline control injection (1 ml/kg). Bottom panel shows responses to 2-mercaptoacetate (MA, 68 mg/kg), 18 h (overnight) food deprivation, and saline control injection. DSAP selectively abolished responses to both glucoprivic agents, but not to food deprivation or MA-induced blockade of fatty acid oxidation. Taken from ref. *64*, Fig. 3, © 2004 by Elsevier.

thalamus, including the ARC and dorsomedial nucleus of the hypothalamus, and injections targeting the ARC specifically also impaired the glucoprivic feeding response *(26)*, as discussed in the following section. Additional

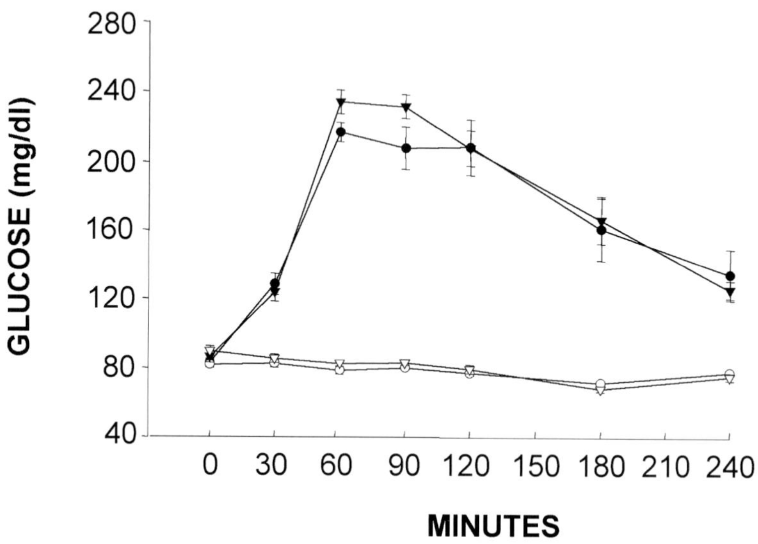

Fig. 6. Blood glucose concentrations following 2-deoxy-D-glucose (2DG, 250 mg/kg) and saline (SAL, 0.9% 1 mL/kg) in rats injected previously into the paraventricular nucleus of the hypothalamus with unconjugated saporin (SAP) control solution or anti-DβH-saporin (DSAP). DSAP injection at this site did not impair the hyperglycemic response to 2DG. Adapted from ref. *61*, Fig. 2, © 2003 by the Endocrine Society.

localization studies will be required to identify the catecholamine terminal areas specifically involved in the feeding response.

NE/E Projections Are Necessary for Induction of NPY and AGRP mRNAs by Glucoprivation

Glucoprivation activates hypothalamic circuits associated with stimulation of appetite. In particular, the peptides NPY and AGRP have been implicated in the glucoprivic control. AGRP is expressed exclusively in ARC NPY neurons, and both peptides possess potent orexigenic effects when injected into the brain *(67–71)*. Feeding induced by 2DG is attenuated by immunoneutralization of endogenous NPY in the PVH *(21)*. In addition, NPY peptide levels *(72)* and levels of both NPY *(24)* and AGRP *(24,25)* mRNA are increased in the ARC by 2DG. The effect of 2DG on NPY and AGRP neurons appears to be specifically related to glucose deficit because MA, which blocks fatty acid oxidation and stimulates food intake, does not produce these effects *(24,72)*.

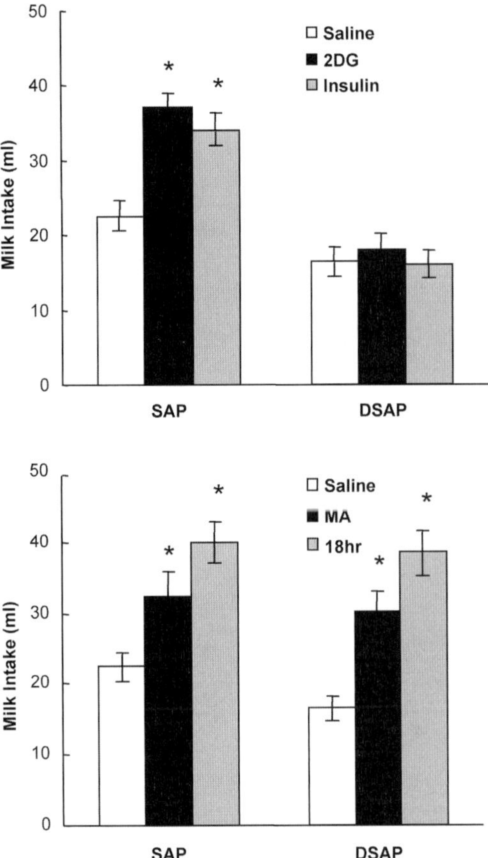

Fig. 7. Consummatory responses of rats injected previously with unconjugated saporin (SAP) control solution or anti-DβH-saporin (DSAP) in the paraventricular nucleus of the hypothalamus in response to insulin and 2-deoxy-D-glucose-induced glucoprivation and saline control (top panel) and to mercaptoacetate (MA) and 18 h (overnight) food deprivation (bottom panel). *See* Fig. 5 caption for drug doses. Consummatory responses were tested using an intraortal fistula connected to a syringe pump for delivery of 40% lactose-free milk directly into the mouth. A delivery schedule of 5 min infusion followed by 1 min rest was repeated until the rat allowed the milk to drip out of its mouth for 30 s. DSAP selectively abolished consummatory feeding responses to both glucoprivic agents, but not to food deprivation or MA-induced blockade of fatty acid oxidation. Taken from ref. *64*, Fig. 4, © 2004 by Elsevier.

The responsiveness of hypothalamic AGRP and NPY neurons to glucose deficit is a highly significant finding because these peptides are very potent orexigens *(67,70,71,73)*. Their responsiveness to glucose deficit may therefore be a mechanism that couples appetite to metabolic need. However, the coupling mechanism and the basis for the responsiveness of these neurons to glucose deficit until recently has not been clear. One possibility is that the activity of NPY and AGRP neurons is directly altered by glucose availability. Neurons that change their electrical activity in response to alterations in glucose availability are widely distributed in the hypothalamus and elsewhere in the brain *(74–78)*. Alternatively, the responsiveness of AGRP and NPY neurons to glucoprivation may be determined by their afferent inputs, which include a heavy innervation by hindbrain NE and E neurons *(50,79,80)*.

We used anti-DβH-sap lesions to test the hypothesis that the response of AGRP and NPY neurons to glucoprivation requires afferent input from hindbrain catecholamine neurons. We found that injections of anti-DβH-sap that eliminate NE/E terminals in the ARC of the hypothalamus, where cell bodies coexpressing NPY and AGRP are located *(81)*, not only impaired glucoprivic feeding, but also blocked the 2DG-induced increase in NPY and AGRP mRNA expression in the ARC. Thus, the AGRP and NPY neurons in the ARC appear to be a downstream link in a circuit originating in the hindbrain that is activated by glucoprivation and driven by catecholamine neurons. This circuitry may also be influenced during basal functioning by the catecholamine inputs because the basal gene expression was significantly increased by removal of these inputs.

With respect to NPY, it is also important to note that this peptide is coexpressed in catecholamine afferents to the PVH and ARC and is synthesized by neurons in the ARC and elsewhere. The anti-DβH-sap lesion, because it selectively removes the hindbrain NPY contribution to the medial hypothalamus, promises to be useful for chemical dissection of the distinct roles and patterns of innervation of the hypothalamic and hindbrain NPY systems.

PVH Anti-DβH-Sap Injection Selectively Impairs the Glucoprivic Control of Corticosterone Secretion

Despite the recognized potential of catecholaminergic neurons for altering hypthalmo–pituitary–adrenal (HPA) axis function, major questions still exist regarding the precise nature of their involvement in the reactions to stress and homeostatic challenges *(82,83)*. A major question is whether NE and E neurons activate the HPA axis only in response to specific modalities of sensory information or whether they contribute in a more general way to HPA activation by responding to and transmitting many or all forms of stress-related sensory information. The functional complexity of the hindbrain catecholamine cell groups and the physiological complexity of many stressors have impeded the resolution of these questions. Another major obstacle has been the lack of sufficiently selective tools for lesioning these neurons, which has made it difficult to attribute lesion-associated disruption of HPA function specifically to loss of PVH catecholamine terminals. This seemed to us an ideal question to pursue using anti-DβH-sap immunolesions of catecholamine inputs to the neuroendocrine CRH neurons in the PVH.

We tested rats with bilateral anti-DβH-sap injections into the PVH under basal conditions and in response to two qualitatively distinct challenges: systemic glucoprivation and 5 min of forced swimming in tepid (37°C) water *(61)*. Glucoprivation is an internal metabolic stress, and forced swim has been described as an external aversive stress. By using these two very different stressors, we hoped to determine the degree to which each depends on catecholamine afferents. This information in turn would begin to reveal the degree of stimulus specificity of the catecholamine afferents to the CRH neurons.

We found that anti-DβH-sap lesions that virtually eliminated the NE and E innervation of neuroendocrine CRH neurons severely attenuated the corticosterone responses to both insulin-induced hypoglycemia and systemic 2DG. Integrated plasma corticosterone levels *(84)* of anti-DβH-sap rats following 2DG were only 34% of the response of the SAP-injected rats. In response to insulin, the response of anti-DβH-sap rats was only 28% of the response of the SAP controls (Fig. 8).

Despite the profound impairment of the response to glucoprivation, the corticosterone response of the same anti-DβH-sap-lesioned rats to a 5-min forced swim was not impaired. Responses of the two groups were virtually identical. In addition, the basal circadian secretion of corticosterone was not altered by anti-DβH-sap. Thus, hindbrain NE or E neurons are essential for the glucoprivic stimulation of neuroendocrine CRH neurons but are not essential for the daily corticosterone surge or during swim stress. Our results, therefore, support the hypothesis that the HPA axis is controlled by stimulus-specific pathways and further reveal the close functional relationship between catecholamine neurons and glucoregulatory responses.

In collaboration with Dr. Alan Watts at University of Southern California, we analyzed basal and transcriptional activity of medial parvicellular CRH neurons in these same anti-DβH-sap- and SAP-treated rats *(61)*. Results showed clearly that basal expression of CRH mRNA did not differ between SAP and anti-DβH-sap, providing additional evidence that CRH neurons are not functionally impaired by the anti-DβH-sap injection. However, anti-DβH-sap lesions profoundly impaired the induction of CRH heteronuclear RNA

INSULIN
CORTICOSTERONE (ng/ml)
500
400
300
200
100
0
SAP/INSULIN
SAP/SAL
DSAP/INSULIN
DSAP/SAL
0 30 60 90 120 150 180 210 240

SWIM
CORTICOSTERONE (ng/ml)
350
300
250
200
150
100
50
0
SAP/SWIM
SAP/NO SWIM
DSAP/SWIM
DSAP/NO SWIM
-30 0 30 60 90 120 150 180 210 240

BASAL CIRCADIAN SECRETION
CORTICOSTERONE (ng/ml)
160
140
120
100
80
60
40
20
0
DSAP
SAP
9 13 17 21 1 5 9
CLOCK TIME

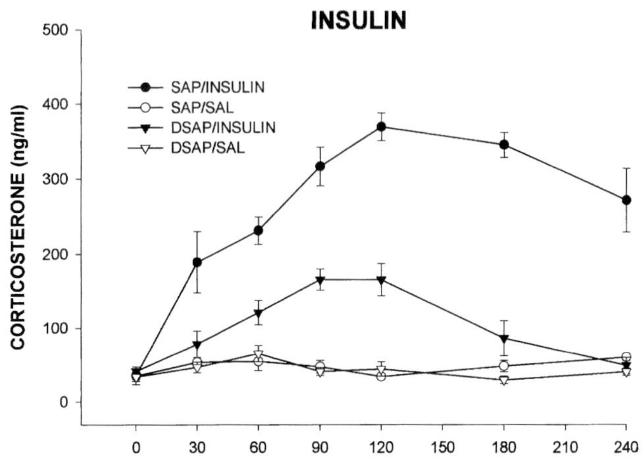

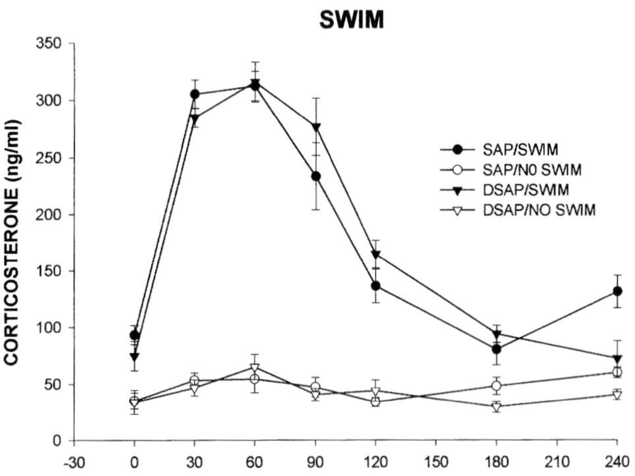

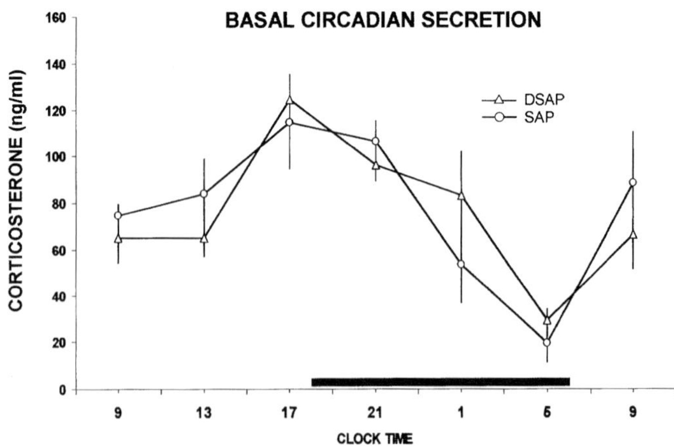

Fig. 8

(hnRNA) and c-*fos* mRNA in the PVH by glucoprivation (Fig. 9). Thus, both indices of activation showed that NE/E denervation of the PVH resulted in the failure of glucoprivation to activate CRH neurons, further confirming the hypothesis that glucoprivation controls these neurons through NE/E neurons.

Because anti-DβH-sap was microinjected into the vicinity of the CRH-secreting neurons, it was important to evaluate carefully the effect of the anti-DβH-sap injection on these neurons. We found that the CRH-immunoreactive neurons in the PVH were indistinguishable in SAP and anti-DβH-sap rats. In addition, the basal levels of CRH mRNA expression in the PVH did not differ between groups as noted here. These histological findings were supported by the results of the swim test and circadian rhythm study, which indicated that the CRH neurons are functionally intact, although their response to glucoprivation was profoundly reduced.

Intraspinal Anti-DβH-Sap Injections Impair the Glucoprivic Control of Adrenal Medullary Secretion

Hindbrain catecholamine cell groups C1–C3 and A5–A7 contain neurons that project spinally to innervate a variety of neuronal cell types. Cell group C1 predominantly innervates neurons in the intermediolateral column. As discussed in the section on destruction of NE and E neurons, injection of anti-DβH-sap into the intermediolateral gray matter at cord levels T2–T4 destroys these spinally projecting catecholamine neurons *(59)*. Intraspinal anti-DβH-sap injections abolished expression of Fos in the adrenal medulla in response to 2DG 200 mg/kg and eliminated the hyperglycemic response to 2DG, which is mediated primarily by adrenal medullary secretion of epinephrine (Fig. 10). Glucoprivic feeding was not impaired by the intraspinal anti-DβH-sap injections, providing functional evidence that injections at this site do not impair the rostrally projecting catecholamine cell populations.

Fig. 8. Corticosterone concentrations in remotely sampled blood collected from rats injected previously with unconjugated saporin control solution (SAP) or anti-DβH-saporin (DSAP) in the paraventricular nucleus of the hypothalamus. Samples were collected between 0 and 240 min following insulin (1.5 U/kg) at time 0 (top) or a 5-min swim in 37° water from 0 to 5 min (middle). Basal secretion over a 24-h period (bar indicates lights off) is shown in the bottom panel. DSAP caused profound reduction of the corticosterone response to insulin-induced hypoglycemia. The response to 2-deoxy-D-glucose (not shown) was also severely impaired by DSAP. However, the response to forced swimming and the basal corticosterone secretory rhythm were not impaired. Blood glucose concentrations of DSAP rats did not differ from those of SAP rats for any condition. Adapted from ref. *61*, Figs. 3–5, © 2003 by the Endocrine Society.

SAP/saline
SAP/2DG
DSAP/saline
DSAP/2DG
CRH hnRNA
CRH mRNA
c-fos mRNA

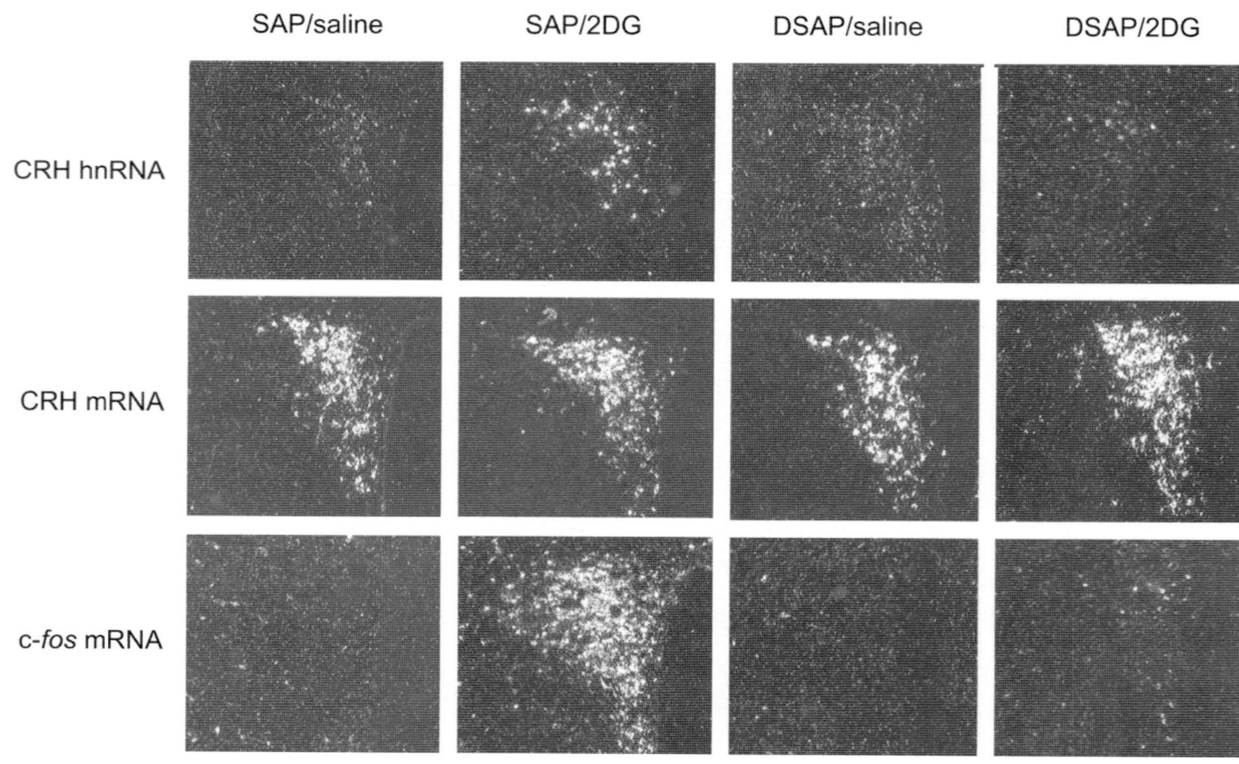

Fig. 9

200

Blood glucose is an indirect measure of adrenal medullary secretion. We confirmed the loss of the adrenal medullary response to glucoprivation in intraspinal anti-DβH-sap-injected rats using direct measurement of plasma NE and E responses (unpublished data). In the rat, plasma E is an indicator of adrenal medullary secretion, whereas NE is reflective primarily of sympathetic neuronal activation. Blood for high-performance liquid chromatographic analysis of NE and E was sampled remotely between 0 and 240 min after 2DG or insulin administration.

We found that plasma levels of E were elevated by both 2DG and insulin in SAP controls, but not in anti-DβH-sap rats (Fig. 11). Glucoprivation did not increase plasma NE in either SAP or anti-DβH-sap-treated rats. The 5-min forced swim did not elevate plasma E in either group, but did increase NE in both SAP and anti-DβH-sap rats. The preferential control of adrenal medullary secretion by glucoprivation in comparison to other stressors, which more strongly activate sympathetic neurons, was noted previously by several investigators *(84,85)*. Because catecholamine terminals were reduced throughout the extent of the intermediolateral column, the fact that the NE response to swim was not eliminated by anti-DβH-sap highlights the contribution of noncatecholaminergic innerveration of the intermediolateral column to the activation of sympathetic preganglionic neurons by the swim stress.

The deficits in the adrenal medullary secretory response were consistent with the loss of adrenal medullary Fos expression in the anti-DβH-sap rats treated with 2DG and with the loss of the hyperglycemic response. Together, they demonstrated an essential role of descending catecholamine afferents in the adrenal medullary response to glucoprivation. Taken together with

---

Fig. 9. Darkfield photomicrographs showing corticotropin releasing hormone (CRH) heteronuclear (hn) RNA (top row), CRH mRNA (middle row), and c-*fos* mRNA (bottom row) hybridization signal in the paraventricular nucleus of the hypothalamus (PVH) from representative rats previously given bilateral PVH microinjections of unconjugated saporin (SAP, columns 1 and 2) or anti-DβH-saporin (DSAP, columns 3 and 4) to selectively eliminate norepinephrine and epinephrine terminals in the PVH area. Saline (0.9%) or 2-deoxy-D-glucose (2DG, 250 mg/kg) was administered by remote intravenous injection 30 min before death. 2DG-induced glucoprivation did not induce CRH hnRNA or c-*fos* mRNA in DSAP-treated rats. The expression of CRH mRNA, which was not altered at this early time point by 2DG, was similar in both SAP and DSAP rats, indicating that the CRH-expressing neurons were not damaged by the DSAP injection. Reprinted from ref. *61*, Fig. 9.

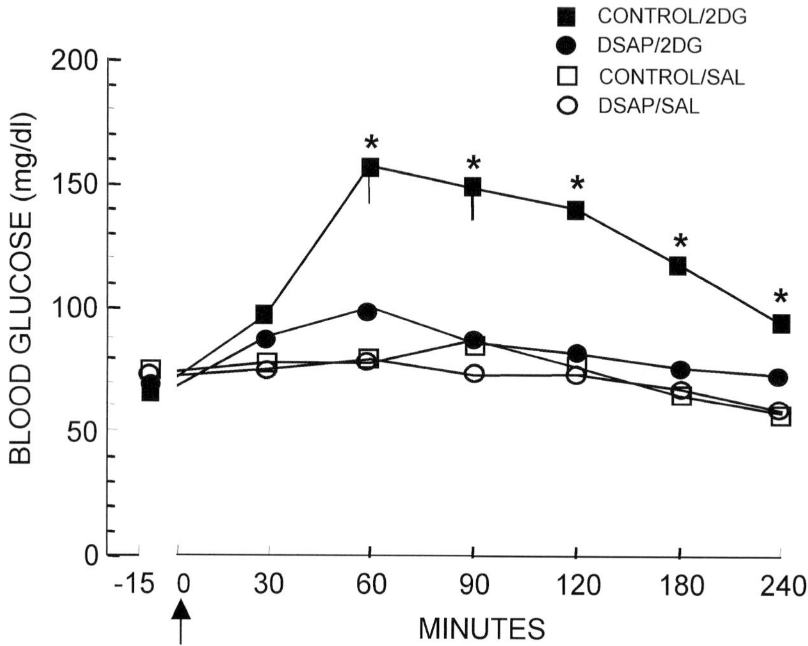

Fig. 10. Blood glucose concentrations following subcutaneous administration of 2-deoxy-D-glucose (2DG, 200 mg/kg) or saline (0.9% 1 ml/kg) in rats previously given intraspinal injections of rats anti-DβH-saporin (DSAP) or control solutions. Food was withheld during the experiment. Saline (0.9%) or 2DG was given at time 0 (arrow). Intraspinal DSAP virtually eliminated the hyperglycemic response to 2DG, but the feeding response (not shown) was not impaired. Means and standard errors (≥ 10 mg/dL) are indicated. *, $p < 0.001$ compared to saline baseline at the same time point for the same group. SAL, saline. Adapted from ref. 59, Fig. 8. © 2001 by Wiley-Liss, Inc.

the results of the PVH anti-DβH-sap injection, which abolished the feeding response but did not impair the hyperglycemic response, these results also demonstrated a division of labor among the catecholamine neurons responsive to glucoprivation.

PVH Anti-DβH-Sap Impairs the Glucoprivic Control of the Estrous Cycle

Glucose availability is now known to be of primary importance for maintenance of mammalian reproductive function. Chronic 2DG-induced glucoprivation (2–3 d) causes a decrease in reproductive behaviors in hamsters *(87)* and lengthened estrous cycles in both hamsters *(87)* and rats *(88,89)*. In sheep and in rats, acute 2DG-induced glucoprivation decreases the pulse frequency of luteinizing hormone secretion *(90,91)*. The delay of ovulation caused by glucose deficit can be broadly viewed as an adaptive glucoregulatory response with similarities to those discussed above. By delaying pregnancy, it conserves metabolic fuels for maternal survival and delays pregnancy until it is more likely to result in viable offspring.

As with the adrenal medullary, corticosterone, and feeding responses, the sensors responsible for the delay of ovulation also appear to be located in the lower brainstem because infusion of very low doses of 2DG into the fourth ventricle of rats suppresses pulsatile luteinizing hormone secretion *(92)*. Furthermore, catecholamine neurons are known to influence gonadotropin-releasing hormone (GnRH) secretion, although their precise role and relative importance are unclear. These similarities between the reproductive response and the other glucoregulatory responses we have studied stimulated us to examine the effects of glucoprivation on estrous cycles of PVH SAP- and anti-DβH-sap-injected rats.

In collaboration with Dr. Helen I'Anson, we injected anti-DβH-sap, as described, into the PVH of female rats with normal 4- to 5-d estrous cycles *(93)*. Approximately 3 wk after surgery, monitoring of estrous cycles was resumed until rats exhibited two normal cycles. Beginning on the day following the next estrus, rats were injected every 6 h with 2DG (200 mg/kg) for 3 d. We continued to monitor estrous cycles during and after chronic 2DG until estrus was detected. We found that PVH anti-DβH-sap injections did not disrupt normal estrous cycles.

However, SAP and anti-DβH-sap rats differed in their response to chronic glucoprivation. In SAP-injected rats, estrous cycle length increased to a mean of 7 d by the chronic glucoprivation. In contrast, anti-DβH-sap-injected rats did not respond to glucoprivation by increasing cycle length (Fig. 12). These findings suggest that the population of E or NE neurons with projections to the PVH injection site are not required for estrous cycling under normal conditions but contribute to the suppression of estrous cycles when glucose supplies are in deficit. Whether this suppression is directly or indirectly mediated is not yet clear. The role of the catecholamine innervation of the medial preoptic area, where GnRH neurons are distributed, also remains to be investigated. The medial preoptic catecholamine terminals were not typically eliminated by our PVH anti-DβH-sap injections (although they may be reduced in density), suggesting that a separate population of NE or E neurons lacking collaterals into the PVH contribute to innervation of this site. The possibility that these cells may play a very different role in control of GnRH secretion than those that innervate the PVH remains an interesting area of investigation that will benefit from immunotoxin lesion approaches.

INSULIN
DSAP
SAP
NE (pg/ml)
1200
800
400
0
0 30 60 90 120 180
E (pg/ml)
1200
600
0
0 30 60 90 120 180
SWIM
NE (pg/ml)
600
400
200
0
0 30 60 90 120 180
MINUTES
E (pg/ml)
1000
800
600
400
200
0
0 30 60 90 120 180
MINUTES

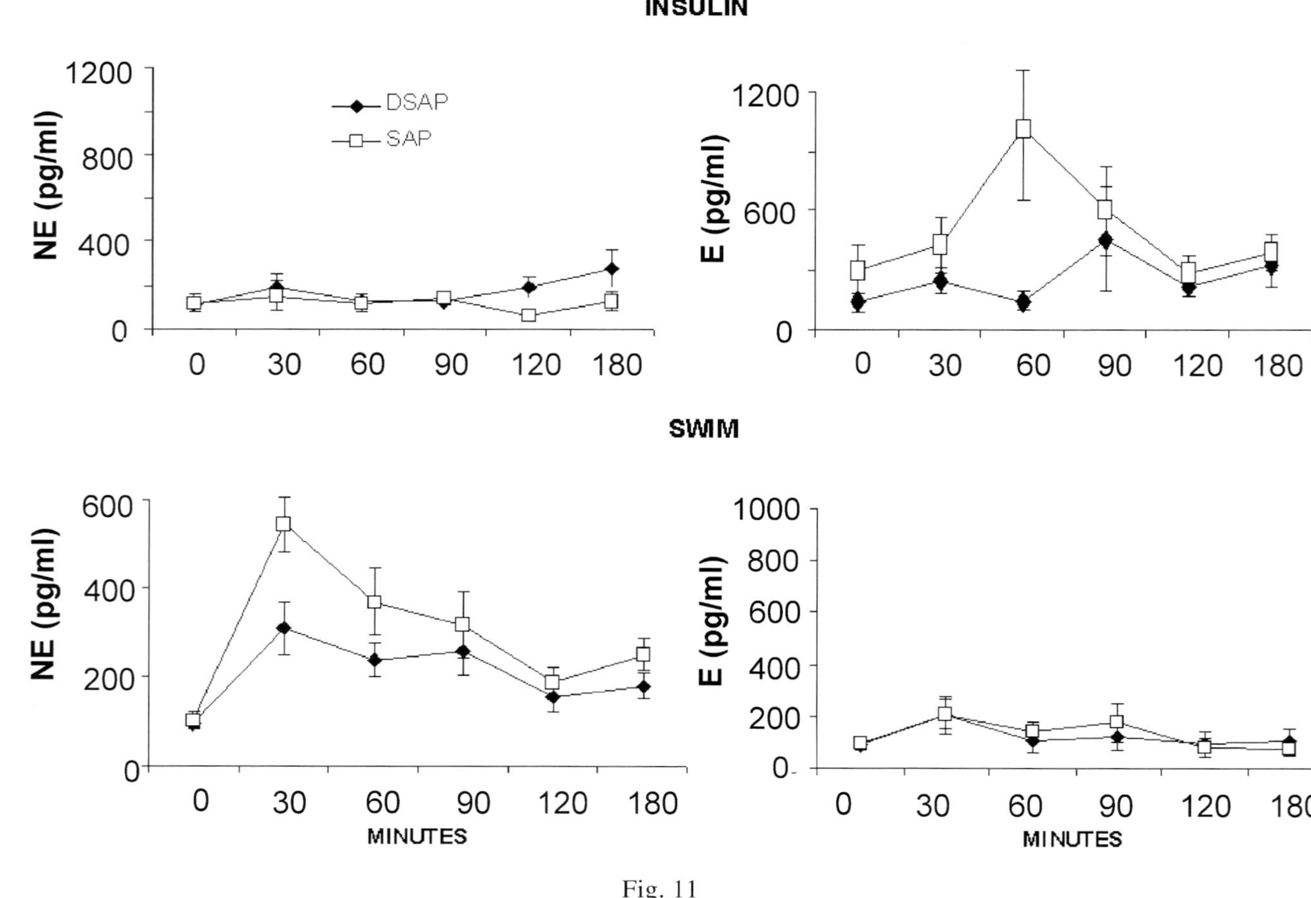

Fig. 11

METHODOLOGICAL AND TECHNICAL ISSUES

Anti-DβH-Sap Administration

Our injections *(26,59,61)* were made acutely using stereotaxic placement of calibrated glass capillary micropipettes pulled to achieve a tip diameter of 30 μm. Solutions were delivered with a Picospritzer using microscopic visualization to confirm drug delivery. Injections contained DβH mouse monoclonal antibody conjugated to saporin (anti-DβH-sap, Advanced Targeting Systems, San Diego, CA, 42 ng/200 nL in phosphate buffer, pH 7.4) or SAP in the same volume of phosphate buffer (pH 7.4). The amount of SAP in the control solution was equated with the amount of saporin present in the anti-DβH-sap conjugate, as indicated in the manufacturer's product information.

In the spinal cord, injections (42 ng anti-DβH-sap per site) were made between T2 and T4 *(59)*. This spinal level was chosen because injections effective in destroying spinally projecting NE and E neurons could be made using an intervertebral as opposed to a transvertebral approach, which is required at more caudal spinal segments. Therefore, the bleeding and trauma associated with transvertebral approaches were avoided, allowing better visualization of tissue, more effective monitoring of injectate delivery, less nonspecific damage, and more rapid recovery of the animal.

Access to the T2–T4 sites was through the intervertebral connective tissue and was facilitated by ventroflexion of the rat's head during the surgery. During intraspinal injections, respiration-associated movements of the spinal cord can cause considerable damage. Therefore, appropriate measures must be taken to stabilize the vertebral column and reduce respiratory movements while the intraspinal injector is in place.

Fig. 11. Plasma norepinephrine (NE, left column) and epinephrine (E, right column) in remotely sampled blood from rats injected intraspinally with unconjugated saporin control solution (SAP) or anti-dopamine β hydroxylase (DβH)-saporin (DSAP). Insulin-induced hypoglycemia did not increase plasma NE in either SAP or DSAP rats, but produced a large E response in the SAP rats (top row). DSAP severely impaired the E response to hypoglycemia. A 5-min swim in 37° water immediately after the 0 time blood sample did not elevate plasma E in either group, but did increase NE in both SAP and DSAP rats. The NE response to swim was present, but attenuated, in DSAP rats, compared to SAP. Results are consistent with studies of adrenal medullary Fos expression and blood glucose after systemic 2-deoxy-D-glucose in indicating impairment of adrenal medullary responses to glucoprivation by intraspinal DSAP.

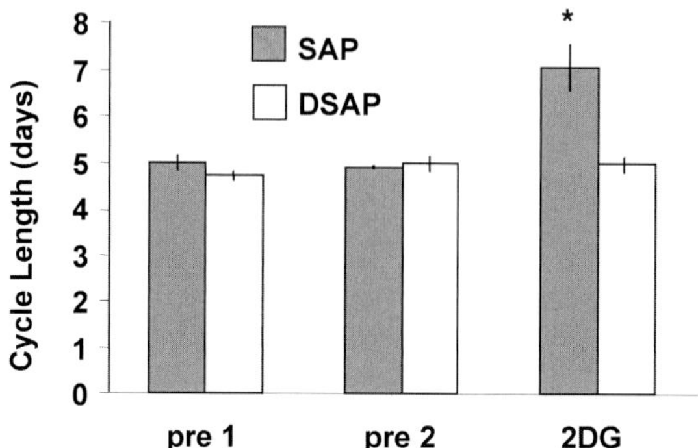

Fig. 12. Estrous cycles under basal conditions and during chronic 2-deoxy-D-glucose (2DG) in rats injected previously into the paraventricular nucleus of the hypothalamus (PVH) with unconjugated saporin control solution (SAP) or anti-DβH-saporin (DSAP). After two normal 4–5-d cycles (pre 1 and pre 2), female rats were injected every 6 h with 2DG (200 mg/kg) for 3 d. Estrous cycles were determined from vaginal cytology until estrus was detected following chronic 2DG. Estrous cycles were extended in SAP controls by chronic 2DG, but were not extended in DSAP-treated rats, suggesting that information related to glucoprivation was not transmitted to forebrain sites controlling reproductive responses to glucose deficit.

We have the impression that the type of anesthesia used during the anti-DβH-sap injection may significantly alter the effectiveness and reproductibility of the resulting lesion, although we have not investigated this systematically, we recommend that a ketamine, xylazine, acepromazine anesthetic cocktail be avoided.

Our choice of SAP as the control injection was made when we began using anti-DβH-sap and choice of control substances was limited. It is still a reasonable choice, although saporin conjugated to preimmune mouse immunoglobulin G antibody (mouse IgG-SAP, Advanced Targeting Systems) is now available and offers an alternative for control injections. To use SAP as our control, we included in our initial studies an examination of the possible nonspecific effects of SAP. We found that animals injected with SAP or sterile 0.9% saline into the PVH or spinal cord did not differ in their responses to glucoprivic challenge, suggesting that SAP *per se* did not introduce confounding effects.

Distribution of Saporin Immunoreactivity After Injection of Anti-DβH-Sap Into the PVH

In our initial efforts to characterize the uptake and distribution of anti-DβH-sap within the brain, Dawna Salter traced its internalization and trans-

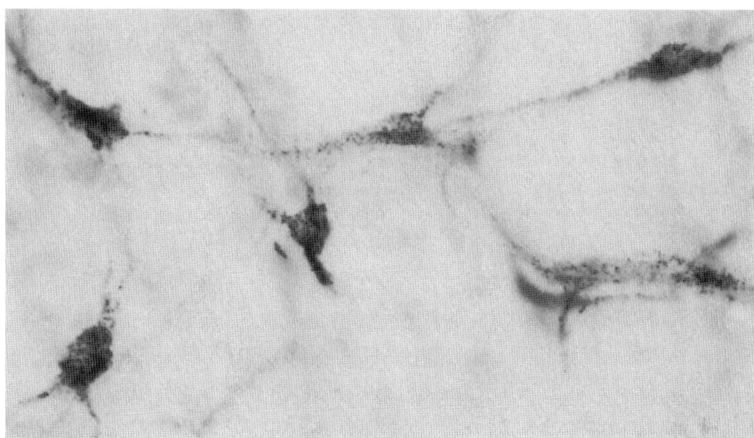

Fig. 13. Photomicrograph showing saporin-immunoreactivity in rat ventrolateral medulla just rostral to the level of area postrema. The section was taken from a rat injected with anti-dopamine β hydroxylase (DβH)-saporin 48 h prior to death in the paraventricular nucleus of the hypothalamus (PVH) and shows saporin-immunoreactive cells in the area of the C1 cell group. Immunoreactive cells were confined to areas containing catecholamine cell bodies with projections to the PVH. Levels of immunoreactivity peaked between 24 and 48 hours after the anti-DβH-saporin injection.

port from a PVH injection site using an antibody directed against SAP. This approach does not necessarily indicate the complete pattern of destruction from the anti-DβH-sap because internalization of undetectably small numbers of SAP molecules may be sufficient to cause cell death. However, this approach was useful to us in showing that the anti-DβH-sap is heavily internalized and retrogradely transported by NE and E neurons, in demonstrating its distribution after injection into a particular site, and in demonstrating the time-course of the subsequent destruction of the affected neurons.

We examined alternate sections of hindbrain for SAP-ir and tyrosine hydroxylase (TH)-ir 2 h and 1, 2, 3, 4, 7, and 14 d after injection of anti-DβH-sap or SAP into the PVH. We found that SAP-ir appears in hindbrain NE and E cell bodies by 24 h after anti-DβH-sap injection. SAP-ir was abundant in cell groups A1, A2, C1, C2, and C3 (close to the floor of the fourth ventricle) and in the main nucleus of A6. Fourteen days after PVH injection, SAP-ir was no longer detectable in the hindbrain, and reduction of TH-ir indicated loss of cell bodies in the PVH-projecting cell groups. The number of SAP-ir cell bodies reached a maximum between 24 and 48 h after anti-DβH-sap injection (Fig. 13) and declined thereafter. In addition, after PVH anti-DβH-sap injection, we did not observe SAP-ir cell profiles at the injection site or in any location in the brain other than those containing NE and E neurons known to innervate the medial hypothalamic area. After injection of SAP, we did not see immunoreactive cell profiles in any location, and we did not detect loss of TH-ir. Thus, except in NE and E neurons, any anti-DβH-sap or SAP that might possibly be internalized was below the level for detection by standard histological procedures.

Assessment of Lesion Specificity

We have evaluated anti-DβH-sap-induced lesions in several ways, and all have revealed remarkable selectivity and absence of tissue disruption. A question that was foremost in our minds when we began using anti-DβH-sap was whether it would produce transynaptic lesions caused by leakage from affected neurons during degeneration. Although spinally and rostrally projecting catecholamine neurons are distinct populations, their cell bodies are closely associated in some hindbrain sites, and many appear to be innervated by other catecholamine neurons.

Therefore, in our quantification of hindbrain cell groups, we considered the possibility that anti-DβH-sap could be liberated from degenerating neurons and internalized by terminals or cell bodies of neighboring, nontargeted catecholamine neurons. However, quantification of spinally and rostrally projecting cell populations indicated this probably does not occur. As noted above, lesions appeared to be limited to cell groups with known projections to the respective spinal or PVH injection sites. A similar anatomic result was reported by Schreihofer and Guyenet, who injected anti-DβH-sap intraspinally *(60)*. This was confirmed by the distribution of SAP-ir after PVH anti-DβH-sap injection, for which SAP-ir was confined to cell groups predicted from tract-tracing studies and was not observed in secondary cell populations.

We have examined noncatecholaminergic neurons in the vicinity of the injection site using a variety of staining procedures to detect and evaluate nonspecific damage from anti-DβH-sap injections. Our use of the microcapillary pipets for anti-DβH-sap injection reduced nonspecific tissue damage from the injection procedure, but also made it difficult to locate the cannula tract and injection site at the end of the experiment. However, the tract and injection site were sometimes visible because of the presence of hemosiderin deposits.

Using cresyl violet stain, we could clearly see that the injection had not disturbed the normal cytoarchitechture of the surrounding tissue *(59)*. We also immunostained identifiable injection sites for TH to observe dopamine cell bodies and for the peptides vasopressin and CRH. Cell bodies containing these substances were present in normal numbers and were normal in appearance at the PVH injection sites (Fig. 14).

In the spinal cord, we coinjected colloidal gold with the anti-DβH-sap in some animals to produce a permanent marker of the injection field and later stained the tissue for choline acetyl transferase to reveal the preganglionic sympathetic neurons of the intermediolateral column *(59)*. In the anti-DβH-sap injection field, indicated by the presence of gold particles, cholinergic neurons were present and were normal in appearance, although DβH-ir terminals had been severely reduced in the same regions by the anti-DβH-sap lesion.

We have used Fos-ir as an indicator of functional integrity of neurons in our anti-DβH-sap denervation zones, as well as verify the loss of stimulus-specific, catecholamine-mediated activation of cells in those regions *(59)*. Fos, the product of the immediate early gene c-*fos*, was increased by cellular activation. Fos expression is widely used as an indicator of cellular activation. In one experiment, we examined the increase in Fos-ir in cells at the PVH anti-DβH-sap injection site in response to intraventricular administration of E. We found that E increased expression of Fos in the PVH to a similar degree in both anti-DβH-sap and SAP rats. Thus, neurons innervated by catecholamine terminals in the vicinity of the anti-DβH-sap injection site were not destroyed by the lesion, although the NE and E innervation itself was virtually eliminated by the anti-DβH-sap. We also found that intraspinal injections of anti-DβH-sap eliminated 2DG-induced Fos expression in the adrenal medulla, and PVH anti-DβH-sap injections reduced 2DG-induced Fos and hnRNA expression in the PVH in response to glucoprivation as discussed previously *(59,61)*.

Selective Anti-DβH-Sap Lesions May Involve Multiple Brain Sites Because of Degeneration of Collateral Projections

Catecholamine neurons are known for their widespread distribution and extensive collateralization. It is important to keep this fact in mind when using anti-DβH-sap to lesion these neurons. When anti-DβH-sap is administered into a catecholamine terminal area, the lesion is not limited to terminals innervating the injection site, but will include all terminals of the affected cell bodies. For this reason, additional experiments may be required to determine which of the denervated sites is (are) responsible for the deficits observed.

SUMMARY

The findings reported here significantly enhance our understanding of the central neural circuitry controlling glucoregulatory responses. These re-

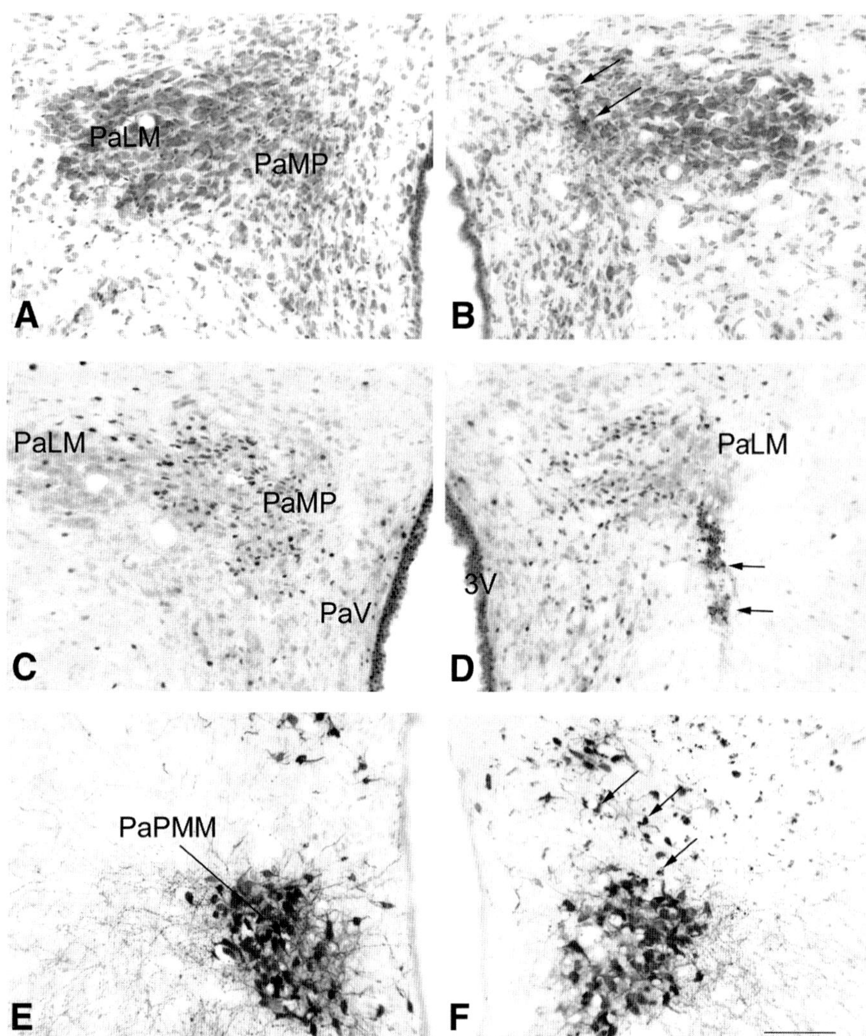

Fig. 14. Photomicrographs showing coronal sections through the medial hypothalamus of control rats (left) and rats injected with anti-dopamine β hydroxylase (DβH)-saporin in the paraventricular nucleus of the hypothalamus (PVH) (right). Sections stained with cresyl violet to reveal the cytoarchitecture of the PVH region are shown in (**A**) and (**B**). The anti-DβH-saporin injection site and tract of the microinjector pipet are indicated by the arrows in B. A slight loss of cellularity is present in the immediate vicinity of the injector tip, but tissue disruption is minimal. Plates (**C**) and (**D**) show Fos-immunoreactive (ir) after injection of L-epinephrine through a chronic lateral ventricular cannula 2 h prior to death. The anti-DβH-saporin microinjection site is shown at the arrow in D. Plates (**E**) and (**F**) show vasopressin-ir cells. In F, anti-DβH-saporin was co-injected with colloidal gold to permanently

sults define a system providing an integrated control of glucose homeostasis by simultaneous activation of downstream neurons stimulating adrenal medullary and corticosterone secretion, food intake, and suppression of reproduction. This system originates with hindbrain glucoreceptor cells and requires ascending and descending NE or E neurons to engage the pertinent downstream circuits for execution of these various responses. Deficits present in rats with selective anti-DβH-sap lesions compellingly revealed that particular subgroups of NE or E neurons are the essential and apparently the sole link connecting hindbrain glucoreceptors with the appropriate downstream sites. Moreover, the profound and selective impairment in glucoregulatory responses after anti-DβH-sap lesions of NE and E neurons provides an equally compelling demonstration that hindbrain glucose-sensing cells make up the key sensory system underlying the elicitation and coordination of multiple regulatory responses that ensure glucose delivery to the brain. A further question to be addressed is whether different populations of PVH-projecting NE or E neurons or different collateral projections of the same neurons mediate the feeding, HPA, and reproductive responses to glucoprivation.

Our current findings suggest that the NE or E neurons lesioned by our anti-DβH-sap injections are not required for daily basal feeding, corticosterone secretion, adrenal medullary function, or estrous cycling because these basal functions do not appear to be impaired in the anti-DβH-sap-lesioned rats. Nevertheless, these NE and E neurons are capable of commandeering the essential circuitry for behavioral, neuroendocrine, and autonomic responses and powerfully activating them when glucose homeostasis is threatened. However, determination of the threshold for activation of these NE/E neurons and their potential influence on physiological responses during normal daily glucose fluctuation remains an important area for further investigation.

Fig. 14. *(continued from opposite page)* mark the injection field. Several examples of gold particulate are indicated by arrows in F. Vasopressin-ir cell bodies within the labeled diffusion field are not different from those shown for the control. Loss of catecholamine cell bodies in the hindbrain and terminals in the medial hypothalamus (not shown) indicated the effectiveness of the anti-DβH-saporin lesions in these same rats. These results provide evidence for the high degree of selectivity and absence of significant nonspecific damage associated with anti-DβH-saporin microinjections. 3V, third ventricle; PaLM, paraventricular nucleus, lateral magnocellular area; PaPMM, paraventricular nucleus, posterior medial magnocellular area; PaMP, paraventricular nucleus, medial parvicellular area; PaV, paraventricular nucleus, ventral. Scale bar = 200 μ*M*. Reprinted from ref. *59*, Fig. 12, © 2001 by Wiley-Liss, Inc.

Investigation of the mechanisms through which the brain provides for its own metabolic needs is important in its own right. However, with the increased prevalence of obesity and diabetes, the ways in which the requirements of brain glucose homeostasis fit within the context of overall energy homeostasis and body weight regulation are related issues that cannot be neglected. In addition, with the increased incidence of insulin-dependent diabetes, the impact of intensive insulin therapy and its potential side effects on mechanisms controlling brain glucose homeostasis are areas in urgent need of investigation. These areas of research will undoubtedly continue to benefit greatly from the availability and innovative uses of selectively targeted chemical lesioning agents such as anti-DβH-sap.

ACKNOWLEDGMENTS

We acknowledge Christi Pedrow for her patience and expertise in conducting the numerous radioimmunoassays required by this work; Trisha Duffy for her expert help with high-performance liquid chromatographic analyses of plasma catecholamines; Shayne Andrew for his meticulous mapping of brainstem sites involved in glucoprivic control of glucagon and corticosterone responses; and grant support from the Juvenile Diabetes Research Foundation International, American Diabetes Association, and National Institutes of Health (DK40498).

REFERENCES

1. Sokoloff L. The metabolism of the central nervous system in vivo. In: Field J, Magoun HW, Hall VE, eds. *Handbook of Physiology–Neurophysiology.* Vol. 3. Washington, DC: American Physiological Society; 1960:1843–1864.
2. Fillenz M, Lowry JP, Boutelle MG, Fray AE. The role of astrocytes and noradrenaline in neuronal glucose metabolism. Acta Physiol Scand 1999; 167:275–284.
3. Picklo MJ, Wiley RG, Lappi DA, Robertson D. Noradrenergic lesioning with an anti-dopamine beta-hydroxylase immunotoxin. Brain Res 1994;666:195–200.
4. Picklo MJ, Wiley RG, Lonce S, Lappi DA, Robertson D. Anti-dopamine β-hydroxylase immunotoxin-induced sympathectomy in adult rats. J Pharmacol Exp Ther 1995;275:1003–1010.
5. Picklo MJ. Methods of sympathetic degeneration and alteration. J Auton Nerv Syst 1997;62:111–125.
6. Wrenn CC, Picklo MJ, Lappi DA, Robertson D, Wiley RG. Central noradrenergic lesioning using anti-DBH-saporin: anatomical findings. Brain Res 1996; 740:175–184.

7. Barthelemy I, Martineau D, Ong M, et al. The expression of saporin, a ribosome-inactivating protein from the plant *Saponaria officinalis*, in *Escherichia coli*. J Biol Chem 1993;268:6541–6548.

8. Ritter RC, Slusser P. 5-Thio-D-glucose causes increased feeding and hyperglycemia in the rat. Am J Physiol 1980;238:E141–E144.

9. Ritter S. Glucoprivation and the glucoprivic control of food intake. In: Ritter RC, Ritter S, Barnes CD, eds. *Feeding Behavior: Neural and Humoral Controls*. Orlando, FL: Academic Press Inc.; 1986:271–313.

10. Epstein AN, Nicolaidis S, Miselis RR. The glucoprivic control of food intake and the glucostatic theory of feeding behaviour. In: Mogenson GJ, Calaresu FR, eds. *Neural Integration of Physiological Mechanisms and Behaviour*. Toronto, Ontario, Canada: University of Toronto Press; 1975:148–168.

11. Slusser PG, Ritter RC. Increased feeding and hyperglycemia elicited by intracerebroventricular 5-thioglucose. Brain Res 1980;202:474–478.

12. Smith GP, Epstein AN. Increased feeding in response to decreased glucose utilization in the rat and monkey. Am J Physiol 1969;217:1083–1087.

13. Brown J. Effects of 2-deoxy-d-glucose on carbohydrate metabolism: review of the literature and studies in the rat. Metabolism 1962;11:1098–1112.

14. Chen M, Whistler RL. Action of 5-thio-D-glucose and its 1-phosphate with hexokinase and phosphoglucomutase. Arch Biochem Biophys 1975;169:392–396.

15. Miselis RR, Epstein AN. Feeding induced by intracerebroventricular 2-deoxy-D-glucose in the rat. Am J Physiol 1975;229:1438–1447.

16. Berthoud HR, Mogenson GJ. Ingestive behavior after intracerebral and intracerebroventricular infusions of glucose and 2-deoxy-D-glucose. Am J Physiol 1977;233:R127–R133.

17. Flynn FW, Grill HJ. Insulin elicits ingestion in decerebrate rats. Science 1983;221:188–190.

18. DiRocco RJ, Grill HJ. The forebrain is not essential for sympathoadrenal hyperglycemic response to glucoprivation. Science 1979;204:1112–1114.

19. Ritter RC, Slusser PG, Stone S. Glucoreceptors controlling feeding and blood glucose: location in the hindbrain. Science 1981;213:451–452.

20. Ritter S, Dinh TT, Zhang Y. Localization of hindbrain glucoreceptive sites controlling food intake and blood glucose. Brain Res 2000;856:37–47.

21. He B, White BD, Edwards GL, Martin RJ. Neuropeptide Y antibody attenuates 2-deoxy-D-glucose induced feeding in rats. Brain Res 1998;781:348–350.

22. Booth DA. Modulation of the feeding response to peripheral insulin, 2-deoxyglucose or 3-*O*-methyl glucose injection. Physiol Behav 1972;8:1069–1076.

23. Muller EE, Cocchi D, Mantegazza P. Brain adrenergic system in the feeding response induced by 2-deoxy-d-glucose. Am J Physiol 1972;223:945–950.

24. Sergeyev V, Broberger C, Gorbatyuk O, Hokfelt T. Effect of 2-mercaptoacetate and 2-deoxy-D-glucose administration on the expression of NPY, AGRP, POMC, MCH and hypocretin/orexin in the rat hypothalamus. Neuroreport 2000;11:117–121.

25. Fraley GS, Dinh TT, Ritter S. Immunotoxic catecholamine lesions attenuate 2DG-induced increase in AGRP mRNA. Peptides 2002;6397:1–8.
26. Fraley GS, Ritter S. Immunolesion of norepinephrine and epinephrine afferents to medial hypothalamus alters basal and 2DG-induced NPY and AGRP mRNA expression in the arcuate nucleus. Endocrinology 2003;144:75–83.
27. Brito NA, Brito MN, Kettelhut IC, Migliorini RH. Intra-ventromedial hypothalamic injection of cholinergic agents induces rapid hyperglycemia, hyperlactatemia and gluconeogenesis activation in fed, conscious rats. Brain Res 1993;626:339–342.
28. Coimbra CC, Migliorini RH. Evidence for a longitudinal pathway in rat hypothalamus that controls FFA mobilization. Am J Physiol 1983;245:E332–E337.
29. Steffens AB, Damsma G, van der Gugten J, Luiten PG. Circulating free fatty acids, insulin, and glucose during chemical stimulation of hypothalamus in rats. Am J Physiol 1984;247:E765–E771.
30. Bellin SI, Ritter S. Insulin-induced elevation of hypothalamic norepinephrine turnover persists after glucorestoration unless feeding occurs. Brain Res 1981;217:327–337.
31. Rowland NE. Effects of glucose and fat antimetabolites on norepinephrine turnover in rat hypothalamus and brainstem. Brain Res 1992;595:291–294.
32. Stricker EM, Friedman MI, Zigmond MJ. Glucoregulatory feeding by rats after intraventricular 6-hydroxydopamine or lateral hypothalamic lesions. Science 1975;189:895–897.
33. Epstein AN, Teitelbaum P. Specific loss of the hypoglycemic control of feeding in recovered lateral rats. Am J Physiol 1967;213:1159–1167.
34. Alheid GF, McDermott L, Kelly J, Halaris A, Grossman SP. Deficits in food and water intake after knife cuts that deplete striatal DA or hypothalamic NE in rats. Pharmacol Biochem Behav 1977;6:273–287.
35. Marshall JF, Richardson JS. Nigrostriatal bundle damage and the lateral hypothalamic syndrome. J Comp Physiol Psychol 1974;87:808–830.
36. Plotsky PM, Cunningham ET Jr, Widmaier EP. Catecholaminergic modulation of corticotropin-releasing factor and adrenocorticotropin secretion. Endocr Rev 1989;10:437–458.
37. Plotsky PM, Otto S, Sutton S. Neurotransmitter modulation of corticotropin releasing factor secretion into the hypophysial-portal circulation. Life Sci 1987;41:1311–1317.
38. Whitnall MH, Kiss A, Aguilera G. Contrasting effects of central alpha-1-adrenoreceptor activation on stress-responsive and stress-nonresponsive subpopulations of corticotropin-releasing hormone neurosecretory cells in the rat. Neuroendocrinology 1993;58:42–48.
39. Whitnall MH. Regulation of the hypothalamic corticotropin-releasing hormone neurosecretory system. Prog Neurobiol 1993;40:573–629.
40. Leibowitz SF. Brain neuropeptide Y: an integrator of endocrine, metabolic and behavioral processes. Brain Res Bull 1991;27:333–337.
41. Smythe GA, Grunstein HS, Bradshaw JE, Nicholson MV, Compton PJ. Relationships between brain noradrenergic activity and blood glucose. Nature 1984;308:65–67.

42. Smythe GA, Edwards SR. A role for central postsynaptic α 2-adrenoceptors in glucoregulation. Brain Res 1991;562:225–229.
43. Smythe GA, Edwards SR. Suppression of central noradrenergic neuronal activity inhibits hyperglycemia. Am J Physiol 1992;263:E823–E827.
44. Leibowitz SF. Hypothalamic paraventricular nucleus: interaction between α 2-noradrenergic system and circulating hormones and nutrients in relation to energy balance. Neurosci Biobehav Rev 1988;12:101–109.
45. Leibowitz SF, Sladek C, Spencer L, Tempel D. Neuropeptide Y, epinephrine and norepinephrine in the paraventricular nucleus: stimulation of feeding and the release of corticosterone, vasopressin and glucose. Brain Res Bull 1988;21:905–912.
46. Curran T, Morgan, JI. Fos: an immediate-early transcription factor in neurons. J Neurobiol 1995;26:403–412.
47. Wesselingh SL, Li YW, Blessing WW. PNMT-containing neurons in the rostral medulla oblongata (C1, C3 groups) are transneuronally labelled after injection of herpes simplex virus type 1 into the adrenal gland. Neurosci Lett 1989;106:99–104.
48. Strack AM, Sawyer WB, Platt KB, Loewy AD. CNS cell groups regulating the sympathetic outflow to adrenal gland as revealed by transneuronal cell body labeling with pseudorabies virus. Brain Res 1989;491:274–296.
49. Tucker DC, Saper CB, Ruggiero DA, Reis DJ. Organization of central adrenergic pathways: I. Relationships of ventrolateral medullary projections to the hypothalamus and spinal cord. J Comp Neurol 1987;259:591–603.
50. Sawchenko PE, Swanson LW. The organization of noradrenergic pathways from the brainstem to the paraventricular and supraoptic nuclei in the rat. Brain Res 1982;257:275–325.
51. Jonsson G. Chemical lesioning techniques: monoamine neurotoxins. In: Bjorklund A, Hokfelt T, eds. *Handbook of Chemical Neuroanatomy: Methods in Chemical Neuroanatomy.* Vol. 1: New York: Elsevier Science Publishers; 1983:463–507.
52. Oltmans GA, Lorden JF, Margules DL. Food intake and body weight: effects of specific and non-specific lesions in the midbrain path of the ascending noradrenergic neurons of the rat. Brain Res 1977;128:293–308.
53. Ahlskog JE, Randall PK, Hoebel BG. Hypothalamic hyperphagia: dissociation from hyperphagia following destruction of noradrenergic neurons. Science 1975;190:399–401.
54. Marshall JF, Richardson JS, Teitelbaum P. Nigrostriatal bundle damage and the lateral hypothalamic syndrome. J Comp Physiol Psychol 1974;87:808–830.
55. Jonsson G, Fuxe K, Hokfelt T, Goldstein M. Resistance of central phenylethanolamine-*n*-methyl transferase containing neurons to 6-hydroxydopamine. Med Biol 1976;54:421–426.
56. Blessing WW, Lappi DA, Wiley RG. Destruction of locus coeruleus neuronal perikarya after injection of anti-dopamine-β-hydroxylase immunotoxin into the olfactory bulb of the rat. Neurosci Lett 1998;243:85–88.
57. Westlund KN, Bowker RM, Ziegler MG, Coulter JD. Noradrenergic projections to the spinal cord of the rat. Brain Res 1983;263:15–31.

58. Cunningham ET Jr, Bohn MC, Sawchenko PE. Organization of adrenergic inputs to the paraventricular and supraoptic nuclei of the hypothalamus in the rat. J Comp Neurol 1990;292:651–667.
59. Ritter S, Bugarith K, Dinh TT. Immunotoxic destruction of distinct catecholamine subgroups produces selective impairment of glucoregulatory responses and neuronal activation. J Comp Neurol 2001;432:197–216.
60. Schreihofer AM, Guyenet PG. Sympathetic reflexes after depletion of bulbospinal catecholaminergic neurons with anti-DβH-saporin. Am J Physiol Regul Integr Comp Physiol 2000;279:R729–R742.
61. Ritter S, Watts AG, Dinh TT, Sanchez-Watts G, Pedrow C. Immunotoxin lesion of hypothalamically projecting norepinephrine and epinephrine neurons differentially affects circadian and stressor-stimulated corticosterone secretion. Endocrinology 2003;144:1357–1367.
62. Ritter S, Taylor JS. Vagal sensory neurons are required for lipoprivic but not glucoprivic feeding in rats. Am J Physiol 1990;258:R1395–R1401.
63. Scharrer E, Langhans W. Control of food intake by fatty acid oxidation. Am J Physiol 1986;250:R1003–R1006.
64. Hudson B, Ritter S. Hindbrain catecholamine neurons mediate consummatory responses to glucoprivation. Physiol Behav 2004;82:241–250.
65. Shor-Posner G, Azar AP, Insinga S, Leibowitz SF. Deficits in the control of food intake after hypothalamic paraventricular nucleus lesions. Physiol Behav 1985;35:883–890.
66. Calingasan NY, Ritter S. Hypothalamic paraventricular nucleus lesions do not abolish glucoprivic or lipoprivic feeding. Brain Res 1992;595:25–31.
67. Stanley BG, Leibowitz SF. Neuropeptide Y injected in the paraventricular hypothalamus: a powerful stimulant of feeding behavior. Proc Natl Acad Sci U S A 1985;82:3940–3943.
68. Stanley BG, Kyrkouli SE, Lampert S, Leibowitz SF. Neuropeptide Y chronically injected into the hypothalamus: a powerful neurochemical inducer of hyperphagia and obesity. Peptides 1986;7:1189–1192.
69. Hagan MM, Benoit SC, Rushing PA, Pritchard LM, Woods SC, Seeley RJ. Immediate and prolonged patterns of agouti-related peptide-(83–132)-induced *c-Fos* activation in hypothalamic and extrahypothalamic sites. Endocrinology 2001;142:1050–1056.
70. Hagan MM, Rushing PA, Pritchard LM, et al. Long-term orexigenic effects of AgRP-(83–132) involve mechanisms other than melanocortin receptor blockade. Am J Physiol Regul Integr Comp Physiol 2000;279:R47–R52.
71. Rossi M, Kim MS, Morgan DG, et al. A C-terminal fragment of agouti-related protein increases feeding and antagonizes the effect of α-melanocyte stimulating hormone in vivo. Endocrinology 1998;139:4428–4431.
72. Akabayashi A, Zaia CT, Silva I, Chae HJ, Leibowitz SF. Neuropeptide Y in the arcuate nucleus is modulated by alterations in glucose utilization. Brain Res 1993;621:343–348.
73. Kalra SP, Dube MG, Pu S, Xu B, Horvath TL, Kalra PS. Interacting appetite-regulating pathways in the hypothalamic regulation of body weight. Endocr Rev 1999;20:68–100.

74. Oomura Y, Ooyama H, Sugimori M, Nakamura T, Yamada Y. Glucose inhibition of the glucose-sensitive neurone in the rat lateral hypothalamus. Nature 1974;247:284–286.
75. Oomura Y. Glucose as a regulator of neuronal activity. Adv Metab Disord 1983;10:31–65.
76. Levin BE. Glucosensing neurons do more than just sense glucose. Int J Obes Relat Metab Disord 2001;25(suppl 5):S68–S72.
77. Levin BE, Dunn-Meynell AA, Routh VH. Brain glucosensing and the K(ATP) channel. Nat Neurosci 2001;4:459–460.
78. Lynch RM, Tompkins LS, Brooks HL, Dunn-Meynell AA, Levin BE. Localization of glucokinase gene expression in the rat brain. Diabetes 2000;49:693–700.
79. Sawchenko PE, Swanson LW. Immunohistochemical identification of neurons in the paraventricular nucleus of the hypothalamus that project to the medulla or to the spinal cord in the rat. J Comp Neurol 1982;205:260–272.
80. Guy J, Pelletier G. Neuronal interactions between neuropeptide Y (NPY) and catecholaminergic systems in the rat arcuate nucleus as shown by dual immunocytochemistry. Peptides 1988;9:567–570.
81. Broberger C, Johansen J, Johansson C, Schalling M, Hokfelt T. The neuropeptide Y/agouti gene-related protein (AGRP) brain circuitry in normal, anorectic, and monosodium glutamate-treated mice. Proc Natl Acad Sci USA 1998;95:15,043–15,048.
82. Herman JP, Cullinan WE. Neurocircuitry of stress: central control of the hypothalamo–pituitary–adrenocortical axis. Trends Neurosci 1997;20:78–84.
83. Van de Kar LD, Blair ML. Forebrain pathways mediating stress-induced hormone secretion. Front Neuroendocrinol 1999;20:1–48.
84. Matthews JN, Altman DG, Campbell MJ, Royston P. Analysis of serial measurements in medical research. BMJ 1990;300:230–235.
85. Levin BE, Sullivan AC. Glucose, insulin and sympathoadrenal activation. J Auton Nerv Syst 1987;20:233–242.
86. Rappaport EB, Young JB, Landsberg L. Effects of 2-deoxy-D-glucose on the cardiac sympathetic nerves and the adrenal medulla in the rat: further evidence for a dissociation of sympathetic nervous system and adrenal medullary responses. Endocrinology 1982;110:650–656.
87. Schneider JE, Goldman MD, Leo NA, Rosen ME. Central vs peripheral metabolic control of estrous cycles in Syrian hamsters. II. Glucoprivation. Am J Physiol 1997;272:R406–R412.
88. Abizaid A, Jafferali S, Pelletier JG, Woodside B. Effect of metabolic fuel availability on fertility varies with reproductive state. Physiol Behav 2001;74:77–83.
89. I'Anson H, Starer CA, Bonnema KR. Glucoprivic regulation of estrous cycles in the rat. Horm Behav 2003;43:388–393.
90. Nagatani S, Bucholtz DC, Murahashi K, et al. Reduction of glucose availability suppresses pulsatile luteinizing hormone release in female and male rats. Endocrinology 1996;137:1166–1170.
91. Bucholtz DC, Vidwans NM, Herbosa CG, Schillo KK, Foster DL. Metabolic interfaces between growth and reproduction. V. Pulsatile luteinizing hormone secretion is dependent on glucose availability. Endocrinology 1996;137:601–607.

92. Murahashi K, Bucholtz DC, Nagatani S, et al. Suppression of luteinizing hormone pulses by restriction of glucose availability is mediated by sensors in the brain stem. Endocrinology 1996;137:1171–1176.
93. I'Anson H, Sundling LA, Roland SM, Ritter S. Immunotoxic destruction of distinct catecholaminergic neuron populations disrupts the reproductive response to glucoprivation in female rats. Endocrinology 2003;144:4325–4331.

9

Cardiovascular Deficits After Lesions of C1 Adrenergic Neurons With a Saporin-Based Immunotoxin

Patrice G. Guyenet, Ruth L. Stornetta, and Ann M. Schreihofer

INTRODUCTION

Central nervous system (CNS) adrenergic neurons are located exclusively in the medulla oblongata *(1)*. The metabolism of CNS adrenaline, its turn-over rate, and its pharmacology were intensely studied in the late 1970s (reviewed in ref. *2*). Since then, the study of CNS adrenergic neurons has been the purview of integrative physiologists interested in stress, autonomic regulations, and the neural control of blood pressure and glucose. The CNS contains three clusters of adrenergic neurons: C1, C2, and C3 *(1)*. The main focus of this chapter is on the C1 neurons, especially those with spinal projections that are most important for sympathetic control and blood pressure regulation *(3–6)*.

Noradrenergic, dopaminergic, and serotonergic neurons have been selectively lesioned since the 1970s using drugs such as 6-hydroxydopamine (6-OHDA) or 5,7-di-OH tryptamine. These neurotoxins contributed greatly to the understanding of the physiological role of these particular aminergic neurons, but they have proven ineffective to lesion CNS adrenergic neurons *(7)*. Antidopamine β-hydroxylase saporin (anti-DβH-sap), an immunotoxin made of the ribosomal toxin saporin conjugated with an antibody to dopamine β-hydroxylase (DβH) is the first tool available for the selective destruction of CNS adrenergic neurons *(8–10)*. This chapter describes how the use of anti-DβH-sap has helped clarify the role of the C1 neurons.

From: *Molecular Neurosurgery With Targeted Toxins*
Edited by: R. G. Wiley and D. A. Lappi © Humana Press Inc., Totowa, NJ

The C1 Adrenergic Neurons, Unusual Members of the Aminergic Family

The defining characteristic of the C1 group is the presence of phenylethylamine *N*-methyl transferase (PNMT) *(1)*, the enzyme that converts noradrenaline into adrenaline *(2)*. The C1 neurons also contain tyrosine hydroxylase (TH), DβH *(11)*, and a vesicular monoamine transporter *(12)*. The C1 neurons are located in the reticular formation of the medulla oblongata caudal to the facial motor nucleus, and their axonal projections are more restricted than that of CNS noradrenergic neurons *(1)*. The rostral half of the C1 cells project to a variety of lower brainstem and midbrain structures involved in autonomic regulations, but their defining characteristic is a spinal projection that targets sympathetic preganglionic neurons with considerable selectivity *(1,13)*. This connection is largely monosynaptic *(14)*.

Although the spinal terminals of C1 cells contain PNMT, evidence that they contain, no less release, adrenaline remains controversial *(2,15)*. The controversy stems from the still-unresolved technical difficulty in detecting very low levels of adrenaline in the presence of high levels of noradrenaline. The caudal group of C1 cells does not project to the cord. Instead, these cells innervate selected regions of the hypothalamus that regulate blood pressure and many endocrine responses associated with stress *(16–18)*. There is excellent evidence that the hypothalamic projections of C1 cells do synthesize adrenaline *(2)*.

Like all monoaminergic neurons, C1 neurons express a variety of neuropeptides (e.g., neuropeptide Y, enkephalins, cocaine- and amphetamine-regulated transcript [CART]) *(19–22)*. The pattern of expression of these peptides varies according to a neuroanatomical code that is still not understood in functional terms. Contrary to noradrenergic neurons, most adrenergic neurons do not express the noradrenaline transporter (NET) *(23)*, and they have no other known catecholaminergic membrane transporter. This peculiarity of C1 neurons is the most likely reason for their resistance to 6-OHDA and related toxins. The selectivity of 6-OHDA relies on the ability of susceptible neurons to concentrate this chemical via their membrane transporter (e.g., NET for noradrenergic cells) to intracellular levels that are high enough to produce toxic levels of reactive oxygen species *(24)*.

Presympathetic Role of Bulbospinal C1 Cells

The earliest evidence that adrenergic cells must play some role in sympathetic tone generation can be traced to the 1973–1974 immunohistochemical work of Hökfelt et al., who demonstrated that, in the spinal cord, PNMT immunoreactivity is almost exclusively confined to the thoracic and lumbar intermediolateral cell column *(1)*. This histological work also established the C1 group of the ventrolateral medulla as one of very few potential sources of adrenergic innervation of the spinal cord.

Physiological research conducted during the late 1970s and early 1980s gradually identified the C1 region as essential for blood pressure regulation and sympathetic tone generation *(3,25)* (for review, *see* chapter 5 in ref. *26*). Soon after, electrophysiologists found that the C1 region contains bulbospinal neurons with a discharge pattern closely related to that of the sympathetic ganglionic neurons that innervate the heart, kidney, or blood vessels of the skeletal muscles and splanchnic area *(27,28)*. These cells are now considered to be excitatory sympathetic premotor neurons that control sympathetic tone to the heart and blood vessels and mediate the baroreflex *(5)*. Definitive evidence that some of these bulbospinal rostral ventrolateral medulla (RVLM) cells are C1 neurons had to await the results of single-cell labeling experiments in vivo *(29–31)*.

These experiments also demonstrated that around 30% of the bulbospinal neurons of the RVLM with discharge properties consistent with a sympathetic premotor role did not contain TH and therefore were not C1 neurons. This observation fueled a controversy over the relative contribution of C1 and noncatecholaminergic neurons to the generation of the vasomotor tone and whether C1 or the other premotor neurons are glutamatergic *(5)*. The theory that bulbospinal presympathetic neurons might be glutamatergic derives from the observation that glutamate receptor antagonists administered into the cord reduce sympathetic outflow and the discharges of preganglionic neurons evoked by stimulation of the RVLM *(32–34)*. The source of the glutamate released by RVLM stimulation has been difficult to ascertain because the bulbospinal projection includes both C1 and noncatecholaminergic neurons *(29,31)*.

The existence of presympathetic neurons devoid of the C1 phenotype opened the door to many alternative interpretations of the role of the RVLM and of the C1 cells. One was that the non-C1 presympathetic neurons were the only glutamatergic neurons in this pathway, and that these cells were the main source of excitatory drive to sympathetic preganglionic neurons. According to this view, the C1 cells could be a gain-setting system, perhaps boosting the effectiveness of the glutamatergic pathway during arousal and stress, a concept derived from parallel speculations concerning the effect of the locus coeruleus *(35)*. This hypothesis was consistent with the fact that C1 cells, like locus coeruleus neurons, are activated by a broad spectrum of behavioral and physical stresses, as judged by Fos expression studies *(36–38)*.

One could also envision that the C1 neurons provide both excitation or inhibition, depending on the type of preganglionic neurons that they target, and thus cause a pattern of cardiovascular responses such as that associated with the fight-or-flight response (splanchnic vasoconstriction, muscle vasodilation, and increased cardiac output). This hypothesis, still not definitively ruled out, was consistent with the fact that catecholamines can produce both inhibition and excitation of preganglionic neurons *(39)*. It also agrees with the fact that C1 neurons target numerous classes of preganglionic neurons *(40)*.

The final alternative was that both C1 and non-C1 RVLM presympathetic cells might be glutamatergic, and that catecholamines are just one of many secondary transmitters differentially expressed by subgroups of these presympathetic neurons. The availability of anti-DβH-sap allowed testing some of these issues by analyzing the nature of the physiological deficits caused by selective lesions of the C1 cells. *(8,9)*.

LESION OF C1 ADRENERGIC NEURONS WITH AN ANTIBODY TO DβH CONJUGATED WITH SAPORIN: THEORY AND PRACTICE

DβH is a membrane-bound enzyme of the dense core vesicles that is transiently exteriorized on the plasma membrane of noradrenergic and adrenergic neurons following exocytotic vesicular fusion. The toxicity of anti-DβH-sap is therefore attributed to the fact that DβH is accessible for binding to anti-DβH-sap present in the extracellular fluid *(41,42)*. The complex between DβH and anti-DβH-sap is then presumably internalized as the vesicle membrane is recycled, providing a means of entry for the ribosomal toxin saporin into the neuron. Neuronal toxicity requires saporin to be transported back to the cell body in its active form.

Experimentation proved that anti-DβH-sap is indeed retrogradely transported over long distances and in sufficient amounts to cause the destruction of noradrenergic and adrenergic cell bodies *(9,43,44)*. Specifically, a single toxin injection of anti-DβH-sap into the olfactory bulb destroyed a substantial fraction of the locus coeruleus neurons *(44)*, and injections into the paraventricular region of the hypothalamus destroyed a large fraction of the A5, A6, and C1 cells of the pontomedullary region *(43)*. Similarly, injections of anti-DβH-sap into the spinal cord destroyed A5, A7, and some A6 noradrenergic neurons, as well as C1 adrenergic neurons with spinal projections *(9,43)*. The sensitivity of C1 cells to spinal injections of anti-DβH-sap is evidence that the spinal terminals of C1 cells exteriorize DβH and therefore is evidence that these cells release catecholamines. Whether noradrenaline or adrenaline is released by C1 cells in the spinal cord is unresolved *(15)*.

In theory, anti-DβH-sap should destroy noradrenergic and adrenergic neurons with a high degree of selectivity because DβH is present exclusively in these two classes of neurons. In practice, the selectivity of anti-DβH-sap against catecholaminergic neurons may not be as large as would be expected *a priori* from a compound with as high affinity and specificity as an antibody, especially when the toxin is injected intraparenchymally. Depending on the report, the selectivity of the lesion caused by intraparenchymal injections of anti-DβH-sap is assessed as very high *(43)*, marginal but adequate *(10)*, or probably inadequate *(8)*. These differing points of view are presented, and an attempt is made to outline potential reasons for these divergent conclusions.

The study of Ritter and colleagues *(43)* described the effect of anti-DβH-sap injection into the region of the paraventricular nucleus of the hypothalamus (PVH). A dose of 42 ng in 200 nL (0.25 pmol assuming a molecular weight of around 210,000) was injected on each, side and the tissue was examined 4 to 6 wk later. Despite extensive loss of TH-immunoreactive terminals in the hypothalamus and massive retrograde degeneration of brainstem noradrenergic or adrenergic neurons, nonspecific tissue damage at the level of the injection site was described as minimal to nonexistent. This assessment was based on the apparent integrity of the cytoarchitecture of the PVH following Nissl staining and the persistence of Fos expression in PVH neurons after hypothalamic injections of epinephrine.

Madden et al. injected anti-DβH-sap directly into the ventrolateral medulla to destroy C1 cell bodies *(10)*. In most experiments, histology was typically performed 2 wk after toxin injection. A dose of 53 ng of anti-DβH-sap (0.25 pmol in 200 nL) produced "obvious necrosis at the injection site" *(10)*. The published illustrations showed severe gliosis and what appears following Nissl stain to be major, if not total, neuronal loss in a region at least 600 μm in diameter surrounding the injection site. Half this dose (21 ng) was required to destroy the bulk of the underlying C1 cells while preserving many surrounding neurons, whereas smaller doses produced C1 cell losses too small to be of use.

Madden et al. provided evidence of toxin selectivity at the 21-ng dose (0.125 pmol), although this dose still caused persistent (>2 wk) gliosis and, in 35% of the subjects, a small necrotic core *(10)*. The evidence for selectivity was based on the observation that Fos immunoreactivity could be induced by arterial pressure elevation in the same number of bulbospinal non-C1 RVLM cells in rats treated with anti-DβH-sap as in control rats treated with saporin conjugated with a non-immune immunoglobulin G (IgG). The non-C1 cells of the RVLM that express Fos after short-term hypertension are noncatecholaminergic sympathetic premotor neurons that are interspersed with the bulbospinal C1 cells *(8,9)*. In short, Madden et al. concluded that anti-DβH-sap could produce selective lesions of C1 cell bodies but only within a very narrow range of dose and at the cost of some nonselective neuronal damage at the injection site.

Our experience with intraparenchymal injections of anti-DβH-sap into the RVLM is more limited but similar to that of Madden and colleagues (unpublished results of AM Schreihofer and PG Guyenet, 1999). We observed large necrotic lesions with doses of 0.25 pmol anti-DβH-sap injected in 50 nL of sterile saline and negligible effects with doses of 0.07 pmol or less. Of note, a long-lasting gliosis (>15 d) was observed following doses (0.07 pmol) that were marginally effective in lesioning C1 neurons. The gliosis was not attributable to the elimination of the damaged local aminergic cell bodies because it was also observed when the toxin was injected in regions of the medulla that contained no catecholaminergic cell bodies. Although we have no evidence that the gliosis has significant physiological consequences on the surrounding neuronal networks, we abandoned the intraparenchymal injection of anti-DβH-sap as a means of destroying C1 cells selectively out of concern that this apparent inflammatory process might have deleterious consequences on the local networks.

Most of our experience is with injections of anti-DβH-sap into the spinal terminal fields of the C1 cells because our purpose was to destroy the C1 cells with spinal projections while sparing the rest of the C1 group *(8,9)*. This goal was achieved using four injections of 0.2 pmol of anti-DβH-sap into the thoracic cord in a volume of 100 or 200 nL. After 2 wk, the number of bulbospinal neurons that contained DβH (C1, A5, A6, A7) was severely reduced, but the rest of the bulbospinal projections of the pontomedullary region, including serotonergic neurons, was intact. Of note, 2 wk after injection, the region that previously contained the bulbospinal C1 cells was gliosis free and histologically intact after Nissl staining *(9)*. Finally, equivalent amounts of saporin conjugated to a nonimmune IgG (control toxin) produced no detectable effect on the bulbospinal projections.

On the negative side, however, both anti-DβH-sap and the control toxin produced a macroscopically obvious necrosis at the spinal injection sites, although behavioral deficits were not readily detectable. Anti-DβH-sap destroyed a slightly larger percentage of bulbospinal pontine noradrenergic neurons than bulbospinal adrenergic ones. The differential sensitivity of these two groups of cells to anti-DβH-sap could be caused by several factors. NE axons may have more collaterals within each spinal segment than the C1 cells. Alternately, NE terminals may exteriorize more DβH on the membrane of their terminals.

The selectivity of the lesions caused by intraprenchymal injections of anti-DβH-sap may be influenced by the volume and speed of injection. The dose of toxin does not seem at issue because all investigators found the same dose was optimal (0.2–0.25 pmol). The volume and speed of injection were identical in two of the studies (200 nL in 30–120 s), but injections were done more quickly in our studies, which raises the most serious selectivity concerns. Slower injections are beneficial to selectivity by limiting the maximal concentration reached at the injection site.

The time at which lesion selectivity is assessed is also probably a factor. The study of Ritter and colleagues *(43)* examined tissue from 6 wk up to months after injection, whereas Madden et al. *(10)* and Schreihofer et al. *(8,9)* examined the tissue after 2 to 3 wk. After very long periods, it is likely that all damaged neurons, whether selectively or nonselectively destroyed, would have been completely eliminated, which could provide an unduly optimistic assessment of the selectivity.

The severe gliosis observed 2 wk after microinjection of anti-DβH-sap directly into the RVLM cannot be accounted simply by glial cell scavenging of the lesioned C1 cells because following toxin injection into the spinal cord, the RVLM region that contained C1 cells was entirely gliosis free *(8,9)*. In our hands, spinal injections of saporin conjugated with a nonimmune IgG produced similar nonspecific lesions as anti-DβH-sap at the level of the injection site, although brainstem catecholaminergic cell bodies were spared by the control toxin. Our interpretation is therefore that nonselective uptake of saporin by local cells (neurons or others) is causing the local damage. Are similar problems encountered with other saporin-based toxins?

We also encountered specificity problems with another saporin conjugate, SSP-SAP (saporin combined to a selective neurokinin-1 receptor agonist) *(45)*, but in this case the problems were surmountable. The ratio between the intraparenchymal dose that selectively lesioned NK1R-expressing neurons (0.31 ng, 0.01 pmol assuming a molecular weight of 31,000) and that which caused a small, nonspecific necrosis at the injection site was around fourfold. The 0.01-pmol dose of SSP-SAP did not cause necrosis and exhibited clear selectivity because it destroyed the vast majority of the NK1R-expressing neurons without causing a detectable loss of an intermingled control population of neurons. Interestingly, the control population in this case was the C1 cells.

The key for the greater selectivity of SSP-SAP vs anti-DβH-sap may be the saporin dose and, ultimately, its concentration in the injectate. Indeed, the dose of SSP-SAP found useful for selective lesion of NK1R-expressing cells was less than a 10th that of anti-DβH-sap needed to destroy the C1 cells on a molar basis (0.01 vs 0.125 pmol). It is logical to assume that the use of much lower concentrations of conjugated saporin in the injectate minimizes the damage caused by nonselective uptake of saporin.

Finally, the fact that the somata of C1 neurons are somewhat more sensitive than surrounding neurons to anti-DβH-sap injections into the RVLM suggests that the C1 cells may exteriorize some DβH *(10)*. By extension, the observation suggests that these neurons may be capable of exocytotic release of catecholamines within the RVLM, either via recurrent collaterals or via dendritic release. This possibility is consistent with the fact that catecholamines are tonically released in the ventrolateral medulla *(46,47)*, but there is no proof that C1 cells are the source of these catecholamines because the ventrolateral medulla contains nerve terminals that originate in the A6 or A5 (pontine) noradrenergic neurons. The difficulty of lesioning C1 cells selectively via intraparenchymal injections of anti-DβH-sap could be because these cells exteriorize relatively little DβH.

In summary, our experience with two different saporin conjugates suggested that the ability of these toxins to destroy a given neuronal type selectively by injecting the toxin in their midst should not be taken on faith. One possible explanation for the surprisingly low selectivity of intraparenchymal injections is that toxin concentrations in the 0.1–1μM range need to be injected for the toxin to spread into a useful volume of tissue. At these high concentrations, nonspecific uptake may occur at the center of the injection site, possibly via ordinary pinocytosis, causing the nonspecific lesion of a variety of cell types, conceivably including vascular and glial cells. Therefore, the intraparenchymal use of these toxins requires careful titration to determine the lowest effective dose, a fairly long process. Selectivity must then be established by injecting unliganded saporin or, preferably, saporin liganded to an inactive form of the conjugate (e.g., saporin conjugated to a nonimmune IgG as a control for anti-DβH-sap).

Finally, appropriate histological controls must be used. In most studies, including ours, toxin selectivity has been established by showing that the conjugate spares a neuronal type other than the targeted one *(8,9,45,48)*. Evidence of this type is the minimum necessary to show that the effect of the toxin is selective, but it does not prove that the toxin destroys the targeted neurons with total specificity, that is, exclusive of any other type.

EFFECTS OF SPINAL INJECTIONS OF ANTI-DβH-SAP ON SYMPATHETIC TONE AND BLOOD PRESSURE

Two weeks after bilateral injections of anti-DβH-sap into the upper thoracic spinal cord, the rats presented with more than more than 85% loss of their bulbospinal C1 projection *(8,9)*. These rats had the same resting blood pressure as control (IgG-saporin-treated) rats under anesthesia, and they still retained an apparently normal sympathetic tone. However, the range of their baroreflex was attenuated, suggesting that they could not increase sympathetic tone to the same extent as the controls in response to hypotensive challenges *(9)*. Lesioned rats also had a reduced ability to elevate their sympathetic tone in response to stimulation of peripheral chemoreceptors *(9)*.

Finally, electrical stimulation of the RVLM in lesioned rats produced greatly reduced evoked responses in the splanchnic nerve *(8)*. Complete destruction of A5 neurons with 6-OHDA injections in the vicinity of their cell bodies did not reproduce the autonomic deficits caused by injections of anti-DβH-sap into the spinal cord, suggesting that these deficits were caused by the loss of the C1 cells, not loss of the A5 pontine noradrenergic neurons *(8)*. A5 neurons innervate the same general spectrum of brain targets as the C1 cells, including the sympathetic preganglionic neurons *(40,49,50)*.

In summary, these experiments not only demonstrated that rats with massive lesions of C1 cells have difficulties coping with conditions that require elevation of sympathetic vasomotor tone, but also showed that the animals maintained a basal sympathetic tone and a normal blood pressure under resting conditions. The data supported the notion that C1 cells exert a stimulating effect on the vasomotor outflow that is especially critical under conditions of stress.

Why is blood pressure unaffected by a massive loss of C1 cells, and why do these rats retain an apparently normal basal sympathetic tone? One possibility is that, after C1 cell lesion, a different brain area takes over the role of generating the sympathetic outflow. This is clearly not the case because the injection of the γ-aminobutyric acid (GABA)-mimetic muscimol into the RVLM produces equally massive drops in sympathetic tone and blood pressure in C1-lesioned as in intact rats *(8)*.

A second possibility is that, under resting conditions, sympathetic tone and resting blood pressure rely primarily on the nonaminergic component of the presympathetic projection from the RVLM. This interpretation is consistent with the data of Madden et al. *(10)*, who showed that, after treatment of the RVLM with anti-DβH-sap, the majority of the remaining RVLM neurons that expressed Fos following sustained hypotension were noncatecholaminergic. This experiment suggested that the toxin might have spared the noncatecholaminergic component of the presympathetic pathway. This interpretation agrees with our electrophysiological evidence. Indeed, treatment with anti-DβH-sap eliminated the vast majority of bulbospinal C1 cells, and the vast majority of the surviving presympathetic neurons that could be identified electrophysiologically were of the noncatecholaminergic variety *(8)*.

The experiments with anti-DβH-sap achieved two objectives. First, they generated much-needed additional evidence for the existence of nonaminergic presympathetic neurons *(29,31)*. Second, they provided a satisfactory explanation for why basal sympathetic tone and blood pressure are maintained after massive lesions of the bulbospinal C1 cells. The probable reason is simply that even massive lesions of the C1 cells spare a large component (about 30%) of the presympathetic neurons consisting largely of neurons that do not express the catecholaminergic phenotype.

SUMMARY

Anti-DβH-sap is a very effective tool to destroy adrenergic neurons in a retrograde fashion following introduction of the toxin into terminal fields. Furthermore, it seems that the toxin is not significantly taken up by noncatecholaminergic nerve terminals exposed to the toxin; therefore, neurons located some distance away from the injection site and projecting to or through the injection site appear to be spared. On the negative side, nonspecific tissue damage occurs at the injection site, making the toxin only minimally selective for the purpose of destroying adrenergic cells by injecting the toxin in their midst. The selectivity of intraparenchymal injections may be increased somewhat by using very slow injections of diluted toxin.

Despite the above caveats, anti-DβH-sap has been a useful tool to investigate the role of the C1 cells. It has provided the first opportunity to examine the consequences of their selective destruction in the adult rat. The results of these studies suggest that C1 presympathetic cells play a major role in raising sympathetic tone and blood pressure under conditions of stress (e.g., hypotension, hypoxia, probably many others), but their integrity appears nonessential under resting conditions.

These results do not contradict established dogma *(38,40,51)*. Their interest is that they provide the first hard evidence of a causal relationship between C1 cell activation and sympathoexcitatory responses. Indeed, the theory that C1 cells are sympathoexcitatory was based on convergent but nevertheless correlative evidence. Specifically, the theory relied on the fact that these cells express Fos under a variety of stresses *(17,38,51–53)*, that they have appropriate axonal projections *(14)*, and that their discharge is profoundly inhibited by baroreceptor stimulation in anesthetized animals *(29,31)*. The use of anti-DβH-sap has also been helpful in supporting the notion that the C1 cells constitute only a portion, albeit significant (around two thirds), of the presympathetic cells of the RVLM *(8,29,31)*. Finally, the use of anti-DβH-saporin has allowed demonstration that maintenance of blood pressure under resting conditions is compatible with the destruction of over 85% of the C1 cells with bulbospinal projections.

EPILOGUE

The bulbospinal C1 cells were recently found to contain vesicular glutamate trasnporter (VGLUT)-2 messenger ribonucleic acid (mRNA), a diagnostic marker of glutamatergic neurons *(54,55)*. The pontine noradrenergic neurons (e.g., locus coeruleus, A5) do not express VGLUT-1 or VGLUT-2 *(55)*, suggesting that, contrary to the C1 cells, these classic noradrenergic cell groups are probably not glutamatergic. Furthermore, the presence of VGLUT-2 mRNA in both C1 and non-C1 presympathetic neurons suggests that both types of neurons are glutamatergic *(55)*.

In light of this evidence, the significance of the C1 phenotype must be reevaluated. The notion that the presympathetic vasomotor neurons of the RVLM consist of C1 catecholaminergic neurons with a modulatory role and non-C1 glutamatergic neurons that provide the basic excitatory glutamatergic drive is clearly no longer tenable *(5,56)*. To accommodate the latest results on VGLUT-2, it is necessary to envision that the presympathetic projection from the RVLM consists of a collection of predominantly glutamatergic neurons that express various combinations of additional neurotransmitters *(20–22)*. The C1 cells are a numerically dominant subgroup of these neurons (about 70%) that express catecholamine biosynthetic enzymes and probably release catecholamines.

ACKNOWLEDGMENT

This work was supported by a National Heart, Lung, and Blood Institute grant (HL28785) to P. G. G.

REFERENCES

1. Hokfelt T, Fuxe K, Goldstein M, Johansson O. Immunohistochemical evidence for the existence of adrenaline neurons in the rat brain. Brain Res 1974;66:235–251.
2. Fuller RW. Pharmacology of brain epinephrine neurons. Annu Rev Pharmacol Toxicol 1982;22:31–55.
3. Ross CA, Ruggiero DA, Joh TH, Park DH, Reis DJ. Adrenaline synthesizing neurons in the rostral ventrolateral medulla: a possible role in tonic vasomotor control. Brain Res 1983;273:356–361.
4. Dampney RAL. Functional organization of central pathways regulating the cardiovascular system. Physiol Rev 1994;74:323–364.
5. Guyenet PG. Neural structures that mediate sympathoexcitation during hypoxia. Respir Physiol 2000;121:147–162.

6. Sun MK. Pharmacology of reticulospinal vasomotor neurons in cardiovascular regulation. Pharmacol Rev 1996;48:465–494.

7. Jonsson G, Fuxe K, Hokfelt T, Goldstein M. Resistance of central phenylethanolamine-*n*-methyl transferase containing neurons to 6-hydroxydopamine. Medical Biol 1976;54:421–426.

8. Schreihofer AM, Stornetta RL, Guyenet PG. Regulation of sympathetic tone and arterial pressure by rostral ventrolateral medulla after depletion of C1 cells in rat. J Physiol (Lond) 2000;529:221–236.

9. Schreihofer AM, Guyenet PG. Sympathetic reflexes after depletion of bulbospinal catecholaminergic neurons with anti-DβH-saporin. Am J Physiol Regul Integr Comp Physiol 2000;279:R729–R742.

10. Madden CJ, Ito S, Rinaman L, Wiley RG, Sved AF. Lesions of the C1 catecholaminergic neurons of the ventrolateral medulla in rats using anti-DβH-saporin. Am J Physiol Regul Integr Comp Physiol 1999;277:R1063–R1075.

11. Phillips JK, Goodchild AK, Dubey R, et al. Differential expression of catecholamine biosynthetic enzymes in the rat ventrolateral medulla. J Comp Neurol 2001;432:20–34.

12. Peter D, Liu YJ, Sternini C, De Giorgio R, Brecha N, Edwards RH. Differential expression of two vesicular monoamine transporters. J Neurosci 1995;15:6179–6188.

13. Ross CA, Armstrong DM, Ruggiero DA, Pickel VM, Joh TH, Reis DJ. Adrenaline neurons in the rostral ventrolateral medulla innervate thoracic spinal cord: a combined immunocytochemical and retrograde transport demonstration. Neurosci Lett 1981;25:257–262.

14. Milner TA, Morrison SF, Abate C, Reis DJ. Phenylethanolamine *N*-methyltransferase-containing terminals synapse directly on sympathetic preganglionic neurons in the rat. Brain Res 1988;448:205–222.

15. Sved AF. PNMT-containing catecholaminergic neurons are not necessarily adrenergic. Brain Res 1989;481:113–118.

16. Tucker DC, Saper CB, Ruggiero DA, Reis DJ. Organization of central adrenergic pathways: I. Relationships of ventrolateral medullary projections to the hypothalamus and spinal cord. J Comp Neurol 1987;259:591–603.

17. Chan RKW, Sawchenko PE. Organization and transmitter specificity of medullary neurons activated by sustained hypertension: implications for understanding baroreceptor reflex circuitry. J Neurosci 1998;18:371–387.

18. Cunningham ET, Jr., Bohn MC, Sawchenko PE. Organization of adrenergic inputs to the paraventricular and supraoptic nuclei of the hypothalamus in the rat. J Comp Neurol 1990;292:651–667.

19. Jansen ASP, Wessendorf MW, Loewy AD. Transneuronal labeling of CNS neuropeptide and monoamine neurons after pseudorabies virus injections into the stellate ganglion. Brain Res 1995;683:1–24.

20. Dun SL, Ng YK, Brailoiu GC, Ling EA, Dun NJ. Cocaine- and amphetamine-regulated transcript peptide-immunoreactivity in adrenergic C1 neurons projecting to the intermediolateral cell column of the rat. J Chem Neuroanat 2002;23:123–132.

21. Stornetta RL, Schreihofer AM, Pelaez NM, Sevigny CP, Guyenet PG. Preproenkephalin mRNA is expressed by C1 and non-C1 barosensitive bulbospinal neurons in the rostral ventrolateral medulla of the rat. J Comp Neurol 2001;435:111–126.
22. Stornetta RL, Akey PJ, Guyenet PG. Location and electrophysiological characterization of rostral medullary adrenergic neurons that contain neuropeptide Y mRNA in rat. J Comp Neurol 1999;415:482–500.
23. Lorang D, Amara SG, Simerly RB. Cell-type-specific expression of catecholamine transporters in the rat brain. J Neurosci 1994;14:4903–4914.
24. Glinka Y, Gassen M, Youdim MB. Mechanism of 6-hydroxydopamine neurotoxicity. J Neural Trans Suppl 1997;50:55–66.
25. Reis DJ, Ross CA, Ruggiero DA, Granata AR, Joh TH. Role of adrenaline neurons of ventrolateral medulla (the C1 group) in the tonic and phasic control of arterial pressure. Clin Exp Hypertension Part A Theory Pract 1984;6:221–241.
26. Blessing WW. *The Lower Brainstem and Bodily Homeostasis.* New York: Oxford University Press; 1997.
27. Brown DL, Guyenet PG. Electrophysiological study of cardiovascular neurons in the rostral ventrolateral medulla in rats. Circ Res 1985;56:359–369.
28. Barman SM, Gebber GL. Axonal projection patterns of ventrolateral medullospinal sympathoexcitatory neurons. J Neurophys 1985;53:1551–1566.
29. Schreihofer AM, Guyenet PG. Identification of C1 presympathetic neurons in rat rostral ventrolateral medulla by juxtacellular labeling in vivo. J Comp Neurol 1997;387:524–536.
30. Lipski J, Kanjhan R, Kruszewska B, Rong WF. Properties of presympathetic neurones in the rostral ventrolateral medulla in the rat: an intracellular study "in vivo." J Physiol (Lond) 1996;490:729–744.
31. Lipski J, Kanjhan R, Kruszewska B, Smith M. Barosensitive neurons in the rostral ventrolateral medulla of the rat in vivo: morphological properties and relationship to C1 adrenergic neurons. Neuroscience 1995;69:601–618.
32. Huangfu D, Hwang LJ, Riley TA, Guyenet PG. Role of serotonin and catecholamines in sympathetic responses evoked by stimulation of rostral medulla. Am J Physiol Regul Integr Comp Physiol 1994;266:R338–R352.
33. Morrison SF, Callaway J, Milner TA, Reis DJ. Glutamate in the spinal sympathetic intermediolateral nucleus: localization by light and electron microscopy. Brain Res 1989;503:5–15.
34. Morrison SF, Callaway J, Milner TA, Reis DJ. Rostral ventrolateral medulla—a source of the glutamatergic innervation of the sympathetic intermediolateral nucleus. Brain Res 1991;562:126–135.
35. Aston-Jones G, Rajkowski J, Kubiak P, Valentino RJ, Shipley MT. Role of the locus coeruleus in emotional activation. Prog Brain Res 1996;107:379–402.
36. Larsen PJ, Mikkelsen JD. Functional identification of central afferent projections conveying information of acute "stress" to the hypothalamic paraventricular nucleus. J Neurosci 1995;15:2609–2627.
37. Ericsson A, Kovacs KJ, Sawchenko PE. A functional anatomical analysis of central pathways subserving the effects of interleukin-1 on stress-related neuroendocrine neurons. J Neurosci 1994;14:897–913.

38. Chan RKW, Sawchenko PE. Spatially and temporally differentiated patterns of c-*fos* expression in the brainstem catecholaminergic cell groups induced by cardiovascular challenges in the rat. J Comp Neurol 1994;34:433–460.

39. Inokuchi H, Yoshimura M, Polosa C, Nishi S. Adrenergic receptors (α1 and α2) modulate different potassium conductances in sympathetic preganglionic neurons. Can J Physiol Pharmacol 1992;70(suppl):S92–S97.

40. Jansen ASP, Nguyen XV, Karpitskiy V, Mettenleiter TC, Loewy AD. Central command neurons of the sympathetic nervous system: basis of the fight-or flight response. Science 1995;270:644–646.

41. Wiley RG, Kline RH. Neuronal lesioning with axonally transported toxins. J Neurosci Methods 2000;103:73–82.

42. Wrenn CC, Picklo MJ, Lappi DA, Robertson D, Wiley RG. Central noradrenergic lesioning using anti-DBH-saporin: anatomical findings. Brain Res 1996;74:175–184.

43. Ritter S, Bugarith K, Dinh TT. Immunotoxic destruction of distinct catecholamine subgroups produces selective impairment of glucoregulatory responses and neuronal activation. J Comp Neurol 2001;432:197–216.

44. Blessing WW, Lappi DA, Wiley RG. Destruction of locus coeruleus neuronal perikarya after injection of anti-dopamine-β-hydroxylase immunotoxin into the olfactory bulb of the rat. Neurosci Lett 1998;243:85–88.

45. Wang H, Germanson T.P., Guyenet PG. Depressor and tachypneic responses to chemical stimulation of the ventral respiratory group are reduced by ablation of neurokinin-1 receptor-expressing neurons. J Neurosci 2002;22:3755–3764.

46. Huangfu D, Goodwin WB, Guyenet PG. Sympatholytic effect of tricyclic antidepressants: site and mechanism of action in anesthetized rats. Am J Physiol Regul Integr Comp Physiol 1995;268: R1429–R1441.

47. Rentero N, Bruandet N, Quintin L. Rostral ventrolateral medulla catechol involvement upon sino-aortic deafferentation—an in vivo voltammetric study. Life Sci 2000;68:177–189.

48. Gray PA, Janczewski WA, Mellen N, McCrimmon DR, Feldman JL. Normal breathing requires pre-Bötzinger complex neurokinin-1 receptor-expressing neurons. Nat Neurosci 2001;4:927–930.

49. Sved AF, Cano G, Card JP. Neuroanatomical specificity of the circuits controlling sympathetic outflow to different targets. Clin Exp Pharmacol Physiol 2001;28:115–119.

50. Byrum CE, Guyenet PG. Afferent and efferent connections of the A5 noradrenergic cell group in the rat. J Comp Neurol 1987;261:529–542.

51. Dampney RAL, Coleman MJ, Fontes MAP, et al. Central mechanisms underlying short- and long-term regulation of the cardiovascular system. Clin Exp Pharmacol Physiol 2002;29:261–268.

52. Horiuchi J, Potts PD, Polson JW, Dampney RAL. Distribution of neurons projecting to the rostral ventrolateral medullary pressor region that are activated by sustained hypotension. Neuroscience 1999;89:1319–1329.

53. Dampney RAL, Li Y-W, Hirooka Y, Potts P, Polson JW. Use of c-*fos* functional mapping to identify the central baroreceptor reflex pathway: advantages and limitations. Clin Exp Hypertension 1995;17:197–208.

54. Takamori S, Rhee JS, Rosenmund C, Jahn R. Identification of differentiation-associated brain-specific phosphate transporter as a second vesicular glutamate transporter (VGLUT2). J Neurosci 2001;21:NIL7–NIL12.
55. Stornetta RL, Sevigny CP, Guyenet PG. Vesicular glutamate transporter DNPI/VGLUT2 mRNA is present in C1 and several other groups of brainstem catecholaminergic neurons. J Comp Neurol 2002;444:191–206.
56. Guyenet PG. Role of the ventral medulla oblongata in blood pressure regulation. In: Loewy AD, Spyer KM, eds. *Central Regulation of Autonomic Functions*. New York: Oxford University Press; 1990:145–167.

10

Saporin Conjugates and Pain

Ronald G. Wiley and Douglas A. Lappi

INTRODUCTION

Several saporin-containing targeted toxins have been used in studies of nociception/pain. This chapter reviews this exciting area, including some of our most recent work. Certainly, substance P-saporin (SP-sap), the first conjugate used for pain research, has generated the most data and interest, but a number of other saporin conjugates have been introduced, and others are on the way. A review discusses this topic *(1)*.

A large body of evidence has long pointed to a role for SP in nociception (*see*, e.g., refs. *2* and *3*). However, this mass of data has not yet resulted in a comprehensive formulation of the exact role of SP in nociception or led to a useful therapeutic strategy based on SP or SP antagonists. The potential for SP antagonists in clinical management of pain remains controversial. A reasonable distillation of the state of knowledge as of 1994 was the conclusion that some primary nociceptive neurons make and release SP, and dorsal horn neurons with neurokinin-1 receptor (NK-1R) are nociceptive. However, SP-secreting dorsal root ganglion neurons release other transmitters, particularly glutamate, which may explain the limited clinical analgesic efficacy of SP antagonists.

Development of SP-sap began in 1994 and was based on evidence for the roles of NK-1R-expressing dorsal horn neurons in nociception coupled with the evidence for receptor-mediated endocytosis of SP. Mantyh and coworkers *(4)* showed that SP is selectively internalized by cells expressing NK-1R, consistent with the general tendency for G protein-coupled receptors to internalize on binding of appropriate ligand. Subsequent studies have shown internalization of SP in neurons of the superficial dorsal horn in response to noxious stimuli *(5)*.

From: *Molecular Neurosurgery With Targeted Toxins*
Edited by: R. G. Wiley and D. A. Lappi © Humana Press Inc., Totowa, NJ

Reasoning that dorsal horn cells that internalize SP were important second-order nociceptive neurons, we set out to make and test the properties of SP conjugated to saporin for selectively destroying dorsal horn neurons that express the NK-1R. At that time, there existed a few reports of other neuropeptide–toxin conjugates *(6–10)*, suggesting the approach was feasible. Initial experiments confirmed that SP-sap was selectively toxic to NK-1R-expressing neurons both in vitro and in vivo *(11)*.

NOCICEPTION AND SP-SAP

SP-Sap Effects on Innate Nocifensive Reflex Behavior

Initial studies using lumbar intrathecal injections of SP-sap showed that NK-1R-expressing neurons in the superficial dorsal horn of the spinal cord were ablated, and that within 3 d, the acute nocifensive responses to hindpaw intradermal injection of capsaicin were profoundly inhibited *(12)*. Thermal hyperalgesia and mechanical allodynia induced by intradermal capsaicin also were strikingly reduced. These results implicated NK-1R-expressing neurons of the superficial dorsal horn in both acute nociception and in the development of hyperalgesia and allodynia. A subsequent series of studies *(13)* reinforced and extended the initial scope and duration of observations, showing that intrathecal SP-sap reduced hyperalgesia and allodynia in a number of different models, including neuropathy and inflammation. Intrathecal SP-sap also attenuated phase II of the response to hindpaw formalin injection, a model of persistent pain. These studies showed that the antinociceptive effects of intrathecal SP-sap were persistent (>200 d).

SP-Sap Effects on Dorsal Horn Electrophysiology

Electrophysiological studies of dorsal horn neurons in rats treated with SP-sap have yielded somewhat surprising results. Suzuki and coworkers *(14)* recorded from nociceptive neurons in deeper laminae of the dorsal horn and found that pretreatment with SP-sap reduced excitability of wide dynamic range neurons. In these studies, receptive field sizes were decreased, as was coding of responses to thermal stimuli and central sensitization. They observed decreased expression of c-*fos* by dorsal horn neurons after intradermal formalin injection. Lumbar SP-sap also prevented activation of diffuse noxious inhibitory controls (DNICs) in response to noxious hindpaw stimulation, as revealed by loss of the usual suppression of c-*fos* expression in the cervical dorsal horn from noxious thermal stimulation of forepaws that occurs when similar noxious stimuli are simultaneously applied to hindpaws. The DNIC response to the opposite sequence, noxious forepaw stimulation to induce DNIC, and test stimulation of the hindpaws in the same rats showed the descending component of the DNIC was intact.

Khasabov and colleagues *(15)* explored the entire dorsal horn with microelectrodes and demonstrated that SP-sap profoundly decreased the number of high-threshold dorsal horn nociceptive neurons (nociception specific, NS). They only were able to record wide dynamic range (WDR) neurons. They also showed decreased excitation of the WDR neurons in response to intradermal capsaicin, along with profoundly decreased capsaicin-induced sensitization of these cells and absence of windup to repetitive C fiber stimulation. Taken together, these results seemed to indicate a pivotal role for lamina I NK-1R-expressing dorsal horn neurons in nociception.

Effects of SP-Sap on Operant Nocifensive Behavior

Anatomic studies showed that the great majority of NK-1R-expressing neurons in the superficial dorsal horn are projection cells that send axons rostrally to innervate multiple supraspinal structures *(16,17)*. Thus, it might be anticipated that NK-1R-expressing lamina I neurons transmit nociceptive information that in turn influences multiple cerebral circuits, and these neurons might be expected to subserve normal baseline pain perception and play a role in development of hyperalgesia and allodynia. The observation of decreased acute electrophysiological and nocifensive responses to intradermal capsaicin seemed consistent with this formulation even though SP-sap did not alter baseline behavioral responses on several innate reflex nociception tests to high-intensity phasic stimuli.

In an attempt to clarify this seeming inconsistency, we studied the effects of lumbar intrathecal SP-sap on operant responses to noxious thermal stimuli *(18)*. Using an operant escape paradigm, we observed that SP-sap-treated rats responded less to a range of noxious temperatures (0.3, 44, and 47°C). This reduction in operant responses lasted longer than 6 mo and was present in spite of normal hot plate (reflex lick/guard) responses in the same animals to the same thermal stimuli. We interpreted these findings to indicate that SP-sap spared acute nocifensive reflex responses while producing long-lasting reduction in pain sensitivity that likely reflects reduced discomfort from noxious thermal stimuli. In addition, the lesion produced by SP-sap may be selective for dorsal horn neurons receiving peripheral C nociceptor inputs and spared the Aδ input that mediates the standard tests of innate nocifensive reflex responses to high-intensity stimuli. If true, this could be a particularly fortuitous circumstance for a pain therapeutic agent: ablation of chronic discomfort with intact protective reflexes.

EXPERIMENTS WITH [SAR^9,MET(O$_2$)^{11}]-SP COUPLED WITH SAPORIN

Anatomic Specificity Issues

Experiments injecting SP-sap directly into brain parenchyma revealed a tendency for the toxin to produce nonspecific damage at the injection site even at minimally effective doses. Figure 1 illustrates some of the competing processes likely to occur when SP-sap is injected.

There is a competition between two uptake processes, the first specific and the second nonspecific:

1. Binding of SP-sap to NK-1R on target cells, which leads to receptor-mediated endocytosis and a specific lesion.
2. Bulk fluid phase pinocytotic uptake by nontarget cells.

This later process would result in a nonspecific lesion when high concentrations of protease-digested SP-sap are present. Peptidases in vivo acting on SP can render the conjugate incapable of binding to NK-1R, but the saporin is still active if taken up nonspecifically by fluid phase pinocytosis. Also, reduction of the disulfide bond between SP and saporin will produce free SP that can compete with the intact conjugate for binding to NK-1R, thus reducing specific uptake of conjugate and again leaving free saporin, which can be taken up nonspecifically. In the case of SP-sap injected into brain parenchyma, the net delivery of saporin to target cells apparently is not very much greater than to nontarget cells, resulting in nonspecific damage even at minimally effective doses.

In an effort to improve on this situation, a congener of SP, [Sar^9,Met(O$_2$)^{11}]-SP was coupled to saporin to make SSP-sap. SSP is more stable, is less readily metabolized by peptidases, and has somewhat higher biological activity toward NK-1R *(19,20)*. As predicted, intraparenchymal injection of SSP-sap was 7–10 times more potent and produced large selective lesions with minimal evidence of nonspecific damage *(21)*.

Specificity of the lesions produced by SP-sap and SSP-sap has been tested to a limited degree. In the striatum, doses of SSP-sap that widely ablated NK-1R-expressing interneurons did not affect parvalbumin-expressing neurons *(21)*. In the spinal cord, intrathecal SP-sap at doses that significantly ablated lamina I NK-1R-expressing neurons did not consistently alter SP or calcitonin gene-related peptide (CGRP) levels in primary afferents or spinal cord staining for CGRP in motor neurons of the ventral horn. Calbindin staining in lamina I and choline acetyltransferase staining in the ventral horn were likewise unaffected *(12,13)*.

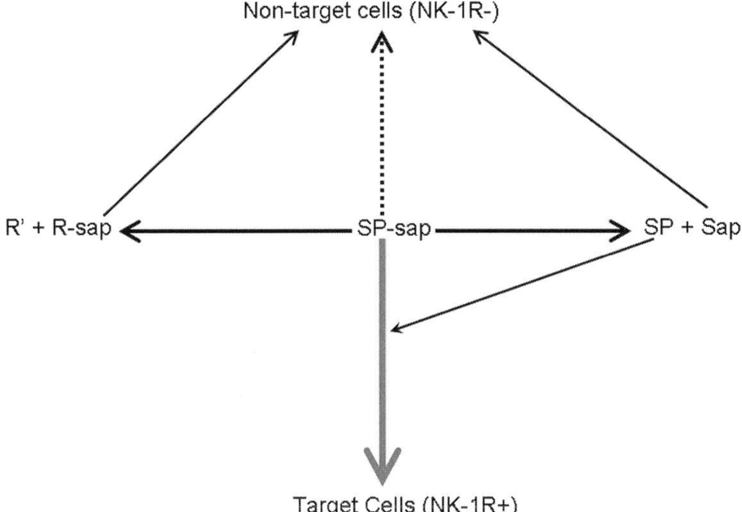

Fig. 1. Simple schematic of competing processes for substance P-saporin (SP-sap) on in vivo injection. The main goal is to deliver intact SP-sap to neurokinin-1 receptor (NK-1R)-expressing cells. However, free SP can compete for binding to NK-1R, and cells without NK-1R can take up saporin as free saporin, SP-sap, or partially peptidase-digested SP-sap (R-sap) by the inefficient process of bulk fluid phase pinocytosis. The more stable the SP-sap conjugate and the higher the affinity for NK-1R, the more conjugate is taken up by the desired target cells (NK-1R+). R + R' = substance P.

Obviously, this limited list of noncolocalized markers does not prove specificity, but currently available results so far support the conclusion that SP-sap and SSP-sap can make selective lesions, with SSP-sap somewhat more potent and selective. In the hippocampus, SSP-sap, at doses sufficient to ablate NK-1R-expressing inhibitory interneurons that colocalize γ-aminobutyric acid , parvalbumin, somatostatin, and cholecystokinin, did not alter adjacent neurons stained for calbindin or GluR2 *(22)*. In this same report, SP-sap did not show the same degree of selectivity, supporting the conclusion that SSP-sap is a superior agent for intraparenchymal injection.

Effects of SSP-Sap on Nocifensive Behavior

In rat experiments using SSP-sap, behavioral effects of the toxin were reliable and identical to those for SP-sap. For example, as reported for SP-sap *(12,13)*, SSP-sap-treated rats showed no long-term change in responses to standard hot plate testing but showed indefinitely persistent decreased operant escape in responding to noxious thermal stimuli *(23)*. In another set of experiments, intrathecal SSP-sap selectively destroyed lamina I/II dorsal horn neurons that expressed NK-1R but left the deeper laminae unaffected. However, c-*fos* expression after hindpaw formalin injection was reduced throughout all laminae of the ipsilateral L_4 dorsal horn in parallel with decreased phase II behavior.

These findings with SSP-sap on c-*fos* expression were interpreted in support of the hypothesis that destroying lamina I NK-1R-expressing neurons prevents activation of descending excitatory/facilitatory projections responsible for phase II behavior *(24)*. Also, similar to SP-sap, SSP-sap treatment blocked secondary thermal hyperalgesia in the operant escape task evoked by application of mustard oil to the dorsal surface of the hindpaws (Wiley et al., unpublished). Just as reported for SP-sap, intrathecal SSP-sap only affected NK-1R-expressing neurons in the superficial laminae (I and II) but not deeper (II–VI) laminae. Preliminary results using intrathecal SSP-sap in monkeys were consistent with the rat data showing decreased operant escape responding to noxious thermal stimuli (Ralston et al., unpublished).

DERMORPHIN–SAPORIN

Anatomic Studies

Following on the successes with SP-sap and SSP-sap, we next made a toxin directed at cells expressing the μ opiate receptor (MOR). The peptide chosen was dermorphin, a selective μ opiate agonist originally found in frog skin *(25)*. Intrastriatal injection of dermorphin–saporin (derm–sap) produced lesions reminiscent of SP-sap (*see* Fig. 2) in that the target neurons indeed diminished, but only at doses that produced some disruption of normal histological appearance.

Porreca and colleagues studied nociception in rats with derm–sap injections of the rostral ventromedial medulla (RVM) *(26)*. In those experiments, anatomic confirmation of the lesion was quite difficult, but pretreatment with the μ opiate antagonist β-funaltrexamine (β-FNA) prevented derm-sap effects on nociception, establishing that derm–sap was acting through binding to MOR.

Lumbar intrathecal injections of derm–sap reduced MOR staining in lamina II of the dorsal horn of the spinal cord (Fig. 3) without affecting primary afferent MOR-expressing neurons *(27)*. In the same animals, derm-sap injections had no effect on calbindin staining. Further anatomic analysis of spinal cords in rats with intrathecal derm–sap injections is in progress.

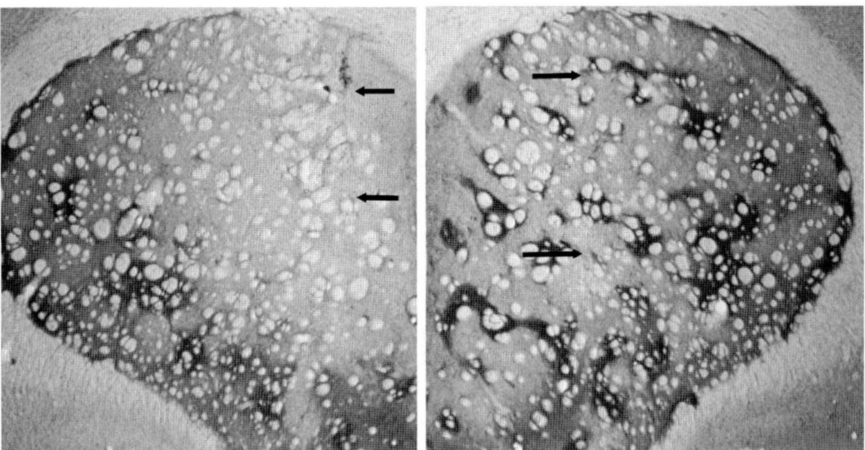

Fig. 2. Intrastriatal derm–sap injection. Left side injected with 30 ng of intact toxin; right side from the same rat injected with 30 ng pretreated with dithiothreitol to break apart toxin (control injection). Arrows indicate track of injection pipet. Tissue stained with immunoperoxidase technique for μ opiate receptor (MOR). Note loss of MOR staining on side injected with intact dermorphin–saporin.

Nociception Studies

Injections of derm–sap into the RVM did not produce any lasting alterations in baseline innate reflex responses to noxious thermal or mechanical stimuli. However, toxin-injected animals demonstrated significantly less enhancement of withdrawal to nonnoxious mechanical and to noxious thermal stimuli that occurs after spinal nerve ligation (SNL) *(26)*. Derm–sap injections into the RVM both prevented development of enhanced withdrawal reflexes after SNL and reversed already enhanced withdrawal from SNL performed before toxin injection. Time-course studies showed that derm–sap-treated rats initially showed enhanced withdrawal responses after SNL but reverted back toward controls after 3–4 d *(28)*. A similar pattern was seen in rats with dorsolateral fasciculus lesions, the presumed pathway from the RVM to the spinal dorsal horn. Last, RVM injections of derm-sap blocked the enhanced in vitro capsaicin-induced spinal release of CGRP in SNL *(29)*. SNL-induced increase in levels of dynorphin in the spinal dorsal horn was also blocked by prior RVM injection of derm–sap. A current hypothesis is that RVM injections of derm-sap destroy medullary "ON" cells thought to facilitate nocifensive reflexes.

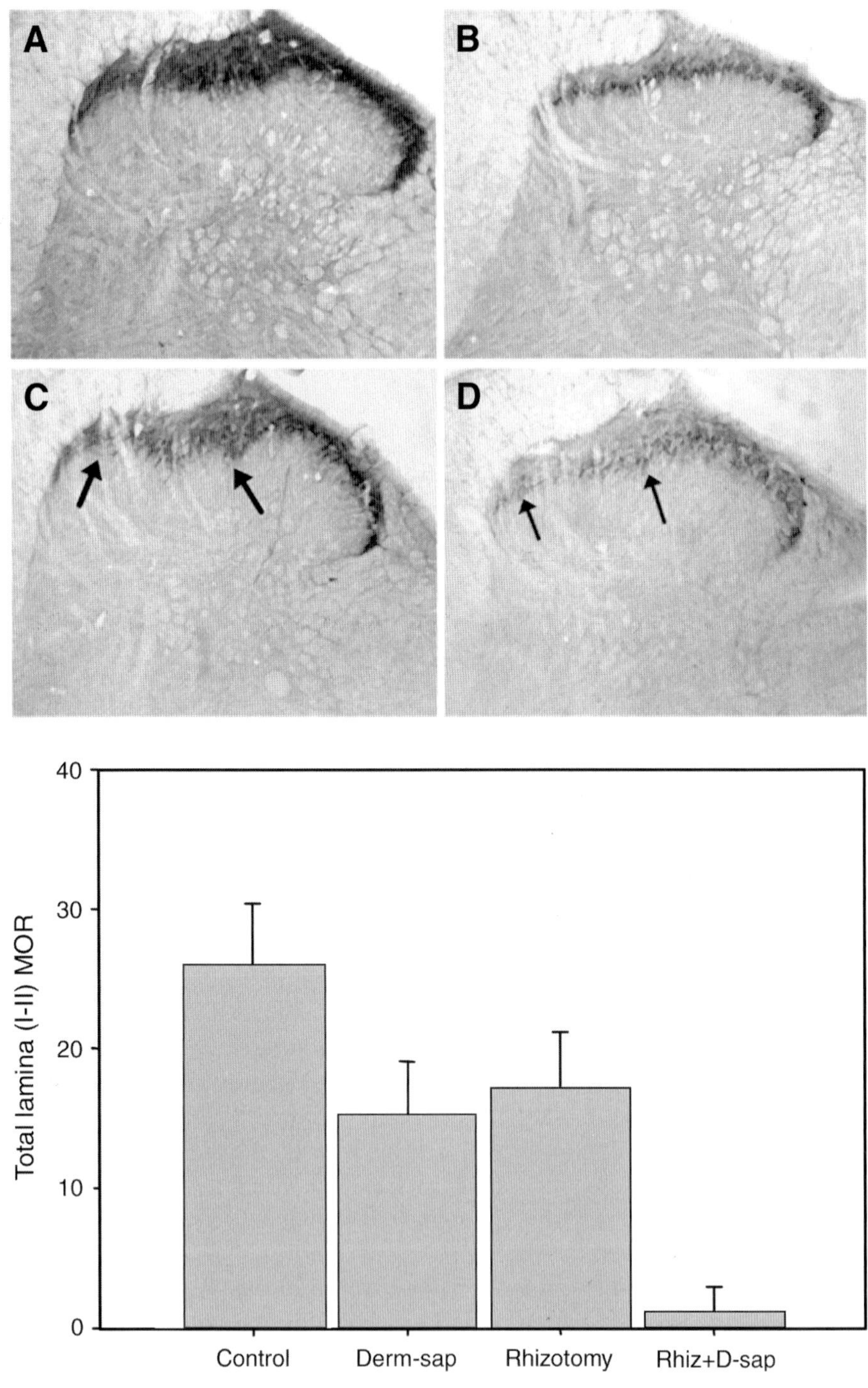

Fig. 3

OTHER NEUROPEPTIDE–TOXIN CONJUGATES AND PAIN

The logic behind the development of derm–sap can be formulated as the use of intrathecal injections to selectively destroy excitatory interneurons in the superficial dorsal horn that express MOR. The next step will be to determine the effect of these injections on behavioral responses to noxious stimuli and morphine analgesia. However, the same logic can be applied to other neuropeptides that act through inhibitory G protein-coupled receptors and are antinociceptive when administered intrathecally. Two such conjugates have been made. Preliminary results indicated that both neuropeptide Y-saporin (NPY-sap) and galanin–saporin (GAL–sap) are antinociceptive when rats are tested on the hot plate using mildly noxious heat (Fig. 4). Additional experiments are under way to characterize further the effects of intrathecal injections of these neuropeptides on the anatomy of the dorsal horn and on other aspects of nociception.

ANTI-DOPAMINE β-HYDROXYLASE-SAPORIN AND NOCICEPTION

The immunotoxin anti-dopamine β-hydroxylase-saporin (anti-DβH-sap) selectively destroys noradrenergic and adrenergic neurons in the central *(30)* and peripheral *(31,32)* nervous systems. Intracerebroventricular injection of anti-DβH-sap has been used to destroy brainstem noradrenergic neurons, primarily the locus coeruleus, and then assess withdrawal from prolonged morphine administration *(33)*. The anti-DβH-sap-injected rats showed more intense withdrawal behavior and more extensive c-*fos* expression in the dorsal horn of the spinal cord, suggesting a role for descending noradrenergic projections in modulating manifestations of opiate withdrawal.

Fig. 3. Changes in μ opiate receptor (MOR) staining of superficial dorsal horn after intrathecal dermorphin–saporin (derm–sap) and/or multilevel lumbar rhizotomies. The photomicrographs in the upper panel show: (**A**) Normal control appearance. (**B**) Two weeks after transection of all ipsilateral lumbar dorsal roots (note particularly severe loss of MOR stain in lamina I consistent with loss of primary afferent terminals [dotted arrows]). (**C**) Two weeks after intrathecal injection of 500 ng of derm–sap showing significant loss of MOR staining particularly in the medial portion of lamina II (arrows). (**D**) Tissue is stained for as in Fig. 2. The lower graph shows the results of quantitative densitometry for MOR. Sections were processed in parallel. Both derm–sap and multilevel lumbar dorsal rhizotomies reduced lamina II MOR stain by about 50% and combined derm–sap and multilevel lumbar dorsal rhizotomies result in more than 90% loss of MOR staining from the dorsal horn. These results are consistent with destruction of lamina II MOR-expressing neurons by derm–sap and loss of MOR-expressing primary afferent terminals after rhizotomies.

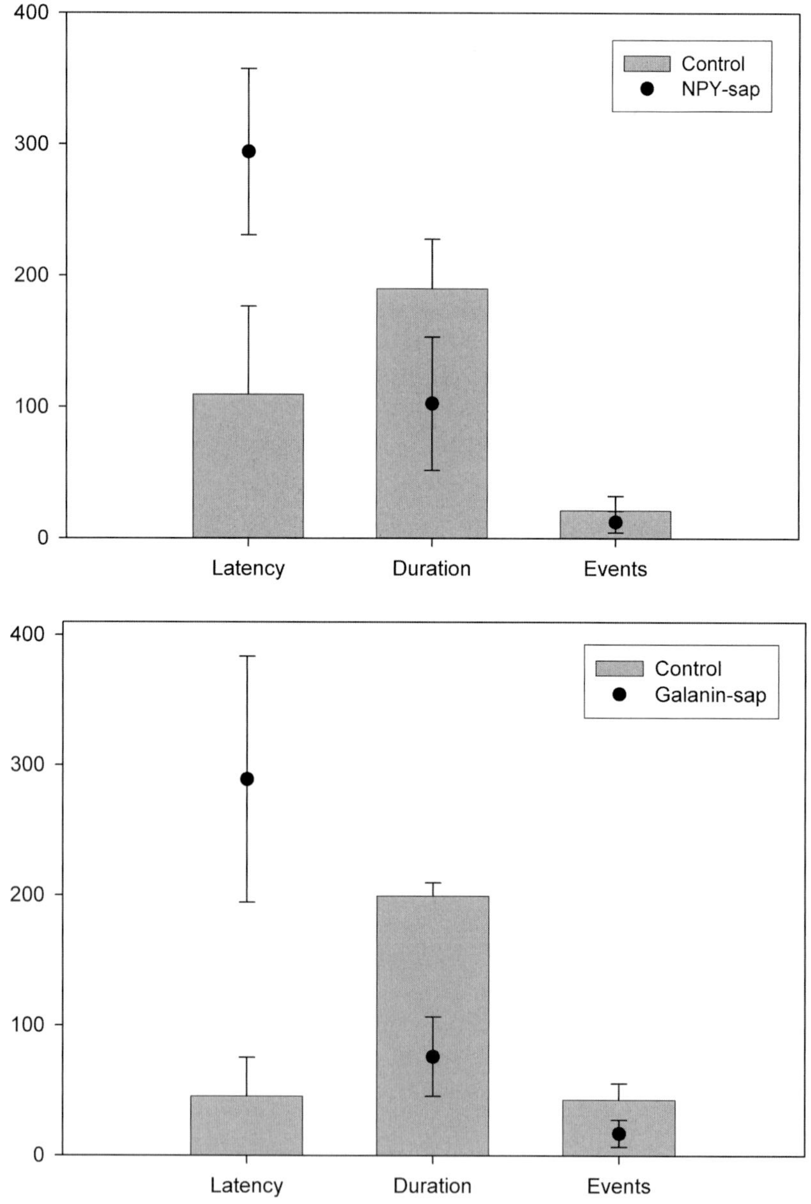

Fig. 4. Effects of galanin–saporin (GAL–sap) and neuropeptide Y (NPY)-sap on hot plate responses. Rats were injected 7 d before testing with either 500 ng GAL–sap, 500 ng NPY-sap, or vehicle. Hot plate testing was performed at 44°C for 10 min. *Latency* refers to the latency to the first hindpaw lick/guard response. *Duration* refers to the total amount of time spent licking and guarding, and *events* refers

In another set of experiments from the same lab, lumbar intrathecal anti-DβH-sap was used to eliminate the noradrenergic innervation to the spinal cord *(34)*. In the formalin test of persistent pain, rats treated with anti-DβH-sap showed decreased phase II behavior and enhanced morphine suppression of phase II behavior. Anti-DβH-sap also reduced expression of c-*fos* in the same rats. These results were interpreted as showing that spinal noradrenergic innervation plays a role in regulating nociceptive sensitivity at the spinal level. Last, intracerebroventricular injections of anti-DβH-sap were used to destroy the locus coeruleus noradrenergic neurons in spontaneously hypertensive (SHR) rats and in Wistar–Kyoto (WKY) rats, the strain from which SHR rats were derived. Toxin injections reduced phase II behavior of the formalin test in WKY but not SHR rats, but toxin-treated SHR rats were more reactive on the hot plate (52.2°C), whereas anti-DβH-sap had no effect on hot plate responses of WKY rats *(35)*. These results were interpreted as evidence in favor of enhanced locus coeruleus noradrenergic activity causing the abnormalities of nociceptive sensitivity seen in SHR rats.

Another approach to analysis of nociception using saporin conjugates is reported by Vulchanova and Honda in Chapter 12. They report on the effects of peripheral nerve injections of the lectin-saporin conjugate isolectin B4-saporin (IB4-sap), which selectively destroys a class of peripheral sensory neurons involved in nociception.

SUMMARY

Although the use of saporin conjugates in pain research is only a few years old, already a number of interesting results have been reported. The attenuation of nociception, hyperalgesia, and allodynia with intrathecal SP-sap and SSP-sap suggests these agents have clinical potential for treating chronic, intractable pain. The potential usefulness of derm-sap as a research tool would seem to go far beyond the initial results, which have been slow in coming because of difficulties establishing the in vivo anatomic effects of

---

Fig. 4. *(continued from opposite page)* to the total number of lick/guard responses. Control means ± standard deviations are shown by the shaded bars. The solid circles with brackets are the toxin means ± standard deviations. Both GAL–sap and NPY-sap rats were slow to react (increased latency to first response) and spent less time licking and guarding (decreased duration). Differences in events were not significant because of the small number in this experimental situation, which emphasized C-nociceptor activation. These results suggested decreased sensitivity to noxious heat in the toxin-injected rats.

the toxin. A number of other neuropeptide–toxin conjugates and immunotoxins are in use in pain experiments and new ones are on the way, extending understanding of the role of spinal neurons that express the appropriate neuropeptide receptors.

REFERENCES

1. Wiley RG, Lappi DA. Targeted toxins in pain. Adv Drug Deliv Rev 2003;55:1043–1054.
2. Yamamoto T, Sakashita Y. The role of the spinal opioid receptor like1 receptor, the NK-1 receptor, and cyclooxygenase-2 in maintaining postoperative pain in the rat. Anesth Analg 1999;89:1203–1208.
3. Quartara L, Maggi CA. The tachykinin NK_1 receptor. Part II: distribution and pathophysiological. Neuropeptides 1998;32:1–49.
4. Mantyh PW, Allen CJ, Ghilardi JR, et al. Rapid endocytosis of a G protein-coupled receptor: substance P evoked internalization of its receptor in the rat striatum in vivo. Proc Natl Acad Sci USA 1995;92:2622–2626.
5. Mantyh PW, DeMaster E, Malhotra A, et al. Receptor endocytosis and dendrite reshaping in spinal neurons after somatosensory stimulation. Science 1995;268:1629–1632.
6. Blackburn RE, Samson WK, Fulton RJ, Stricker EM, Verbalis JG. Central oxytocin and ANP receptors mediate osmotic inhibition of salt appetite in rats. Am J Physiol Regul Integr Comp Physiol 1995;269:R245–R251.
7. Blackburn RE, Samson WK, Fulton RJ, Stricker EM, Verbalis JG. Central oxytocin inhibition of salt appetite in rats: evidence for differential sensing of plasma sodium and osmolality. Proc Natl Acad Sci USA 1993;90:10,380–10,384.
8. Samson WK, Huang FL, Fulton RJ. C-type natriuretic peptide mediates the hypothalamic actions of the natriuretic peptides to inhibit luteinizing hormone secretion. Endocrinology 1993;132:504–509.
9. Samson WK, Alexander BD, Skala KD, Huang FL, Fulton RJ. Ricin-cytotoxin conjugate administration reveals a physiologically relevant role for oxytocin in the control of gonadotropin secretion. Ann NY Acad Sci 1992;652:411–422.
10. Samson WK, Alexander BD, Skala KD, Huang FL, Fulton RJ. Central peptidergic mechanisms controlling reproductive hormone secretion: novel methodology reveals a role for the natriuretic peptides. Can J Physiol Pharmacol 1992;70:773–778.
11. Wiley RG, Lappi DA. Destruction of neurokinin-1 receptor expressing cells in vitro and in vivo using substance P-saporin in rats. Neurosci Lett 1997;230:97–100.
12. Mantyh PW, Rogers SD, Honore P, et al. Inhibition of hyperalgesia by ablation of lamina I spinal neurons expressing the substance P receptor. Science 1997;278:275–279.
13. Nichols ML, Allen BJ, Rogers SD, et al. Transmission of chronic nociception by spinal neurons expressing the substance P receptor. Science 1999;286:1558–1561.

14. Suzuki R, Morcuende S, Webber M, Hunt SP, Dickenson AH. Superficial NK1-expressing neurons control spinal excitability through activation of descending pathways. Nat Neurosci 2002;5:1319–1326.

15. Khasabov SG, Rogers SD, Ghilardi JR, Peters CM, Mantyh PW, Simone DA. Spinal neurons that possess the substance P receptor are required for the development of central sensitization. J Neurosci 2002;22:9086–9098.

16. Todd AJ. Anatomy of primary afferents and projection neurones in the rat spinal dorsal horn with particular emphasis on substance P and the neurokinin 1 receptor. Exp Physiol 2002;87:245–249.

17. Todd AJ, McGill MM, Shehab SA. Neurokinin 1 receptor expression by neurons in laminae I, III and IV of the rat spinal dorsal horn that project to the brainstem. Eur J Neurosci 2000;12:689–700.

18. Vierck CJ, Kline RH, Wiley RG. Intrathecal substance p-saporin attenuates operant escape from nociceptive thermal stimuli. Neuroscience 2003;119:223–232.

19. Drapeau G, D'Orleans-Juste P, Dion S, Rhaleb N-E, Rouissi N-E, Regoli D. Selective agonists for substance P and neurokinin receptors. Neuropeptides 1987;10:43–54.

20. Tousignant C, Guillemette G, Drapeau G, Telemaque S, Dion S, Regoli D. ^{125}I[Sar^9,Met(O$_2$)^{11}]-SP, a new selective ligand for the NK-1 receptor in the central nervous system. Brain Res 1990;524:263–270.

21. Wiley RG, Lappi DA. Targeting neurokinin-1 receptor-expressing neurons with [Sar^9,Met(O$_2$)^{11}]substance P-saporin. Neurosci Lett 1999;277:1–4.

22. Martin JL, Sloviter RS. Focal inhibitory interneuron loss and principal cell hyperexcitability in the rat hippocampus after microinjection of a neurotoxic conjugate of saporin and a peptidase-resistant analog of Substance P. J Comp Neurol 2001;436:127–152.

23. Wiley RG, Lappi DA, Vierck CJ. Inihibition of mustard oil-induced hyperalgesia in an operant escape task by substance P-saporin. Abstr Soc Neurosci 1999;25:1330.

24. Wiley RG, Kline RH, Lappi DA. Dose-dependent effects of intrathecal substance P-saporin and SSP-saporin. Abstr Soc Neurosci 2001;26:281.11.

25. Montecucchi PC, de Castiglione R, Erspamer V. Identification of dermorphin and Hyp6-dermorphin in skin extracts of the Brazilian frog *Phyllomedusa rhodei*. Int J Pept Protein Res 1981;17:316–321.

26. Porreca F, Burgess SE, Gardell LR, et al. Inhibition of neuropathic pain by selective ablation of brainstem medullary cells expressing the μ-opioid receptor. J Neurosci 2001;21:5281–5288.

27. Wiley RG, Miller SA, Kline RH. Selective destruction of MOR expressing dorsal horn neurons using intrathecal dermorphin–saporin. Abstr Soc Neurosci 2003;28:174.15.

28. Burgess SE, Gardell LR, Ossipov MH, et al. Time-dependent descending facilitation from the rostral ventromedial medulla maintains, but does not initiate, neuropathic pain. J Neurosci 2002;22:5129–5136.

29. Gardell LR, Vanderah TW, Gardell SE, et al. Enhanced evoked excitatory transmitter release in experimental neuropathy requires descending facilitation. J Neurosci 2003;23:8370–8379.
30. Wrenn CC, Picklo MJ, Lappi DA, Robertson D, Wiley RG. Central noradrenergic lesioning using anti-DBH-saporin: anatomical findings. Brain Res 1996;740:175–184.
31. Picklo MJ, Wiley RG, Lonce S, Lappi DA, Robertson D. Anti-dopamine β-hydroxylase immunotoxin-induced sympathectomy in adult rats. J Pharmacol Exp Ther 1995;275:1003–1010.
32. Picklo MJ, Wiley RG, Lappi DA, Robertson D. Noradrenergic lesioning with an anti-dopamine β-hydroxylase immunotoxin. Brain Res 1994;666:195–200.
33. Rohde DS, Basbaum AI. Activation of coeruleospinal noradrenergic inhibitory controls during withdrawal from morphine in the rat. J Neurosci 1998;18:4393–4402.
34. Martin WJ, Gupta NK, Loo CM, Rohde DS, Basbaum AI. Differential effects of neurotoxic destruction of descending noradrenergic pathways on acute and persistent nociceptive processing. Pain 1999;80:57–65.
35. Taylor BK, Roderick RE, Basbaum AI. Brainstem noradrenergic control of nociception is abnormal in the spontaneously hypertensive rat. Neurosci Lett 2000;291:139–142.

11

The Use of Saporin Conjugates to Dissect Neurons Responsible for Sleep and Wakefulness

Carlos Blanco-Centurion, Dmitry Gerashchenko, Eric Murillo-Rodriguez, Frank Desarnaud, and Priyattam J. Shiromani

INTRODUCTION

Virtually all organisms manifest regular periods of behavioral quiescence and activity. In mammals and birds, these periods have evolved into regular episodes of wakefulness and sleep. The sleep period itself has further differentiated into two distinct states, slow wave sleep (SWS) and rapid eye movement (REM) sleep. In humans, SWS has further differentiated into four distinct stages, each identified by a specific pattern on the electroencephalogram (EEG). REM sleep is very similar to wakefulness in many ways; the main difference is that there is behavioral quiescence during REM sleep. For this reason, REM sleep is often referred to as *paradoxical sleep.*

The normal human sleep pattern is characterized by a progression through the four SWS stages, followed by REM sleep. This pattern lasts for about 90 min and is repeated about four to five times during the night. Sleep occupies nearly a third of our life. During this period, we are totally unproductive, useless, and defenseless. Yet, we cannot survive without sleep *(1).*

What brain region is responsible for generating these states of consciousness? To answer this question, researchers have relied on the classical "slash-and-burn" method. Historically, the transection and electrolytic lesion method quickly identified the regions of the brain subserving wakefulness, SWS, and REM sleep. The weakness of this method is that it destroys fibers

From: *Molecular Neurosurgery With Targeted Toxins*
Edited by: R. G. Wiley and D. A. Lappi © Humana Press Inc., Totowa, NJ

of passage (transection), and specific neurons cannot be identified. Excitatory amino acids, such as ibotenic and kainic acid, are improvements in that they lesion cells without damaging fibers of passage. However, the disadvantage is that the lesion cannot be limited to a particular cell type, only to a region. Indeed, we have begun to realize that it is necessary to target a specific neuronal phenotype because neurons serving states of consciousness are intermingled with neurons responsible for other functions.

The saporin conjugate is a marked improvement over other lesion methods in that a specific cell type can be targeted *(2,3)*. Elsewhere in this book, other investigators have discussed advantages of saporin, and we respectfully refer the reader to those chapters. In our efforts, we are using saporin-based neurotoxins to lesion specific neuronal phenotypes and thereby create a circuit model of sleep generation. For instance, 192 immunoglobulin G-saporin (192 IgG-sap) lesions basal forebrain (BF) cholinergic neurons, and antidopamine β-hydroxylase-saporin lesions only noradrenergic neurons such as those of the locus coeruleus (LC). Both types of neurons have been proposed as key components to sustain alertness.

HYPOCRETIN–OREXIN–SAPORIN CONJUGATE

We have now created a new saporin conjugate, hypocretin 2-saporin (HCRT-2-sap), to lesion HCRT/OX (orexin) receptor-containing neurons *(4)*. The impetus for creating this neurotoxin was the discovery that the neuropeptide hypocretin, which is also known as orexin (OX), was linked to the sleep disorder narcolepsy *(5,6)*. HCRT/OX was discovered by two independent groups using different approaches *(7–9)*. In the central nervous system, HCRT/OX-containing neurons are located only in the lateral hypothalamus, from where they project to the entire brain and spinal cord, providing especially heavy innervation to the arousal populations.

Two OX receptors have been identified, and the distribution of the receptor messenger ribonucleic acid (mRNA) *(10,11)* and protein *(12)* have been determined. Orexin 1 (HCRT-1) receptor (OX-1R/HCRT-1R) mRNA is more abundant in ventromedial hypothalamic nucleus, hippocampal formation, dorsal raphe, and LC. In the rat, OX-2R mRNA is mainly expressed in cerebral cortex, nucleus accumbens, subthalamic and paraventricular thalamic nuclei, and posterior pretectal nuclei *(10,13)*. In the pontine brainstem, OX-1Rs are located in the LC *(13)*. The LC receives the heaviest projection of OX-containing fibers, and intraventricular administration of OX A or HCRT-2/OX B excites LC neurons *(14,15)*. OX-containing terminals are also found in areas implicated in wakefulness, such as the LC, tuberomammillary nucleus (TMN), the dorsal raphe, and the BF *(7)*. Because of these projections to neuronal populations implicated in wakefulness, it is believed that OX promotes wakefulness *(7)*.

To aid our research efforts, we obtained saporin conjugated to the peptide OX B (HCRT-2), resulting in HCRT-2-sap. OX B is a linear peptide with a free N-terminus that facilitates conjugation to saporin. OX A is much more difficult to couple to saporin because both of its termini are blocked *(8)*. Because of affinity characteristics of OX-1R (also known as HCRT-1 receptor) to bind OX A over OX B and OX2R (HCRT-2R) to bind both peptides at high affinity *(8)*, it is possible that our saporin conjugate binds principally to the OX-2R (HCRT-2R). Our preliminary evidence bore this out *(4)* because LC neurons, which contain OX-1R/HCRT-1R, were more resistant to lesioning by the HCRT-2-sap, whereas TMN neurons, which contain HCRT-2R, were lesioned (Fig. 1). We also used in vitro cell culture assays using Chinese hamster ovary (CHO) cells containing either HCRT-1R or HCRT-2R and found that HCRT-2-sap bound to these cells but not to other peptide receptor-containing cells *(4)*. In other words, the HCRT-2-sap bound to its receptor and not to other peptide receptors.

The use of different saporin conjugates is a tremendous boon to neurobiologists because they facilitate dissection of different neuronal phenotypes, thereby aiding in the creation of better neuronal circuit models. Mice knockouts do not offer this kind of versatility because usually the gene is missing in the entire mouse, which rules out identifying specific brain regions responsible for the behavior. In the case of HCRT/OX, this is a particularly critical issue because the HCRT/OX neurons project widely, and it is not known which projection to which target site regulates which aspect of sleep-wakefulness. Inducible knockouts would be an important step, but there is the associated high cost of producing the knockouts. On the other hand, saporin conjugates provide a quick, easy, and low-cost method of destroying specific neuronal phenotypes, and this is key in testing specific hypotheses.

We have written reviews detailing the neuronal network underlying wakefulness, non-REM, and REM sleep *(16–18)*. Refer to these publications for full information. Here, we summarize the essential points covered in those reviews and summarize our use of saporin conjugate to test specific hypotheses.

BRAIN REGIONS RESPONSIBLE FOR WAKING

Neurons responsible for wakefulness are located in the forebrain and brainstem and include the major neurotransmitters acetylcholine (BF and pons), norepinephrine (LC), histamine (TMN), and serotonin (dorsal raphe). To this mix, the HCRT/OX peptidergic system was added. We are using

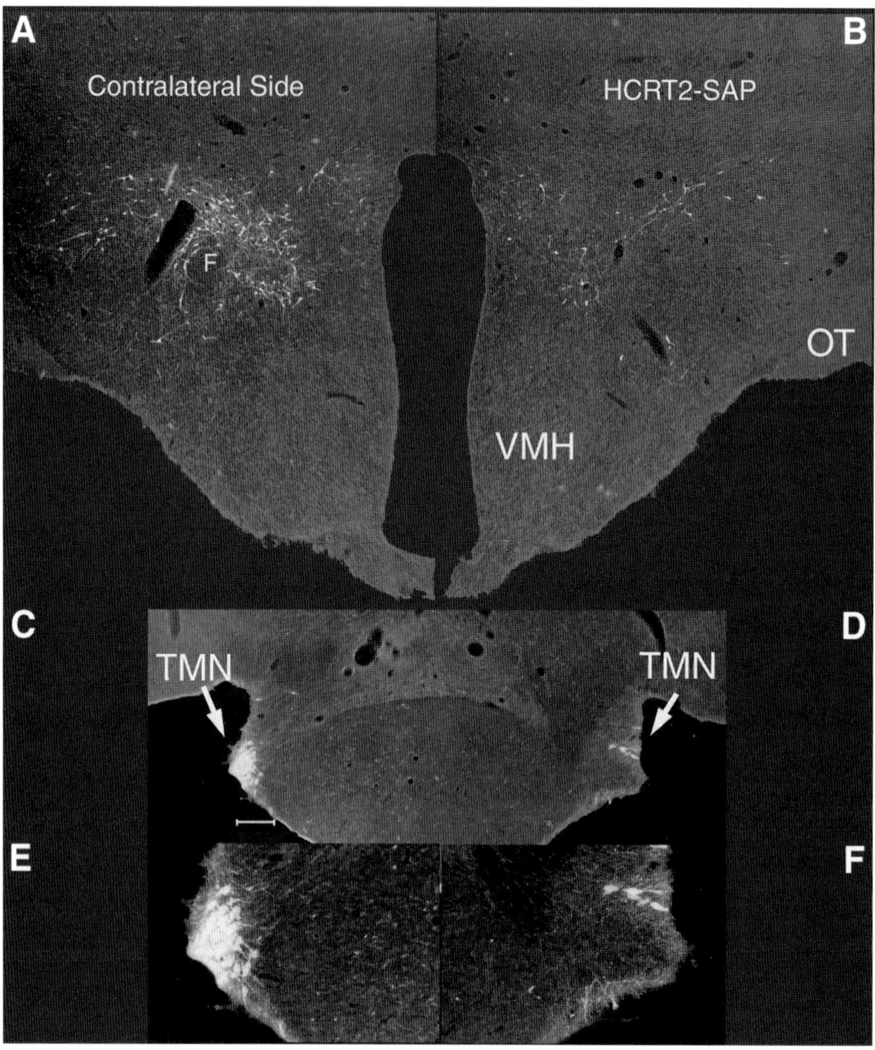

Fig. 1. Photomicrographs depicts loss of hypocretin (HCRT)/orexin (OX) (panels **A** and **B**) and adenosine deaminase (panels **C–F**) immunoreactive neurons after unilateral injection of hypocretin-2-saporin (HCRT-2-sap) into the lateral hypothalamus (panel **B**) or tuberomammillary nucleus (TMN) (panel **D**). HCRT/OX neurons (panel **A**) possess the HCRT/OX receptor, and these are destroyed by the HCRT-2-sap (panel **B**). Panel **C** depicts neurons in the TMN (identified by adenosine deaminase immunoreactivity), which possess the HCRT receptor 2/OX receptor 2, and these are destroyed when the injection is made into the TMN (panel **D**). Panels **E** and **F** represent higher magnification of the TMN in panels **C** and **D**. Bar in panel **C** represents 100 μm. F, fornix; OT, olfactory tubercle; TMN, tuberomammillary nucleus; VMH, ventral medial hypothalamus.

saporin-based conjugates to lesion these specific neuronal phenotypes to determine which aspect of waking behavior is regulated by these neurons.

Basal Forebrain

Cholinergic neurons located in the BF and pons are implicated in waking. The cholinergic BF neurons can be easily destroyed using 192 IgG-sap, but to date there is no effective way of selectively lesioning the pontine cholinergic neurons. Szymusiak reviewed the role of the BF in EEG desynchronization and waking *(19)*.

The BF represents the cholinergic cells in the medial septal nucleus (MS; i.e., Ch1), vertical limb of the diagonal band of Broca (VDB; Ch2), horizontal limb of the diagonal band of Broca (HDB; Ch3), substantia innominata (SI), and the nucleus basalis of Meynert (NBM; Ch4). Each of these cell groups (Ch1–Ch4) has distinct projection patterns. The medial septum and VDB cholinergic groups innervate the hippocampus; the HDB innvervates the olfactory bulb, entorhinal cortex, and piriform cortex; and the SI/NBM innervate the neocortex. These groups receive ascending influence from the pontine cholinergic cells (Ch5–Ch6) as noted below. In fact, it has been suggested that the BF represents a telencephalic extension of the reticular core *(20)*.

Sleep–wake-related firing of BF neurons has been examined. The predominant (50% of recorded cells) firing pattern of SI/NBM and HDB neurons is increased activity during waking and REM sleep, and these cells project to the thalamus and cortex (reviewed in ref. *19*). The wake-REM active BF cells decrease their firing in response to local warming, which is somnogenic *(21)*. The SI/NBM-HDB area also contains cells (25%) that discharge only during non-REM sleep *(19,22)*. To separate the sleep-active from wake-active cells, we used c-fos expression and found increased numbers of cholinergic cells that are c-fos positive in awake animals *(12)*.

Unfortunately, the cholinergic BF neurons are intermingled with γ-aminobutyric acid (GABA) neurons, and it is not clear which or both of these cell types is relevant for maintaining waking behavior. One research group has hypothesized that the increased activity of the BF cholinergic cells during wakefulness produces adenosine, which then inhibits these cells, and sleep may occur *(23)*. Increased adenosine levels, as measured by microdialysis, are found in the BF during wakefulness *(23)*. During sleep, the adenosine levels decline *(23)*. Indeed, the BF cholinergic pathway is active during waking and REM sleep *(24)*. Increased acetylcholine is found in cortex during waking and REM sleep *(25,26)*, indicating activation of underlying cholinergic neurons. Stimulation of the cholinergic cells in BF (SI/NBM) increases

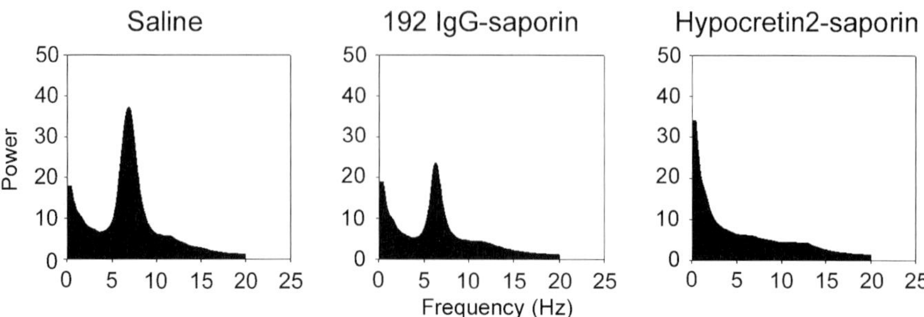

Fig. 2. Hippocampal τ activity during rapid eye movement (REM) sleep in rats given saline, 192 immunoglobulin G-saporin , or hypocretin-2-saporin (HCRT-2-sap). Results from a rat representative for each drug treatment are depicted. In saline-treated rats, there was hippocampal τ activity during REM sleep; this is identified by a single peak at 6–8 Hz. This peak was diminished, but present, in rats with cholinergic lesions of the medial septum and vertical limb of the diagonal band of Broca. With HCRT-2-sap injections to the same area, there was complete loss of hippocampal τ during REM, although the percentage of REM sleep was unchanged. In other words, REM sleep still occurred normally, but without hippocampal τ. We can identify that it is REM sleep because of the complete loss of muscle tone and the cortical desynchronization. A complete description of these findings is given in Gerashchenko et al., 2001.

acetylcholine release in cortex *(27)*. Lesions of SI/NBM produce slow waves in the EEG *(28,29)* and decrease cortical acetylcholine levels *(30)*.

However, destruction of the BF cholinergic neurons using 192 IgG-sap does not increase sleep, suggesting that noncholinergic neurons might be relevant for promoting wakefulness *(31,32)*. To shed light on this controversy, we utilized HCRT-2-sap vs 192 IgG-sap. Our initial efforts were limited to the MS and VDB. We applied HCRT-2-sap to lesion HCRT-R/OX-R-containing neurons in the MS and VDB and discovered that τ activity was completely abolished, but there was no overall change in the percentage of sleep and wakefulness *(33)* (Fig. 2). When 192 IgG-sap was applied to the same area, the cholinergic neurons were lesioned, but there was only a diminution of τ activity. Previously, other researchers had found diminution of τ following 192 IgG-sap application *(31,32)*. However, our finding of complete loss of τ following HCRT-2-sap lesion suggests that the noncholinergic cells in the medial septal and VDB were triggering τ. Another research group also reached this conclusion but using the in vitro slice preparation *(34,35)*. The use of the two types of saporin conjugates was instrumental in separating the two phenotypes in production of theta activity.

Lateral Hypothalamus

The posterior hypothalamus was implicated in promoting wakefulness because of the pioneering studies of von Economo and Nauta *(36)*. The HCRTs are located in a part of the brain regarded as a "wake" center following von Economo's observations that patients suffering from the viral encephalitis epidemic of 1918 were excessively sleepy, and postmortem analysis revealed damage to the posterior hypothalamus. However, the role of the posterior hypothalamus in promoting wakefulness has remained largely unexplored except for a few lesion studies, which to date have yielded results that are not entirely consistent with the emerging evidence linking HCRT with narcolepsy.

For instance, behavioral signs of sleepiness following electrolytic lesions of the posterior hypothalamus were observed *(36,37)*, but neither study reported the daily amounts of sleep. McGinty *(38)* recorded sleep EEG from rats with large electrolytic lesions of the posterior hypothalamus that included the lateral hypothalamus and observed hypersomnia in two of seven lesioned rats for 5–8 d after the lesion, followed by increased wakefulness in all rats; REM sleep was suppressed or decreased. Other reports have also found increased wakefulness and reduced REM sleep after electrolytic lesions of the lateral hypothalamus *(39)*. Excitotoxic lesions that theoretically spare fibers of passage have also produced inconsistent effects. In two studies from the same laboratory *(40,41)*, ibotenic acid applied to the posterior hypothalamus increased sleep for 1–4 d, but then increased wakefulness; REM sleep was increased only during the first 3–21 h.

The inconsistent effects on sleep following electrolytic or excitotoxic lesions might have occurred because the lesion methods did not destroy the appropriate neurons. In our experiments *(4,42)*, we administered HCRT-2-sap to the lateral hypothalamus and found that it lesioned the HCRT-R-bearing neurons, including the HCRT-immunoreactive neurons. The HCRT/OX neurons contain the receptor *(14)* and as such were lesioned. These lesions produced sleep fragmentation, excessive sleepiness, increase in REM sleep, and sleep-onset REM periods. All these symptoms are characteristic of narcolepsy in humans, dogs, and HCRT/OX null mice. The application of the toxin to caudal regions that do not contain HCRT-containing neurons lesioned HCRT-R-bearing neurons but did not produce narcolepticlike sleep behavior, further reinforcing the primary role of the HCRT-containing neurons in the disease.

For almost 80 yr, only a few studies investigated the lateral hypothalamus, and this was partly because the appropriate tools were not brought to bear on the problem. There are still many unanswered questions. For instance, are HCRT/OX neurons the only neurons absent in narcoleptics? We think not because lesion of other adjacent non-HCRT/OX neurons might be responsible for the hypersomnia in narcolepsy *(42)*.

Tuberomammillary Nucleus

Antihistamines have a potent somnogenic effect. The TMN represents the only collection of histamine neurons in the brain *(43)*. TMN neurons have the highest discharge rate during waking and are virtually silent during sleep *(44–46)*. In this respect, these neurons are similar to the LC and dorsal raphe cells. Histamine microinjections into the BF produce a dose-dependent increase in wakefulness *(47)*. The blockage of histamine synthesis in the preoptic area (POA) increases sleep and decreases wakefulness *(47)*. Histamine H1 and H2 receptors are postulated to mediate the arousal *(47)*.

The TMN by itself has never been selectively damaged, and we suspect that the reason is because it is difficult to approach. Moreover, it appears to be resistant to damage by excitatory amino acids, much in the same way that suprachiasmatic nucleus neurons cannot be lesioned by ibotenic or kainic acid. The HCRT-2-sap provides a ready solution to lesioning the TMN neurons.

In preliminary studies *(4)*, HCRT-2-sap lesioned TMN neurons but did not produce hypersomnolence. This is consistent with emerging data from histamine decarboxylase knockout mice studies *(48)*, which did not show an overall change in sleep in knockout mice. However, the histamine decarboxylase knockout mice fell asleep faster in a novel environment, indicating that histamine may be important in maintaining vigilance and arousal in new environments. HCRT/OX neurons innervate the TMN and stimulate the histamine neurons *(49)*. This could be via a histamine receptor 1 because direct application of HCRT/OX onto TMN neurons increases wakefulness in wild-type mice but not in histamine receptor 1-null mice *(50)*. There could also be a histamine influence onto HCRT/OX neurons, although a recent article showed no direct effect of histamine on identified HCRT/OX neurons *(51)*.

BRAIN REGIONS RESPONSIBLE FOR SLEEP

Nauta's experiments led him to conclude that there was a sleep center because discrete lesions of the POA produced insomnia. In the succeeding years, a great body of evidence has accumulated to support Nauta's conclusions *(52–58)*.

Sleep-active neurons are found in the POA and adjacent BF in rats, cats, and rabbits *(59–62)*. These neurons begin to fire during drowsiness, and peak activity is seen during non-REM sleep. The sleep-active cells comprise about 25% of the recorded cells in the BF POA and are intermixed with wake-active cells, which predominate *(62)*.

We have used c-fos to identify sleep-active neurons, which are located in the ventral lateral preoptic area (VLPO) *(63)*. The VLPO Fos-immunoreactive cells project to the histaminergic TM cells. We hypothesize that the VLPO cells are inhibitory, and our preliminary evidence showed numerous GABA and galanin-positive cells in VLPO. The likelihood that the VLPO cells play an important role in sleep was further substantiated by findings that a majority of cells in this region are sleep active *(64)*.

The current hypothesis is that sleep occurs as a result of increased activity of POA and VLPO GABA neurons, which project to posterior hypothalamic wake-active neurons and inhibit these neurons. Unfortunately, we do not know which receptors are on sleep-active neurons, and as such the saporin method has not been used.

BRAIN REGIONS RESPONSIBLE FOR REM SLEEP

Transection and lesion studies have identified the pontine brainstem as critically important for the generation of REM sleep. The specific neurons include the serotonergic dorsal raphe, the noradrenergic LC, the cholinergic pontine neurons, GABA interneurons, and glutamatergic neurons. These neuronal phenotypes overlap each other, making it difficult to lesion specific neurons. The serotonergic neurons can be lesioned using 5,7-dihydroxytryptamine (5,7-DHT), and the LC neurons can be lesioned using dopamine β-hydroxylase-saporin (DβH-sap). However, the other neuronal phenotypes have been difficult to lesion selectively. With the discovery of HCRT/OX, it is necessary to determine whether elimination of neurons containing HCRT/OX receptor results in a phenotype with narcolepsy. This would be an important advance because it will permit identification of a circuit from the lateral hypothalamus to the pons and to the spinal cord that could be relevant to maintaining motor control during waking behavior.

The LC

The LC has played a central role in theories of REM sleep generation. It is hypothesized that REM sleep begins in the pons when the activity of neurons in the dorsal raphe and LC stops. Indeed, LC and dorsal raphe neurons do cease firing only during REM sleep and are referred to as REM-off neurons. When these REM-off neurons become silent, the cholinergic neurons of the lateral dorsal tegmental and pedunculopontine nuclei become disinhibited, and they begin high discharge rates. A subset of these cells innervates medial pontine reticular formation (PRF) and activates possibly glutaminergic cells, which in turn activate lateral dorsal tegmental-pedunculopontine cholinergic cells. Medial PRF neurons might also activate GABA neurons, which hyperpolarize dorsal raphe serotonergic neurons.

The discovery of OX/HCRT and the finding that loss of the ligand HCRT/OX, which is located in neurons rostral to the pons, can trigger cataplexy and REM sleep onset in mice demonstrates that forebrain mechanisms also control REM sleep. The LC receives an especially heavy innervation of HCRT fibers. Narcoleptic canines and HCRT/OX knockout mice display cataplexy and rapid onset to REM sleep. In the dogs, the HCRT-2R/OX2R is mutated *(65)*, whereas in the mice the ligand is absent. Both findings indicate that cataplexy and REM sleep can be obtained by manipulating the HCRT/OX pathway, at either the ligand or the receptor level. It is very likely that ligand–receptor interaction in the dorsolateral pons is the site of action for the REM sleep and cataplexy because of the extensive literature implicating this region in these behaviors.

The findings associating loss of HCRT/OX with REM sleep and cataplexy provide a possible mechanism that could stop LC neuronal firing. The peptide HCRT/OX is excitatory *(66)*, increasing the activity of LC neurons *(15,67)*. Thus, HCRT/OX firing would secrete the peptide onto LC neurons and maintain LC firing. This in turn would maintain muscle tone and inhibit REM sleep. Loss of the ligand (OX knockout) or mutation of the receptor (narcoleptic canines) would impair LC firing, resulting in cataplexy and REM sleep.

Siegel proposed this model *(68)*, which can be directly tested. Indeed, if the HCRT/OX innervation of LC neurons is critical for maintaining muscle tone, one can very easily destroy the LC and determine whether cataplexy or REM sleep occurs. This can be directly tested by lesioning the LC and determining if it triggers cataplexy or increases REM sleep. We have used the DβH-sap in combination with the HCRT-2-sap to determine changes in sleep after pontine lesions.

When we applied HCRT-2-sap to the pontine brainstem region implicated in REM sleep generation, total sleep time increased *(69)*. During the third week after injection, HCRT-2-sap lesions increased total sleep time by 31.1% over controls ($p < 0.008$). Both non-REM and REM sleep percentages were increased. In the third week, nighttime non-REM sleep was 30% above control levels ($p = 0.011$ vs saline). HCRT-2-sap also increased overall nocturnal REM sleep by 57.5% ($p < 0.001$). Medullary lesions with

HCRT-2-sap also significantly increased nighttime amounts of REM sleep percentage during each of the 3 wk of recording (+22% vs saline, $p = 0.003$).

When the LC was destroyed with DβH-sap, no long-term increase in sleep was found, indicating that HCRT/OX projection to the LC neurons is not key to promoting wakefulness or inhibiting REM sleep. This is consistent with data that LC neurons contain the HCRT/OX receptor 1, whereas it is only the HCRT/OX receptor 2 that is mutated in canine narcolepsy.

Our findings are very interesting in that, in over 60 yr of research in the PRF, no lesion has ever been shown to increase REM sleep or total sleep time. With HCRT-2-sap lesions, we obtained an increase in both non-REM and REM sleep, which again argues for targeting specific neuronal phenotypes.

SUMMARY

Transection, lesion, and electrophysiology studies determined that wakefulness, non-REM sleep, and REM sleep are generated from specific brain areas. However, in these areas neurons responsible for sleep and wakefulness are intermingled with neurons subserving other behaviors. With the aid of saporin conjugates, we are lesioning specific neuronal phenotypes and determining the role of specific neurons in sleep and wakefulness. For instance, by conjugating the ligand HCRT-2 (OX B) to saporin (HCRT-2-sap), HCRT-R/OX-R-bearing neurons can be selectively lesioned. When this conjugate is applied to the lateral hypothalamus, the HCRT/OX neurons are lesioned, and rats demonstrate narcolepticlike behavior. Previously, investigators had made electrolytic or excitotoxic lesions of the lateral hypothalamus, but consistent changes in sleep/wakefulness were never obtained. Now, with targeted application of the saporin conjugate, specific neurons can be lesioned, resulting in behaviors that had not been seen in other nonspecific lesion experiments.

The saporin-based neurotoxins provide an inexpensive, easy, and reliable method to lesion specific cell types. Investigators can test specific hypotheses across species to determine whether the network is the same in all animals. Our use of these neurotoxins has significantly aided our understanding of the neuronal circuit underlying sleep.

ACKNOWLEDGMENTS

This work was supported by grants from the National Institutes of Health and Veterans Administration Medical Research Service.

REFERENCES

1. Rechtschaffen A, Gilliland MA, Bergmann BM, Winter JB. Physiological correlates of prolonged sleep deprivation in rats. Science 1983;221:182–184.
2. Mantyh PW, Rogers SD, Honore P, et al. Inhibition of hyperalgesia by ablation of lamina I spinal neurons expressing the substance P receptor. Science 1997;278:275–279.
3. Waite JJ, Wardlow ML, Chen AC, Lappi DA, Wiley RG, Thal LJ. Time course of cholinergic and monoaminergic changes in rat brain after immunolesioning with 192 IgG-saporin. Neurosci Lett 1994;169:154–158.
4. Gerashchenko D, Kohls MD, Greco M, et al. Hypocretin-2-saporin lesions of the lateral hypothalamus produce narcoleptic-like sleep behavior in the rat. J Neurosci 2001;21:7273–7283.
5. Peyron C, Faraco J, Rogers W, et al. A mutation in a case of early onset narcolepsy and a generalized absence of hypocretin peptides in human narcoleptic brains. Nat Med 2000;6:991–997.
6. Thannickal TC, Moore RY, Nienhuis R, et al. Reduced number of hypocretin neurons in human narcolepsy. Neuron 2000;27:469–474.
7. Peyron C, Tighe DK, Van den Pol AN, et al. Neurons containing hypocretin (orexin) project to multiple neuronal systems. J Neurosci 1998;18:9996–10,015.
8. Sakurai T, Amemiya A, Ishii M, et al. Orexins and orexin receptors: a family of hypothalamic neuropeptides and G protein-coupled receptors that regulate feeding behavior [comment]. Cell 1998;2:573–585.
9. De Lecea L, Kilduff TS, Peyron C, et al. The hypocretins: hypothalamus-specific peptides with neuroexcitatory activity. Proc Natl Acad Sci USA 1998;95:322–327.
10. Trivedi P, Yu H, MacNeil DJ, Van der Ploeg LH, Guan XM. Distribution of orexin receptor mRNA in the rat brain [published erratum appears in FEBS Lett 1999;442:122]. FEBS Lett 1998;438:71–75.
11. Marcus JN, Aschkenasi CJ, Lee CE, et al. Differential expression of orexin receptors 1 and 2 in the rat brain. J Comp Neurol 2001;435:6–25.
12. Greco MA, Shiromani PJ. Hypocretin receptor protein and mRNA expression in the dorsolateral pons of rats. Mol Brain Res 2001;88:176–182.
13. Date Y, Ueta Y, Yamashita H, et al. Orexins, orexigenic hypothalamic peptides, interact with autonomic, neuroendocrine and neuroregulatory systems. Proc Natl Acad Sci USA 1999;96:748–753.
14. Horvath TL, Diano S, Van den Pol AN. Synaptic interaction between hypocretin (orexin) and neuropeptide Y cells in the rodent and primate hypothalamus: a novel circuit implicated in metabolic and endocrine regulations. J Neurosci 1999;19:1072–1087.
15. Hagan JJ, Leslie RA, Patel S, et al. Orexin A activates locus coeruleus cell firing and increases arousal in the rat. Proc Natl Acad Sci USA 1999;96:10,911–10,916.
16. Shiromani P, Rapaport MH, Gillin JC. The neurobiology of sleep: basic concepts and clinical implications. In: Hales RE, Frances AJ, eds. *Psychiatry Up-*

date: The American Psychiatric Association Annual Review. Vol. 6. Washington, DC: American Psychiatric Press; 1987:235–259.

17. Shiromani PJ, Scammell TE, Sherin JE, Saper CB. Hypothalamic regulation of sleep. In: Lydic R, Baghdoyan HA, eds. *Handbook of Behavioral State Control: Cellular and Molecular Mechanisms.* Boca Raton, FL: CRC Press; 1998:311–325.

18. Shiromani PJ. Sleep circuitry, regulation and function: lesson from c-fos, leptin and timeless. In: Morrison A, Fluharty C, eds. *Progress in Psychobiology and Physiological Psychology.* San Diego, CA: Academic Press; 1998:67–90.

19. Szymusiak R. Magnocellular nuclei of the basal forebrain: substrates of sleep and arousal regulation. Sleep 1995;18:478–500.

20. Mesulam MM. Human brain cholinergic pathways. In: Aquilonius SM, Gillberg PG, eds. *Cholinergic Neurotransmission: Functional and Clinical Aspects.* Amsterdam, The Netherlands: Elsevier Science; 1990:231–241.

21. Alam MN, Szymusiak R, McGinty D. Local preoptic/anterior hypothalamic warming alters spontaneous and evoked neuronal activity in the magno-cellular basal forebrain. Brain Res 1995;696:221–230.

22. Koyama Y, Hayaishi O. Modulation by prostaglandins of activity of sleep-related neurons in the preoptic/anterior hypothalamic areas in rats. Brain Res Bull 1994;33:367–372.

23. Porkka-Heiskanen T, Strecker RE, Thakkar M, Bjorkum AA, Greene RW, McCarley RW. Adenosine: a mediator of the sleep-inducing effects of prolonged wakefulness. Science 1997;276:1265–1266.

24. Vanderwolf CH. Cerebral activity and behavior control by central cholinergic and serotonergic systems. Int Rev Neurobiol 1988;30:225–340.

25. Jasper HH, Tessier J. Acetylcholine liberation from cerebral cortex during paradoxical (REM) sleep. Science 1971;172:601–602.

26. Szerb JC. Cortical acetylcholine release and electroencephalographic arousal. J Physiol (London) 1967;192:329–345.

27. Rasmusson DD, Clow K, Szerb JC. Frequency-dependent increase in cortical acetylcholine release evoked by stimulation of the nucleus basalis magnocellularis in the rat. Brain Res 1992;594:150–154.

28. Buzsaki G, Bickford R, Ponomareff G, Thal LJ, Mandel R, Gage FH. Nucleus basalis and thalamic control of neocortical activity in the freely moving rat. J Neurosci 1998;8:4007–4026.

29. Ray P, Jackson W. Lesions of nucleus basalis alter ChAT activity and EEG in rat frontal neocortex. Electroencephalogr Clin Neurophysiol 1991;79:62–68.

30. Dekker AJ, Thal LJ. Independent effects of cholinergic and serotonergic lesions on acetylcholine and serotonin release in the neocortex of the rat. Neurochem Res 1993;18:277–283.

31. Bassant MH, Apartis E, Jazat-Poindessous FR, Wiley RG, Lamour YA. Selective immunolesion of the basal forebrain cholinergic neurons: effects on hippocampal activity during sleep and wakefulness in the rat. Neurodegeneration 1995;4:61–70.

32. Kapas L, Obal FJ, Book AA, Schweitzer JB, Wiley RG, Krueger JM. The effects of immunolesions of nerve growth factor-receptive neurons by 192 IgG-saporin on sleep. Brain Res 1996;712:53–59.

33. Gerashchenko D, Salin-Pascual R, Shiromani PJ. Effects of hypocretin-saporin injections into the medial septum on sleep and hippocampal τ. Brain Res 2001;913:106–115.

34. Alreja M. Excitatory actions of serotonin on GABAergic neurons of the medial septum and diagonal band of Broca. Synapse 2000;22:15–27.

35. Wu M, Shanabrough M, Leranth C, Alreja M. Cholinergic excitation of septohippocampal GABA but not cholinergic neurons: implications for learning and memory. J Neurosci 2000;20:3900–3908.

36. Nauta WJH. Hypothalamic regulation of sleep in rats. An experimental study. J Neurophysiol 1946;9:285–316.

37. Shoham S, Teitelbaum P. Subcortical waking and sleep during lateral hypothalamic "somnolence" in rats. Physiol Behav 1982;28:323–333.

38. McGinty DJ. Somnolence, recovery and hyposomnia following ventromedial diencephalic lesions in the rat. Electroencephalogr Clin Neurophysiol 1969;26:70–79.

39. Jurkowlaniec E, Trojnar W, Tokarski J. The EEG activity after lesions of the diencephalic part of the zona incerta in rats. Acta Physiol Pol 1990;41:85–97.

40. Denoyer M, Sallanon M, Buda C, Kitahama K, Jouvet M. Neurotoxic lesion of the mesencephalic reticular formation and/or the posterior hypothalamus does not alter waking in the cat. Brain Res 1991;539:303.

41. Sallanon M, Sakai K, Buda C, Puymartin M, Jouvet M. Increase of paradoxical sleep induced by microinjections of ibotenic acid into the ventrolateral part of the posterior hypothalamus in the cat. Arch Ital Biol 1988;126:87–97.

42. Gerashchenko D, Blanco-Centurion C, Greco MA, Shiromani PJ. Effects of lateral hypothalamic lesion with the neurotoxin hypocretin2-saporin on sleep in Long Evans rats. Neuroscience 2003;116:223–235.

43. Senba E, Daddona PE, Watanabe T, Wu JY, Nagy JI. Coexistence of adenosine deaminase, histidine decarboxylase, and glutamate decarboxylase in hypothalamic neurons of the rat. J Neurosci 1985;5:3392–3402.

44. Vanni-Mercier G, Sakai K, Jouvet M. Neurones specifiques de l'eveil dans l'hypothalamus posterieur. CR Acad Sci 1984;298:195–200.

45. Szymusiak R, Iriye T, McGinty D. Sleep-waking discharge of neurons in the posterior lateral hypothalamic area of cats. Brain Res Bull 1989;23:111–120.

46. Sakai K, El Mansari M, Lin JS, Zhang G, Vanni-Mercier G. The posterior hypothalamus in the regulation of wakefulness and paradoxical sleep. In: Mancia M, Marini G, eds. *The Diencephalon and Sleep.* New York: Raven Press; 1990:171–198.

47. Lin JS, Sakai K, Jouvet M. Hypothalamo-preoptic histaminergic projections in sleep-wake control in the cat. Eur J Neurosci 1994;6:618–625.

48. Parmentier R, Ohtsu H, Djebbara-Hannas Z, Valatx J-L, Watanabe T, Lin J-S. Anatomical, physiological, and pharmacological characteristics of histidine decarboxylase knock-out mice: evidence for the role of brain histamine in behavioral and sleep-wake control. J Neurosci 2003;22:7695–7711.

49. Eriksson KS, Sergeeva O, Brown RE, Haas HL. Orexin/hypocretin excites the histaminergic neurons of the tuberomammillary nucleus. J Neurosci 2001;21:9273–9279.
50. Huang ZL, Qu WM, Li WD, et al. Arousal effect of orexin A depends on activation of the histaminergic system. Proc Natl Acad Sci USA 2001;98:9965–9970.
51. Li Y, Gao XB, Sakurai T, Van den Pol AN. Hypocretin/orexin excites hypocretin neurons via a local glutamate neuron- a potential mechanism for orchestrating the hypothalamic arousal system. Neuron 2002;35:1169–1181.
52. Lucas EA, Sterman MB. Effect of a forebrain lesion on the polycyclic sleep-wake cycle and sleep-wake patterns in the cat. Exp Neurol 1975;46:368–388.
53. Szymusiak R, McGinty D. Sleep suppression following kainic acid-induced lesions of the basal forebrain. Exp Neurol 1986;94:598–614.
54. Sallanon M, Denoyer M, Kitahama K, Aubert C, Gay N, Jouvet M. Long-lasting insomnia induced by preoptic neuron lesions and its transient reversal by muscimol injection into the posterior hypothalamus in the cat. Neuroscience 1989;32:669–683.
55. Shoham S, Blatteis CM, Krueger JM. Effects of preoptic area lesions on muramyl dipeptide-induced sleep. Brain Research Brain Res 1989;476:396–399.
56. Asala SA, Okano Y, Honda K, Inoue S. Effects of medial preoptic area lesions on sleep and wakefulness in unrestrained rats. Neurosci Lett 1990;114:300–304.
57. John J, Kumar VM, Gopinath G, Ramesh V, Mallick H. Changes in sleep-wakefulness after kainic acid lesion of the preoptic area in rats. Jpn J Physiol 1994;44:231–242.
58. Sterman MB, Clemente C. Forebrain inhibitory mechanisms: sleep patterns induced by basal forebrain stimulation in the behaving cat. Exp Neurol 1962;6:103–117.
59. Szymusiak R, McGinty D. Sleep-related neuronal discharge in the basal forebrain of cats. Brain Res 1986;370:82–92.
60. Kaitin K. Preoptic area unit activity during sleep and wakefulness in the cat. Exp Neurol 1984;83:347–351.
61. Findlay ALR, Hayward JN. Spontaneous activity of single neurones in the hypothalamus of rabbits during sleep and waking. J Physiol 1969;201:237–258.
62. Koyama Y, Hayaishi O. Firing of neurons in the preoptic/anterior hypothalamic areas in rat: its possible involvement in slow wave sleep and paradoxical sleep. Neurosci Res 1994;19:31–38.
63. Sherin JE, Shiromani PJ, McCarley RW, Saper CB. Activation of ventrolateral preoptic neurons during sleep. Science 1996;271:216–219.
64. Szymusiak R, Alam MN, Steininger TL, McGinty D. Sleep–waking discharge patterns of ventrolateral preoptic/anterior hypothalamic neurons in rats. Brain Res 1998;803:178–188.
65. Lin L, Faraco J, Li R, et al. The sleep disorder canine narcolepsy is caused by a mutation in the hypocretin (orexin) receptor 2 gene. Cell 1999;98:365–376.
66. Horvath TL, Peyron C, Diano S, et al. Hypocretin (orexin) activation and synaptic innervation of the locus coeruleus noradrenergic system. J Comp Neurol 1999;415:145–159.

67. Bourgin P, Huitron-Resendiz S, Spier AD, et al. Hypocretin-1 modulates rapid eye movement sleep through activation of locus coeruleus neurons. J Neurosci 2000;20:7760–7765.
68. Siegel JM. Narcolepsy. Sci Am 2000;282:76–81.
69. Blanco-Centurion C, Gerashchenko D, Salin-Pascual R, Shiromani PJ. Effects of hypocretin2-saporin and antidopamine-beta-hydroxylase saporin neurotoxic lesions of the dorsolateral pons on sleep and muscle tone. Eur J Neurosci 2004;19:2741–2752.

Isolectin IB4-Mediated Cytotoxic Targeting of Sensory Neurons

Lucy Vulchanova and Christopher N. Honda

INTRODUCTION

Lectins are carbohydrate-binding proteins that recognize distinct oligosaccharide moieties of glycoproteins and glycolipids. In vertebrates, endogenous lectins serve a variety of functions, including cell adhesion, cell recognition, signal transduction, and endocytosis, in both neuronal and non-neuronal cells *(1–5)*. A role for cell surface carbohydrate recognition has been described in processes, such as fertilization, development, leukocyte homing, and the innate immune response *(1,2)*. Among the known classes of vertebrate carbohydrate-binding proteins are some cytokines (e.g., interleukin 1β [IL-1β]) and growth factors, which possess a receptor-binding domain and a carbohydrate recognition domain *(4,5)*.

A number of exogenous lectins that recognize cell surface carbohydrates in vertebrates are used as research tools. Among these is isolectin I-B4 from *Bandaireae simplicifolia* (IB4), which recognizes terminal α-D-galactose residues of glycosphingolipids and glycoproteins. In rodents, IB4 binds to a number of cell types, including sensory neurons, activated microglia, endothelial cells, and macrophages *(6–9)*. In most cases, the identity or function of the IB4-binding site is unknown. For example, in sensory neurons, there is evidence for the existence of an IB4-binding glycolipid *(10)*, as well as IB4-binding glycoproteins *(11)*, whereas in macrophages, IB4 binds to a glycoprotein, eliciting signal transduction that leads to modulation of gene transcription *(7)*.

One of the most common research applications of IB4 is its use as a histochemical marker and neuronal tracer in dorsal root ganglia (DRG). We and

From: *Molecular Neurosurgery With Targeted Toxins*
Edited by: R. G. Wiley and D. A. Lappi © Humana Press Inc., Totowa, NJ

others have extended these applications to cytotoxic targeting of IB4-binding neurons in DRG using a conjugate of IB4 and saporin (IB4-sap) *(12–14)*. These studies were designed as a "loss-of-function" approach exploring the role of IB4-binding sensory neurons in acute and persistent pain. This chapter presents a discussion of the application of IB4-sap in pain studies.

OVERVIEW OF IB4-BINDING SENSORY NEURONS

The subset of IB4-binding DRG neurons is neurochemically, and most likely functionally, heterogeneous. The majority (85%) of these neurons also contain the enzyme fluoride-resistant acid phosphatase (FRAP) *(9,15,16)*. Although FRAP neurons are often referred to as nonpeptidergic, it has been shown indirectly that many of them contain calcitonin gene-related peptide *(16)*. A detailed characterization of the subpopulation of IB4-binding neurons showed that it includes nearly all (95%) FRAP-positive DRG neurons, all somatostatin-positive neurons, and 40% of the substance P (SP)-positive neurons *(16)*.

It has been shown that a large proportion of IB4-binding neurons express other proteins linked to nociception or chronic pain, such as the adenosine triphosphate-gated ion channel P2X3, the capsaicin receptor VR1, cyclooxygenase-1, and tetrodotoxin-resistant sodium channels *(17–22)*. Based on double-labeling experiments reported in some of these studies, it can be deduced that the presence or absence of FRAP, SP, somatostatin, P2X3, and VR1 can define as many as six neurochemical subtypes of IB4-binding neurons; the largest is FRAP/IB4/VR1/P2X3 positive.

It should be noted that histological characterization of IB4-binding neurons has been done almost exclusively in the rat, and reports have pointed out that the neurochemical signature of IB4-binding neurons in the mouse is different. For example, mouse IB4-binding neurons do not appear to express VR1 *(23)*.

Based on studies in culture, the functional properties of IB4-binding neurons are consistent with the idea that they represent a heterogeneous population, which includes nociceptors *(24–26)*. Finally, IB4-binding neurons are glial cell line-derived neurotrophic factor-dependent in adulthood, but there is functional and histochemical evidence that a fraction is also nerve growth factor responsive *(26,27)*.

When injected into the sciatic nerve, IB4 recognizes binding sites on axons and undergoes endocytosis, followed by retrograde transport to the cell body and central terminals of IB4-binding sensory neurons *(16,28–30)*. It has been demonstrated that the axons that internalize IB4 are from the same neurons that bind IB4 in histological experiments *(16)*. Cholera toxin B and wheat germ agglutinin (WGA), which recognize the glycosphingolipid GM1 and *N*-acetyl-D-glucosamine sugar residues and sialic acid, respectively, are also internalized and transported retrogradely. In sensory ganglia, WGA and cholera toxin B label predominantly small- and large-diameter neurons, respectively. The IB4-binding neurons are most likely a subset of the WGA neurons *(29)*.

ADMINISTRATION OF IB4-SAP TO IB4-BINDING NEURONS

Based on the evidence for retrograde transport of IB4, we have used sciatic nerve injection to deliver IB4-sap to IB4-binding neurons *(12)*. The injection is administered at the level of the thigh, proximal to the branching of the peroneal and tibial nerves. Because there is variability in the specific location of this branching, it is possible that inadvertent targeting of one of these branches rather than the entire sciatic nerve contributes to variability in the outcome of the treatment.

To deliver the injection, the sciatic nerve is exposed and teased apart from connective tissue. A strip of parafilm (~10 mm wide) is threaded under the nerve to provide support. The needle (16-gage Hamilton syringe) is inserted as parallel to the nerve as possible to minimize nerve damage, and 5 µL of test solution are injected slowly. Although this delivery approach is inevitably associated with some degree of nerve damage, the injection alone does not contribute to abnormal nociceptive responses. Signs of a successful injection include a slight swelling of the nerve, as well as lack of leakage following needle retraction.

Because IB4 binding sites are present in the central (spinal cord) and peripheral (skin) processes of IB4-binding neurons, theoretically it should be possible to deliver IB4 and IB4 conjugates by intrathecal or intradermal injections. To our knowledge, there are no reports of lectin uptake into DRG neurons after intrathecal injection. However, we have observed retrograde transport of IB4 after an intradermal injection. This route of administration would avoid the damage associated with direct injection into the nerve and may also be advantageous in studies using IB4-sap in combination with certain models of neuropathic pain. However, intradermal delivery of IB4-sap may be associated with widespread targeting of non-neuronal cells (e.g., epidermis, endothelium) and with variability in the subset of targeted neurons because of the challenge to deliver consistent injections.

Table 1
Experimental Groups and Treatment Doses

Experimental groups	Treatment doses
IB4-sap conjugate[a] (IB4-sap)	400 µg/mL
IB4[b]	280 µg/mL[c]
Saporin[a]	120 µg/mL[c]
Mixture of unconjugated IB4 and saporin (IB4 + saporin)	280 µg/mL IB4 and 120 µg/mL saporin
Vehicle (PBS)	—

[a]Advanced Targeting Systems, San Diego, CA.
[b]Sigma Chemical Co., St. Louis, MO.
[c]These concentrations were based on the fact that IB4 (MW 114,000) accounts for 71% of the molecular weight of the conjugate (MW 160,000). There are approx 1.3 molecules of saporin per molecule of IB4. PBS, phosphate buffered saline; IB4, isolectin I-B4.

The volume of all injections and the concentrations of IB4 are similar to those previously reported for injections of IB4 into sciatic nerve *(16)*. For retrograde labeling, Wang et al. tested concentrations from 0.02 to 20% in a 5-µL volume and concluded that the labeling was optimal at 0.2–2%. The dose dependence of IB4-sap effects has not been examined in vivo. We have administered IB4-sap as a 0.04% or 400 µg/mL solution in 5 µL (equivalent to 2 µg/injection). The extent of depletion of IB4-binding neurons suggested that treatment with this dose affected all neurons with axons that were exposed to the conjugate, achieving a maximal effect. Therefore, higher doses would not be recommended because they may compromise the selectivity of IB4-sap for IB4-binding sensory neurons, whereas lower doses may be beneficial in reducing non-neuronal cytotoxicity at the injection site. The study of the dose dependence of IB4-sap effects may be complicated by the fact that lower doses can reduce the number of affected neurons or delay the onset of cytotoxicity, which behaviorally would be manifested as reduction in maximal effect and changes in time-course, respectively. Finally, the doses of control treatments of unconjugated IB4 and saporin should correspond to their molar ratio in the conjugate (Table 1).

VISUALIZATION OF IB4-BINDING SITES AND IB4-SAP INTERNALIZATION IN DRG NEURONS

Histologically, IB4 binding sites on neurons can be detected with IB4 conjugated to a compound permitting visualization, such as biotin, a fluorophore, or horse radish peroxidase. Alternately, binding of unconjugated IB4 can be followed by visualization with an antiserum (anti-BSI) that recognizes all type I isolectins from *Bandaireae simplicifolia* (i.e., A4, A3B1, etc.). These methods differ in their sensitivity and the number of steps involved in the procedure.

Fluorophore conjugates of IB4 allow visualization of binding sites in a single step and have been very useful in the in vitro studies of IB4-binding neurons *(24–26)*. In sections of fixed DRG, we have observed the following order of labeling intensity at the commonly used IB4 concentration of 10 μg/mL: fluorophore-IB4 less than biotin-IB4, visualized by fluorophore-conjugated streptavidin, visualized less than IB4, by anti-BSI and secondary antiserum. As the optimal combination of sensitivity and efficiency, we routinely use biotinylated IB4 followed by Cyanine 3.18 (Cy3)- or FITC(DTAF)-conjugated streptavidin for detection of IB4 binding in fixed tissue (*see* Table 2 for details).

Reports of the proportion of DRG neurons that bind IB4 vary considerably, most likely because of technical differences in detection methods, tissue-processing methods, or approaches to counting of neurons. Studies reporting higher proportions of IB4-binding neurons (up to 65% of total neurons in lumbar DRG) have described three different patterns of IB4 labeling (Fig. 1) *(16,19,27)*:

1. Small cells (approx 40% of total) with intense labeling along the cell membrane and on coarse granules surrounding the nucleus.
2. Small cells with weaker labeling along the cell membrane and on coarse granules surrounding the nucleus.
3. Larger cells with fine granular labeling distributed throughout the cytoplasm but weak or no labeling along the cell membrane.

Less sensitive detection methods may limit the ability to visualize reliably the last two categories.

Following injection into the sciatic nerve, IB4 can be detected in DRG cell bodies as early as 12 h, and the staining intensity is maximal between 3 and 8 d after injection. We examined the transport of IB4-sap, unconjugated IB4, and unconjugated saporin in DRG 3 d after sciatic nerve injection. Anti-BSI was used to detect transported IB4 following injections of IB4 (not shown), IB4-sap, and IB4 plus saporin (not shown), whereas biotinylated IB4 was used to visualize IB4-binding sites in the DRG independent of IB4 uptake (Fig. 2, green). A saporin antibody was used to visualize saporin after injections of IB4-sap, saporin, and IB4 plus saporin (*see* Table 2 for details). In IB4-sap-treated rats, anti-BSI (not shown) and anti-saporin (Fig. 2, red) staining was observed in L4 and L5 DRG. Transported IB4 was also observed in L4 and L5 DRG following injections of IB4 alone and IB4 plus saporin (not shown). Anti-saporin labeling was not detected in DRG of any

Table 2
Materials and Methods: Histochemistry

Primary reagent	Concentration	Vendor	Secondary reagent	Concentration	Vendor
Biotinylated IB4	10 µg/mL	Sigma	FITC- or Cy3-conjugated streptavidin	1:200–400	Jackson Immuno-Research
Goat anti-BSI	1:1000	Vector Laboratories	All secondary antisera were obtained from Jackson ImmunoResearch and used diluted		
Goat anti-saporin	1:1000	Advanced Targeting Systems	1:100–200 Single labeling: cyanine 3.18-conjugated secondary antisera (Cy3).		
Rabbit anti-PGP9.5	1:1000	Biogenesis	Double labeling: a combination of lissamine rhodamine[a]–fluorescein isothiocyanate-conjugated secondary antisera		
Mouse anti-myelin basic protein	1:1000	Chemicon			

[a]The currently available fluorophore is rhodamine Red-X.

Tissues were obtained after perfusion fixation. Rats were deeply anesthetized and perfused through the heart with phosphate buffered saline (PBS) followed by fixative (4% paraformaldehyde and 0.2% picric acid in $0.1M$ phosphate buffer at pH 6.9) for 30 min. Dissected tissues were immersed in 20% (skin) or 10% (DRG, spinal cord) sucrose in PBS for at least 24 h prior to cryostat sectioning. Slide-mounted cryostat tissue sections (14 μM for spinal cord and sciatic nerve; 14, 20, or 30 μM for DRG) and free-floating 30-μM sections of glabrous skin were processed for immunohistochemistry as previously described (62). Tissue sections were surveyed with conventional fluorescence microscopy, and images were obtained using laser scanning confocal microscopy (MRC-1024, BioRad Laboratories, Hercules, CA).

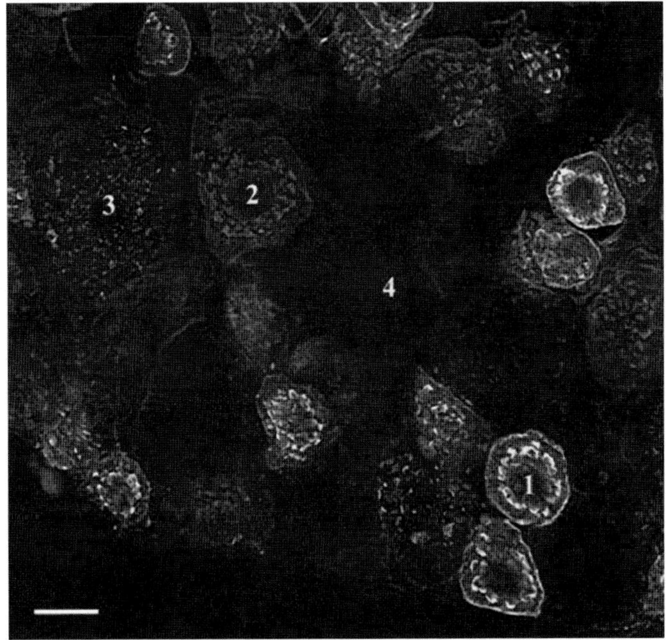

Fig. 1. Three distinct patterns of isolectin I-B4 binding in dorsal root ganglia neurons. The numbers correspond to the description in the text. An unlabeled neuron is indicated by 4. Scale bar = 60 μM.

group of animals except for those receiving IB4-sap, suggesting that unconjugated saporin was not internalized and transported by axons of sensory neurons. Anti-saporin staining was not present in all IB4-binding neurons (Fig. 2) as would be expected based on the fact that not all of the neurons in L5 DRG have axons in the sciatic nerve at the injection level *(31,32)*.

EVALUATION OF THE DEPLETION OF IB4-BINDING NEURONS

The rationale for using IB4-sap for selective cytotoxic targeting was based on the assumption that IB4-sap would retain the binding properties of unconjugated IB4 and would be taken up by the same neurons that take up unconjugated IB4. The affinity of IB4 for its carbohydrate ligand in DRG has not been determined experimentally. We have tested the binding properties of IB4-sap by comparing staining of fixed DRG with equivalent concentrations of IB4-sap and unconjugated IB4. Although the binding activity of IB4-sap (judged by intensity and signal-to-noise ratio of staining)

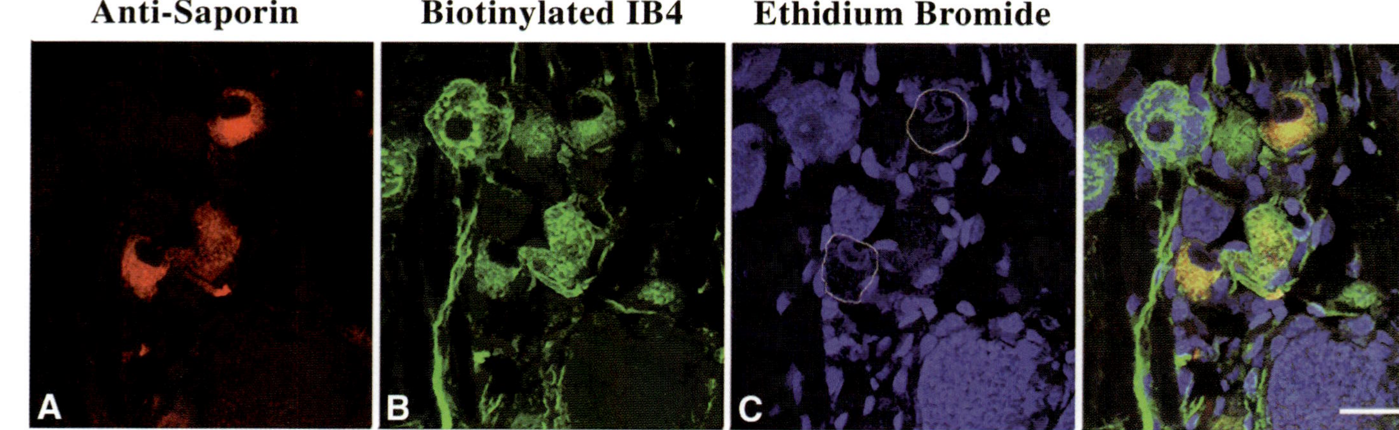

Fig. 2. Uptake of isolectin I-B4 saporin (IB4-sap) in dorsal root ganglion neurons 3 d after a sciatic nerve injection. Labeli with (**A**) anti-saporin and (**B**) biotinylated IB4 showed that the conjugate was transported to the cell bodies of a subset of IB binding neurons, which have eccentric nuclei and appear shriveled. (**C**) Conjugate-containing neurons (outlined in white) are n labeled by ethidium bromide, which binds to ribosomal RNA in the cytoplasm of neurons, suggesting disruption of protein synth sis by IB4-sap. (**D**) Digital overlay of the three markers. Scale bar = 25 µ*M*.

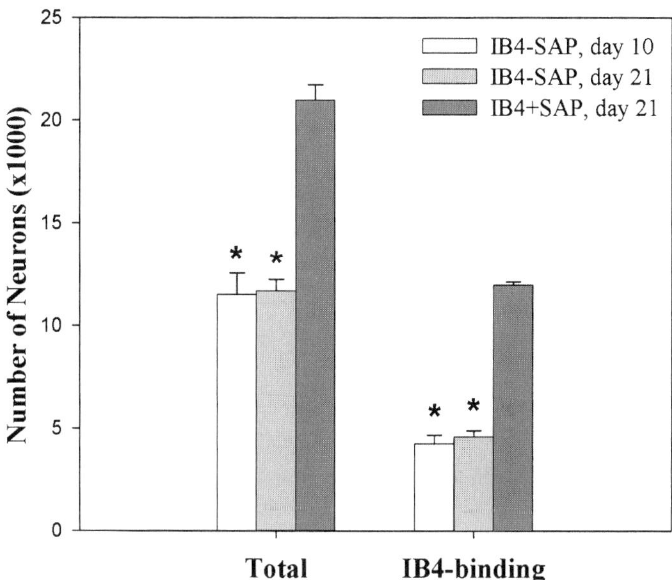

Fig. 3: Depletion of sensory neurons after isolectin I-B4 saporin (IB4-sap) treatment. L5 dorsal root ganglia (DRG) were double labeled with ethidium bromide (EB; 5 µg/mL) and biotinylated IB4. EB was used to determine the total number of neurons, and biotinylated IB4 was used to determine the number of IB4-binding neurons. At 10 and 21 d after IB4-sap treatment, the total number of neurons and the number of IB4-binding neurons in ipsilateral L5 DRG ($n = 4$) was decreased compared to control ($n = 6$) treatment with unconjugated mixture of IB4 and saporin ($p < 0.001$; one-way analysis of variance, followed by Tukey test for multiple comparisons). *Significant difference from control.

appeared to be decreased compared to IB4, the pattern of staining obtained with IB4-sap and IB4 was the same. Based on these observations we concluded that the binding properties of IB4-sap were adequate for cytotoxic targeting of IB4-binding neurons.

We used qualitative and quantitative histological analysis to assess the cytotoxicity of IB4-sap after internalization in sensory neurons. Varying degrees of cytotoxic damage were evident in DRG somata 3 d after sciatic nerve injection of the IB4-sap conjugate. The majority of conjugate-containing neurons showed signs of disrupted protein synthesis and had irregular nuclei and irregular cell perimeters (Fig. 2). At 10 and 21 d after IB4-sap treatment, the total number of neurons in the ipsilateral L5 DRG was reduced by 37% when compared to a control injection of unconjugated IB4, and the number of IB4-binding neurons decreased by approx 65% (Fig. 3).

The quantitative analysis of IB4-sap cytotoxicity is based on determining the number of neurons that die after IB4-sap treatment. There are two general approaches for estimating the total number of cells in a tissue of interest; these approaches are based on profile counting and stereology *(33,34)*. It has been argued that the interpretation of the effects of an experimental treatment using profile counts may be misleading *(35)*. For example, differences in numbers of profiles between two groups may result from morphological changes rather than changes in total number of cells. Because determining the changes in numbers of DRG neurons was critical for the evaluation of IB4-SAP cytotoxicity, we used a stereological approach based on the principles of the optical dissector *(19)*.

L5 DRG were sectioned perpendicular to their long axis into 30-μM cryostat sections. The length of each ganglion was estimated based on the number of sections that contained neurons. Five sections, equally spaced throughout the length of each ganglion, were selected using systematic random sampling *(34,36)* and were double labeled with biotinylated IB4 and ethidium bromide (EB), which was used to visualize all neurons. In each of the selected tissue sections, all neurons within a depth of 12 or 10 μm were imaged by collecting serial optical sections at 2-μM intervals with a krypton–argon laser confocal microscope that allowed imaging of IB4 binding and ethidium bromide staining within the same sample. The stacks of optical sections were examined using the MetaMorph Imaging system (Universal Imaging Corp., West Chester, PA), but the same analysis can be performed with public domain software, such as the US National Institutes of Health (NIH) developed at the NIH (http://rsb.info.nih.gov/nih-image). The first optical section in each stack was used as a "lookup" section in which cells containing nuclei were marked but not counted. In the subsequent optical sections, cells with nuclei that came into focus were marked and counted. Each tissue section was analyzed in its entirety by imaging adjacent, nonoverlapping fields of view.

This approach provided direct counts of the total number of neurons and the number of IB4-binding neurons within the 12 or 10 μM spanned by the optical sections. The counts satisfied the requirement for a sample size of 100 cells per ganglion for adequate estimate of total cell number *(34)*. An estimate of the numbers of labeled neurons per ganglion was obtained by multiplying the counts by the separation of the sampled tissue sections and correcting for the total volume of the ganglion (estimated by the number of sections containing cells and the thickness of the sections). The accuracy of the results from this analysis was affected by tissue processing (e.g., shrinkage caused by fixation and slide mounting, tissue penetration for labeling). However, this did not compromise the comparison between experimental

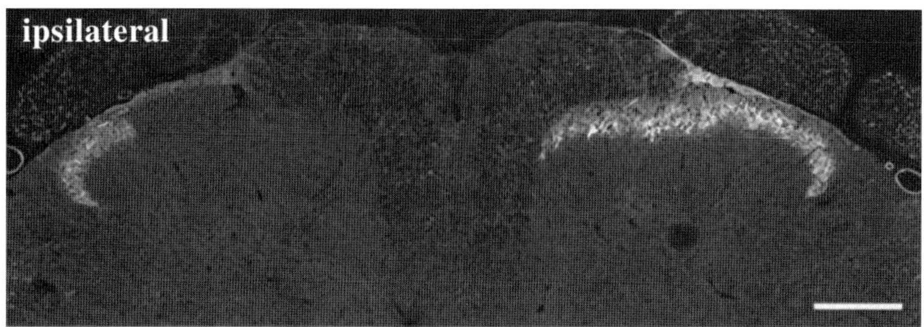

Fig. 4. Depletion of central terminals of isolectin I-B4 (IB4)-binding sensory neurons. At 21 d after unilateral IB4-saporin injection, IB4 binding was absent from the ipsilateral sciatic nerve terminal field in dorsal horn of the spinal cord. Scale bar = 200 μM.

groups because the effects of tissue processing are uniform across samples. Thus, taking advantage of confocal microscopy, this approach allowed evaluation of IB4-sap cytotoxicity based on direct counts of sensory neurons.

The depletion of IB4-binding neurons can also be evaluated at the level of their central and peripheral processes. IB4-sap treatment results in nearly complete loss of IB4 binding in the medial portion of the ipsilateral superficial dorsal horn (Fig. 4). Consistent with administration of the conjugate through sciatic nerve, this effect is restricted to the L4–L5 levels of spinal cord, and its mediolateral distribution corresponds to the terminal fields of sensory neurons projecting in sciatic nerve *(28)*. The loss of labeling was evident 10 d after IB4-sap treatment (the first time-point examined) and persisted for up to 42 d (the latest time-point examined).

The loss of IB4 binding in superficial dorsal horn can be assessed by quantitative image analysis based on measuring the area of labeling on slide-mounted cryostat sections *(37)*. To decrease variability caused by tissue processing, it is recommended that all experimental groups be represented on each tissue block used to generate sections. The imaging parameters are determined using a control sample and are set so that the labeling in the control image is not saturated. The parameters are held constant for each individual slide. The images can be analyzed using NIH Image or MetaMorph.

First, the area of interest within the dorsal horn of spinal cord is defined by manual outlining or using a standard box. For IB4-sap evaluation, the selected area included the medial two-thirds of dorsal horn, which corresponds to the projection site of sciatic nerve. Next, the image is thresholded to eliminate background staining. The optimal threshold for the control samples is used as the threshold for all measurements. Finally, the area of staining is measured either as number of labeled pixels or as percentage thresholded area, depending on the software program. For each slide, the area of staining of each sample (including control treated) is normalized to the mean of the area of staining of the control samples on the same slide. The final value for each sample is obtained by averaging the normalized measurements of the images from the three slides representative of a particular spinal cord segment.

When we used this approach to evaluate the depletion of IB4 binding in spinal cord, we found a decrease of 80% or more in IB4 binding ipsilateral to the injection compared to the contralateral side. In control animals or animals in which the IB4-sap injection was unsuccessful, the difference between the two sides was consistently within 20%. This quantitative analysis correlated well with qualitative evaluation of IB4 binding. Therefore, we have used qualitative evaluation of binding in spinal cord as a routine confirmation of cytotoxicity in behavioral studies.

Evaluation of depletion of IB4-binding peripheral processes in skin is more challenging than in DRG and spinal cord. In the skin, it is harder to achieve adequate sampling and to control conditions of tissue processing, such as the angle of cutting. Furthermore, the quantitative analysis of labeling in skin, whether it is based on the number of branching points of the nerve fibers or on their length, is very labor intensive and time consuming. Finally, the skin contains a number of non-neuronal IB4-binding sites (e.g., endothelial cells, epidermis), which interfere with the reliable identification of IB4-binding nerve fibers.

Our evaluation of IB4 binding in the skin of IB4-sap-treated rats was based on qualitative analysis. We created montages of slightly overlapping fields of view to obtain images of entire sections of footpads, ensuring that observed effects were not limited to isolated fields of view. To differentiate between IB4-binding nerve fibers and non-neuronal structures, we used double labeling with biotinylated IB4 and PGP9.5 (*see* Table 2). Images from the double-labeled preparations were processed in Adobe Photoshop (Adobe Systems Inc., San Jose, CA) to yield a thresholded image containing only IB4-binding nerve fibers (Fig. 5). Footpads from control rats exhibited a distinct plexus of IB4-binding fibers that was conspicuously absent 21 d after IB4-sap treatment. Moreover, in conjugate-treated rats, IB4-binding associated with the epidermis and blood vessels persisted, and PGP9.5 staining indicated the presence of surviving axons that did not bind IB4. Because the area of staining in the thresholded images is technically quantifiable, this approach has the potential for more automated analysis of labeling in

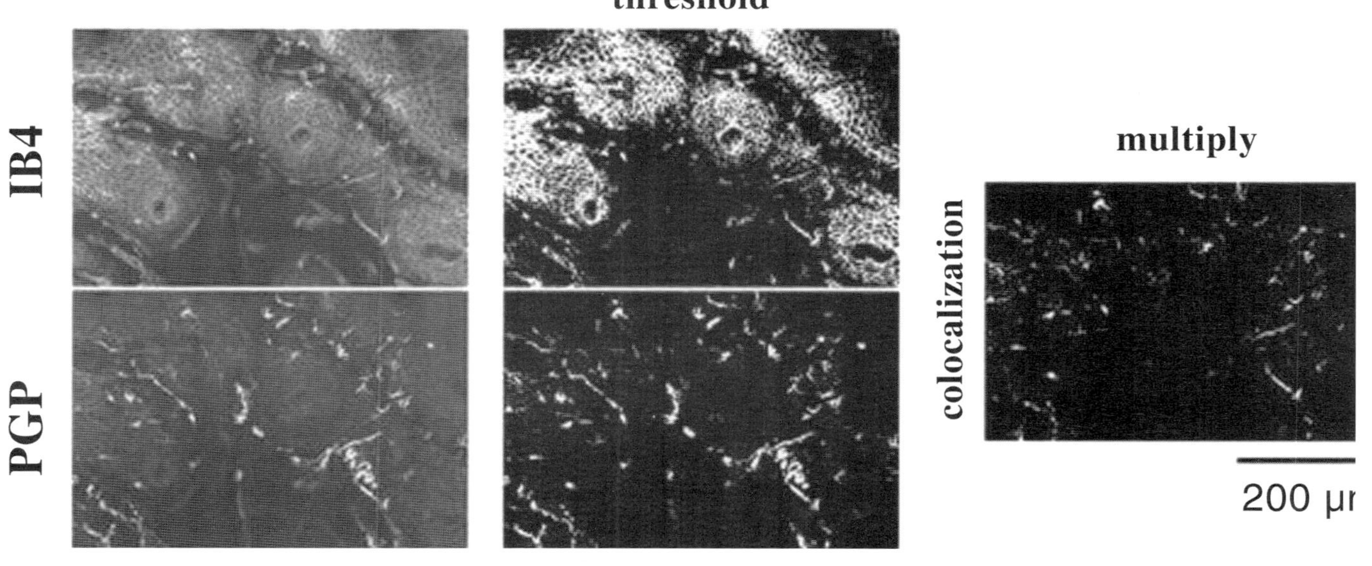

Fig. 5. Image processing of double labeling with anti-PGP9.5 and biotinylated isolectin I-B4 (IB4) in skin. Anti-PGP9 labels all nerve fibers, and biotinylated IB4 labels some nerve fibers, as well as other structures, such as blood vessels. To visualize clearly IB4-binding nerve fibers, the IB4 and PGP9.5 images were processed in Adobe Photoshop 5.0. First, the images were thresholded to separate the specific staining from background noise. Then, the thresholded images for IB4 and PGP9.5 were combined using the function "multiply." Corresponding pixels in the two thresholded images were multiplied so that pixels that were white (above threshold) in both images appeared white in the resulting image, whereas pixels that were black in one or both images appeared black in the resulting image. Therefore, the multiplication of the IB4 and PGP9.5 images showed the colocalization of the two markers. Scale bar = 200 μ*M*. Reprinted from ref. *12* with permission. Copyright 200 Elsevier.

skin, as well as colocalization of labeling in nerve fibers in the periphery or the central nervous system.

SELECTIVITY OF IB4-SAP TREATMENT FOR IB4-BINDING NEURONS

The utility of IB4-sap for the study of sensory neurons depends on its selectivity for IB4-binding neurons. The issue of selectivity arises at two levels. First, it is necessary to demonstrate that the treatment is restricted to IB4-binding sensory neurons and that it does not affect the non-IB4-binding subsets. Second, it is necessary to evaluate the potential contribution of non-neuronal IB4-binding sites to the observed treatment effects.

We used two approaches to test the selectivity of the IB4-sap conjugate for IB4-binding neurons. We determined first whether IB4-sap internalization and transport were restricted to IB4-binding DRG neurons. If the internalization of the conjugate is restricted to axons of IB4-binding neurons, then all IB4-sap-containing cell bodies in DRG should express IB4-binding sites. Using profile counting, we examined the colocalization of the conjugate and IB4-binding sites in L5 DRG 3 d after IB4-sap injection. Ipsilateral L5 DRG were sectioned in the plane parallel to their long axis, and five sections, equally spaced throughout each ganglion, were selected and processed histochemically. The sections were double labeled with anti-saporin (Fig. 2, red) to visualize the conjugate and biotinylated IB4 (Fig. 2, green) to visualize all IB4-binding sites independent of the internalization of IB4-sap.

In each section, one to three nonoverlapping images were collected with a confocal microscope. Only cells with nuclei were counted. For each marker, the counts from all images taken from the same ganglion were added. The percentage colocalization was determined for each ganglion, and the results were averaged. This approach allows assessment of the variability between individual ganglia and the consistency of the counting procedures. Nearly all (93.1 ± 1.3%) of the neurons that were labeled with anti-saporin also bound biotinylated IB4. Cells not showing colocalization generally appeared shriveled and disfigured, suggesting that the necrotic processes in these cells were more advanced.

We also evaluated the selectivity of IB4-sap for IB4-binding neurons by testing whether the number of neurons that died after IB4-sap treatment was similar to the number of neurons that internalized unconjugated IB4. At 3 d after injection of unconjugated IB4, we counted the number of DRG neurons immunoreactive for anti-BSI (Fig. 6, IB4 internalization). This number was then subtracted from the total number of neurons in L5 DRG as determined by EB staining to estimate the number of neurons that did not inter-

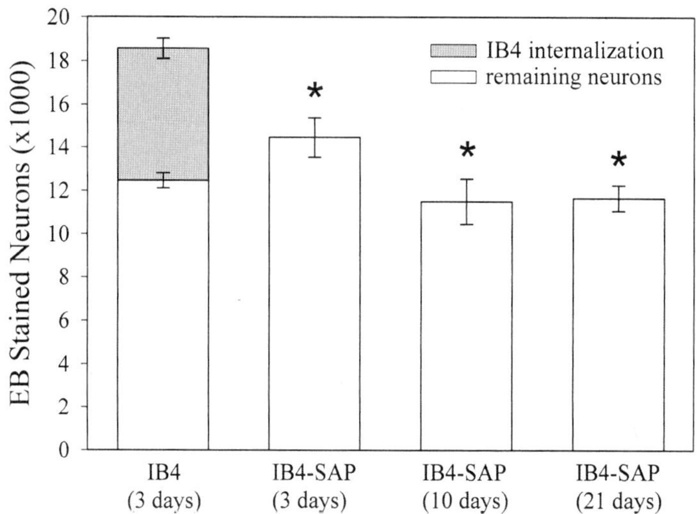

Fig. 6. Number of neurons in the ipsilateral L5 dorsal root ganglia (DRG) 3 d after injection of unconjugated isolectin I-B4 (IB4) ($n = 6$) and 3 ($n = 3$), 10 ($n = 4$), and 21 ($n = 4$) d after injection of IB4-saporin (sap). L5 DRG were labeled with ethidium bromide (EB; 5 μg/mL) and anti-BSI. EB was used to determine the total number of neurons. Anti-BSI was used to determine the number of neurons that internalized IB4 after a sciatic nerve injection At all three time-points, the number of neurons in IB4-sap-treated DRG was significantly decreased compared to the total number of neurons in DRG treated with unconjugated IB4 ($p < 0.01$; one-way analysis of variance and Tukey multiple comparisons test) but was not different from the number of neurons that did not internalize unconjugated IB4. *Significant difference from total number of neurons after treatment with unconjugated IB4.

nalize IB4. The number of cells that did not internalize IB4 after 3 d was similar to total numbers of EB-labeled cells 3, 10, and 21 d after IB4-sap treatment (Fig 6), suggesting that only neurons that internalized IB4 were affected by treatment with conjugate. These counts were obtained using the modified optical dissector method.

Nonneuronal IB4-binding sites in the rat are present on a number of cell types, including macrophages, activated microglia, endothelial cells, and Schwann cells *(6–9,38)*. Because IB4-sap is delivered by a sciatic nerve injection, Schwann cells and possibly endothelial cells in the vicinity of the injection are exposed to the conjugate. The cytotoxic effects of IB4-sap on a particular cell type depend on the ability of the IB4-binding entity in that cell type to deliver and release saporin at its site of action. In sensory neurons, saporin reaches the cell body as a result of active endocytosis and retrograde transport following binding of IB4 to its carbohydrate ligand. Moreover, the appearance of distinct IB4-positive and saporin-positive granules in conjugate-containing cells (Fig. 2, overlay) indicated that the toxin was separated from its carrier.

It is unknown whether IB4 is endocytosed on binding to non-neuronal cells, and addressing this question would generally be beyond the scope of projects using IB4-sap to study sensory neurons. Nevertheless, it is important to assess the potential contribution to the overall conjugate effects of cytotoxic damage to non-neuronal cells. Demyelination following the loss of Schwann cells is particularly relevant to studies of nociception because it may interfere with the withdrawal reflex and may be associated with the development of neuropathic pain *(39)*.

We evaluated the integrity of Schwann cells based on the degree of myelination in the sciatic nerve after IB4-sap treatment (Fig. 7). Myelination was assessed using an antibody to myelin basic protein, a myelin sheath component synthesized by Schwann cells. IB4-sap (Fig. 7B), and to a lesser extent unconjugated saporin treatment (Fig. 7C) was associated with signs of demyelination in the portion of the nerve that included the injection site. Our approach to distinguishing between IB4-sap effects caused by sensory neurons and loss of Schwann cells was to examine the consequences of treatment with the antimitotic agent doxorubicin, which only affects Schwann cells *(12)*. A study of the dose dependence of IB4-sap cytotoxicity after sciatic nerve injection may enable dissociation between the effects of IB4-sap on sensory neurons and Schwann cells.

PAW ABNORMALITY ASSOCIATED WITH IB4-SAP TREATMENT

IB4-sap-treated animals develop curling of the ipsilateral paw and often exhibit skin lesions on the plantar surface (Fig. 8). Paw curling is also present in animals treated with unconjugated saporin or doxorubicin, suggesting that it is most likely related to Schwann cell rather than sensory neuron effects of IB4-sap.

The paw-curling develops within the first week of treatment and is similar to that observed in some neuropathic pain models. The use of multiple control groups allowed us to rule out confounding effects of the curling on the behavioral testing because control saporin- and IB4-plus-saporin-injected rats (which both developed curling) had nociceptive thresholds similar to control IB4- and phosphate buffered saline (PBS)-injected rats (which did not develop curling) (Fig. 9).

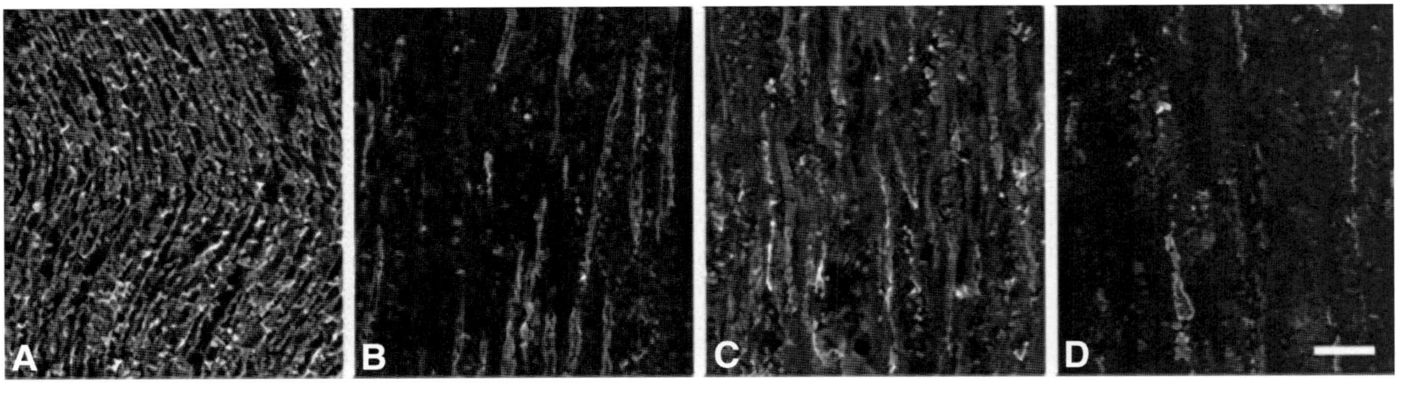

Fig. 7. Schwann cell damage associated with isolectin I-B4 saporin (IB4-sap) treatment. (**A**) Staining for myelin basic protein, a myelin sheath component synthesized by Schwann cells, in normal sciatic nerve. (**B**) Staining for myelin basic protein was reduced 21 d after IB4-sap treatment, suggesting that IB4-sap may have toxic effects on Schwann cells in the vicinity of the injection. (**C**) Decreased staining for myelin basic protein was also seen after control treatment with unconjugated IB4 plus saporin, suggesting IB4-independent uptake of saporin by Schwann cells. (**D**) Decreased staining for myelin basic protein after sciatic nerve injection of the antimitotic agent doxorubicin, which causes Schwann cell death accompanied by decreased axonal conduction velocity. Scale bar = 50 µ*M*. Modified from ref. *12* with permission. Copyright 2001, Elsevier.

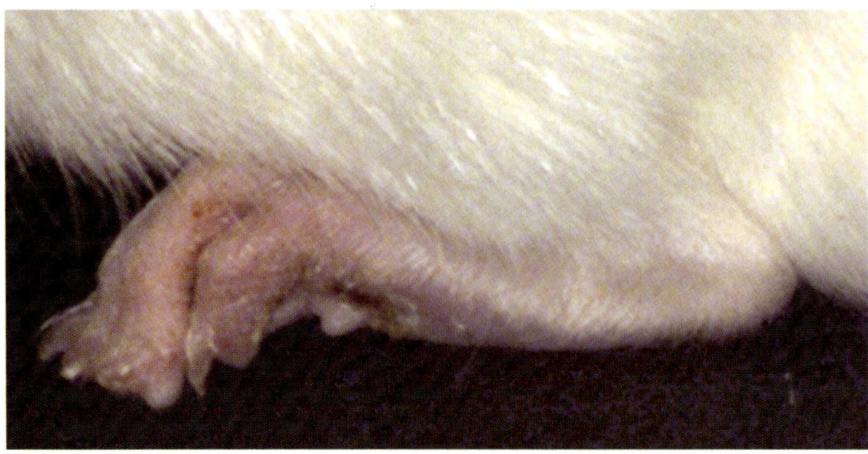

Fig. 8. Curling of the ipsilateral paw and skin lesions on the plantar surface of an isolectin I-B4 saporin-treated rat.

The skin lesions developed 7–10 d after IB4-sap treatment and were not observed in any of the control groups. Their severity ranged from slight discolorations of a small area in the medial part of the plantar surface to open sores with scabs. Healing of the skin was evident by day 21. The presence of skin lesions did not correlate with any aspect of the nociceptive behavior of IB4-sap-treated rats. The lesions may have been a result of the loss of sensory fibers because there was evidence of trophic effects of sensory fibers on the epidermis *(40)*. The appearance of skin lesions in IB4-sap-treated rats may be a result of mechanisms similar to those causing skin sores in diabetic neuropathy.

MEASUREMENT OF NOCICEPTIVE THRESHOLDS IN IB4-SAP-TREATED RATS

The thermal (Fig. 9) and mechanical nociceptive thresholds of IB4-sap-treated rats were increased 7–14 d post-treatment *(12)*. Maximum increase was usually observed at d 10, although for some animals the maximum increase occurred at d 7 or d 14. By d 21, the thresholds returned to the levels of the control groups, suggesting compensatory changes in nociceptive signaling in response to the loss of IB4-binding neurons. Based on their thermal thresholds relative to the control group in each experiment ($LATENCY_{IB4\text{-}sap\ treated} >$ [mean + standard deviation] of $LATENCY_{PBS\ treated}$), approx 65% (42–83%; 83 animals from eight experiments) of IB4-

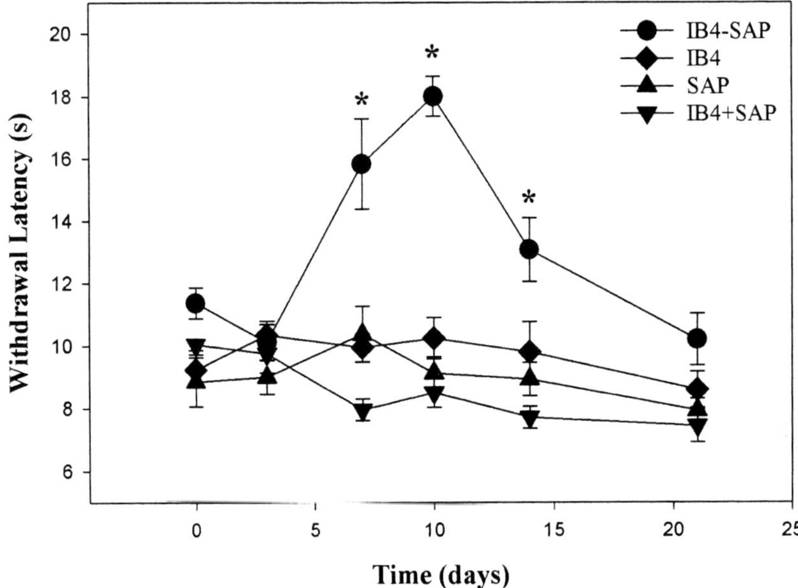

Fig. 9. Increased thermal nociceptive thresholds of isolectin I-B4 saporin (IB4-sap)-treated animals 7–14 d after treatment. Asterisks indicate significant difference from the three control groups ($p < 0.01$, two-way analysis of variance [ANOVA] for repeated measures, Tukey multiple comparisons test). The nociceptive thresholds of the contralateral paws of IB4-sap-treated rats were not significantly different from those of control treated rats (two-way ANOVA for repeated measures). The thresholds of control animals treated with IB4 alone, saporin alone, or unconjugated IB4 plus saporin were not different from the thresholds of phosphate buffered saline-treated animals (not shown) throughout the 21-d test period (two-way ANOVA for repeated measures).

sap-treated animals developed this behavioral phenotype. The variability appeared to be largely attributable to individual differences in the level of segregation of the sciatic nerve into tibial and peroneal nerves, which was not always apparent during the injection. If the injection was delivered distal to this segregation, there was a 50% chance of targeting only neurons that projected in the peroneal nerve and did not contribute substantially to the innervation of the plantar surface.

We have used withdrawal latency in response to radiant heat stimuli delivered to the plantar surface of the hindpaws *(41)* as a measurement of nociceptive thermal thresholds. The stimulus intensity was adjusted in the beginning of each experiment to produce baseline withdrawal latency of approx 10 s and kept constant for the duration of the experiment. Care was taken to direct the stimulus consistently at the middle of the plantar surface. For each paw, the withdrawal latency was determined by averaging three measurements separated by at least 1 min.

A number of studies have suggested that different thermal tests or test parameters may activate distinct functional subsets of thermal nociceptors *(42–45)*. Therefore, evaluation of heat nociception of IB4-sap-treated animals with radiant heat delivered at different heating rates or with other methods, such as the hot plate, may provide additional insight into the involvement of IB4-binding neurons.

The order of the thermal and mechanical testing was random, but the two tests were always separated by at least 15 min. Mechanical sensitivity was evaluated with von Frey filaments using the up–down method, which measures the 50% withdrawal threshold *(46)*. However, this method is not optimal for the assessment of analgesia or hypoalgesia. Measurement of increased thresholds requires the use of high filaments, which often push up the paw without eliciting a response. Furthermore, the withdrawal threshold is likely to be determined by activation of both noxious and innocuous mechanoreceptors, complicating the interpretation of behavioral changes in terms of effects of IB4-sap on mechanical nociception. The use of an algesimeter may provide a more adequate approach for determining the mechanical sensitivity of IB4-sap-treated rats.

IB4-SAP TREATMENT AND MODELS OF CHRONIC PAIN

IB4-sap treatment has been applied in models of neurogenic inflammation and neuropathic pain *(13,14)*. The use of IB4-sap for the study of the role of IB4-binding neurons in chronic pain should take into account the compatibility of the time courses of IB4-sap treatment and the particular chronic pain model. The impact of time-course was illustrated by our studies of the effects of IB4-sap treatment on capsaicin-induced neurogenic inflammation. In this model, inflammation was induced by an intradermal injection of capsaicin *(47)*. The injection resulted in acute nocifensive behavior, which was most intense in the first 3 min; short-lasting thermal hyperalgesia that peaked at 5 min; and mechanical hypersensitivity that peaked at 10 min and lasted for several hours. These effects appeared to be mediated by the capsaicin receptor VR1 *(44)*.

After measuring baseline thermal and mechanical thresholds, neurogenic inflammation was induced by the injection of 10 µg of capsaicin in a 10-µL volume in the plantar surface of the treated hindpaw at 10 and 21 d after IB4-sap treatment (Fig. 10A). Nocifensive behavior was measured for the first 3 min, thermal thresholds were measured at 5 min and mechanical

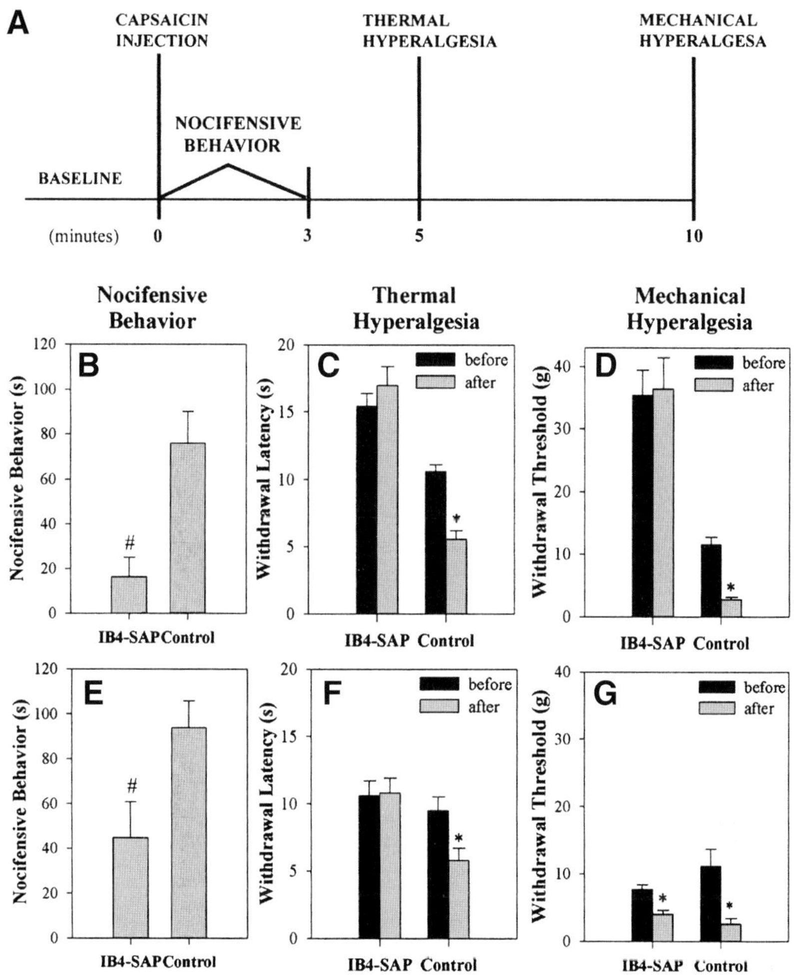

Fig. 10. Effect of isolectin I-B4 saporin (IB4-sap) treatment on capsaicin-induced nocifensive behavior and hyperalgesia. **(A)** Experimental design. **(B–G)** Effects of IB4-sap treatment of capsaicin-induced neurogenic inflammation. At 10 d after treatment **(B–D)**, IB4-sap-treated rats exhibited thermal and mechanical hypoalgesia, which was resolved by day 21 **(E–G)**. Nocifensive behavior at day 10 was 21% of control (**B**; $p < 0.01$, t-test), whereas at day 21 it increased to 48% of control (**E**; $p < 0.05$, t-test). Control phosphate buffered saline (PBS)-treated animals developed thermal ($p < 0.001$, paired t-test) and mechanical ($p < 0.001$ at day 10, $p < 0.01$ at day 21, paired t-test) hyperalgesia at both 10 **(C,D)** and 21 d **(F,G)** after treatment. IB4-sap-treated animals did not develop thermal hyperalgesia at either 10 **(C)** or 21 **(F)** d after treatment. In contrast, mechanical hyperalgesia was absent at day 10 **(D)** but recovered at day 21 **(G)** ($p < 1110.01$, paired t-test). *Significant differences before and after capsaicin treatment. # Significant difference from control.

thresholds at 10 min. Different animals were tested at the two time-points (10 and 21 d) because of the lasting effects of intradermal capsaicin on cutaneous innervation *(48)*.

At 10 d after treatment, intradermal capsaicin injection in IB4-sap-treated rats induced only 20% of the nocifensive behavior of control PBS rats (Fig. 10B). In addition, IB4-sap rats did not develop thermal (Fig. 10C) and mechanical (Fig. 10D) hyperalgesia. These results suggested that IB4-binding neurons are required for the development of capsaicin-induced nocifensive behavior and hyperalgesia. They are consistent with the fact that, in rat, the majority of VR1-expressing neurons (~70%) also bind IB4, and that the behavioral effects observed in this model depended on the activation of VR1. At 21 d after treatment, intradermal capsaicin injection in IB4-sap-treated rats induced 50% of the nocifensive behavior of control rats (Fig. 10E), suggesting potentiation of VR1-mediated signaling in surviving neurons. IB4-sap-treated rats still failed to develop thermal hyperalgesia (Fig. 10F), but they did develop mechanical hyperalgesia (Fig. 10G). These results suggested that the compensatory mechanism responsible for the recovery of acute nociceptive thresholds after IB4-sap treatment enabled the development of mechanical but not thermal hyperalgesia.

Neurogenic inflammation induced by capsaicin at different time-points after IB4-sap treatment demonstrated that the effects of the loss of IB4-binding neurons on the development or maintenance of chronic pain states can only be assessed around the time of maximal hypoalgesia (~10 d post-treatment) because at later time-points they would be masked by the compensatory processes. Moreover, after the time-point of recovery of nociceptive thresholds (21 d), the effects of IB4-sap on chronic pain models may be uninterpretable because of the possibility that the compensatory mechanisms may be analogous to mechanisms underlying chronic pain. Therefore, for questions related to the development of chronic pain, IB4-sap treatment would be expected to be more compatible with chronic pain models with a shorter time-course, in which hypersensitivity develops within the few days of IB4-sap-mediated hypoalgesia (e.g., capsaicin-induced neurogenic inflammation, nerve growth factor-induced hyperalgesia).

Conversely, models with a longer time-course (e.g., spinal nerve ligation) may be more suitable for the study of the effects of IB4-sap on the maintenance of chronic pain. In this case, IB4-sap would be administered following the establishment of the chronic pain model. However, the interpretation of such studies may be complicated by the possibility of "interaction" between the effects of IB4-sap treatment and the mechanisms underlying the chronic pain state.

The usefulness of IB4-sap in chronic pain studies is also affected by the compatibility of administration of the conjugate by sciatic nerve injection with the specific pain model. This is particularly relevant to models of neuropathic pain that are based on some form of sciatic nerve injury. For example, the injection site nearly overlaps with the location of ligatures in the chronic constriction model *(49)*, and an appropriate alternative injection site may be the tibial nerve. From this point of view, it may be beneficial to explore intradermal injection as a route of administration of IB4-sap. It should also be noted that there is evidence for a decrease in IB4 binding after nerve injury *(31,50)*, which would compromise the delivery of IB4-sap in models of neuropathic pain.

Finally, an interesting and so far unexplored application of IB4-sap in chronic pain studies is the potential use of IB4-sap treatment itself as a model of injury-induced hypersensitivity. There is accumulating evidence for a role of uninjured neurons projecting in the injured nerve in the development and maintenance of neuropathic pain *(51–55)*. The nerve injury-induced plasticity of intact sensory neurons is thought to be related to exposure to high levels of cytokines associated with the degeneration of injured nerve fibers *(56–58)*.

Evaluation of the effects of IB4-sap treatment from the perspective of nerve injury raises the possibility that the behavioral recovery of nociceptive thresholds represents a state of hypersensitivity of surviving neurons. It is conceivable that the massive degeneration of IB4-binding neurons after IB4-sap treatment may result in activation of glia and recruitment of immune cells in a manner similar to nerve injury. These effects would be associated with altered levels of growth factors and proinflammatory cytokines at the level of the cell body of the affected neurons, as well as at the level of their central and peripheral processes. Centrally, growth factors and proinflammatory cytokines may contribute to increased excitability of spinal cord neurons that normally receive input from the affected primary afferent neurons *(59)*, whereas in DRG and peripheral processes they can affect the response properties of surviving neurons or stimulate their sprouting in the partially denervated area *(22,26,60,61)*.

All of these effects are likely to contribute to a state of hypersensitivity. In the context of the hypoalgesia resulting from the loss of nociceptive IB4-binding neurons, this hypersensitivity would be manifested behaviorally as recovery of nociceptive thresholds. Thus, IB4-sap treatment may offer a very unique model of neuronal plasticity that combines elements of neurodegeneration, nerve injury, and sensory dysfunction.

ACKNOWLEDGMENT

This work was supported by the National Institutes of Health (DA09641 to Christopher N. Honda and DE07288 to Lucy Vulchanova).

REFERENCES

1. Apostolopoulos V, McKenzie IF. Role of the mannose receptor in the immune response. Curr Mol Med 2001;1: 469–474.
2. Jessell TM, Hynes MA, Dodd J. Carbohydrates and carbohydrate-binding proteins in the nervous system. Annu Rev Neurosci 1990;13:227–255.
3. Kimura M, et al. Engagement of endogenous ganglioside GM1a induces tyrosine phosphorylation involved in neuron-like differentiation of PC12 cells. Glycobiology 2001;11:335–343.
4. Rusnati M, et al. Cell membrane GM1 ganglioside is a functional coreceptor for fibroblast growth factor 2. Proc Natl Acad Sci USA 2002;99:4367–4372.
5. Zanetta JP. Structure and functions of lectins in the central and peripheral nervous system. Acta Anat (Basel) 1998;161(1–4):180–195.
6. Palmetshofer A, Robson SC, Bach FH. Tyrosine phosphorylation following lectin mediated endothelial cell stimulation. Xenotransplantation 1998;5:61–66.
7. Tabor DR, et al. Macrophage membrane glycoprotein binding of *Griffonia simplicifolia* I-B4 induces TNF-alpha production and a tumoricidal response. J Cell Physiol 1992;152:500–506.
8. Dailey ME, Waite M. Confocal imaging of microglial cell dynamics in hippocampal slice cultures. Methods 1999;18:177, 222–230.
9. Silverman JD, Kruger L. Selective neuronal glycoconjugate expression in sensory and autonomic ganglia: relation of lectin reactivity to peptide and enzyme markers. J Neurocytol 1990;19:789–801.
10. Chou DK, et al. Identification of alpha-galactose (alpha-fucose)-asialo-GM1 glycolipid expressed by subsets of rat dorsal root ganglion neurons. J Biol Chem 1989;264:3409–3415.
11. Fullmer JM, Riedl MS, Elde R. Evidence the isolectin IB4 binds to glycoproteins in the nervous system. Soc Neurosci Abstr 2002;46:18.
12. Vulchanova L, et al. Cytotoxic targeting of isolectin IB4-binding sensory neurons. Neuroscience 2001;108:143–155.
13. Tarpley JW, Martin WJ, Baldwin BS, Forrest MJ, MacIntyre DE. Contribution of IB4-positive sensory neurons to NGF-induced hyperalgesia in the rat. Soc Neurosci Abstr 2000;633:18.
14. Tarpley JW, MacIntyre E, Martin WJ. Loss of IB4-positive neurons mitigates the consequences of nerve injury in the rat. Abstracts, IASP Tenth World Congress on Pain, San Diego, CA. IASP Press, 2002.

15. Nagy JI, Hunt SP. Fluoride-resistant acid phosphatase-containing neurones in dorsal root ganglia are separate from those containing substance P or somatostatin. Neuroscience 1982;7:89–97.
16. Wang H, et al. Transganglionic transport and binding of the isolectin B4 from *Griffonia simplicifolia* I in rat primary sensory neurons. Neuroscience 1994;62:539–551.
17. Guo A, et al. Immunocytochemical localization of the vanilloid receptor 1 (VR1): relationship to neuropeptides, the P2X3 purinoceptor and IB4 binding sites. Eur J Neurosci 1999;11:946–958.
18. Bradbury EJ, Burnstock G, McMahon SB. The expression of P2X3 purinoreceptors in sensory neurons: effects of axotomy and glial-derived neurotrophic factor. Mol Cell Neurosci 1998;12:256–268.
19. Vulchanova L, et al. P2X3 is expressed by DRG neurons that terminate in inner lamina II. Eur J Neurosci 1998;10:3470–3478.
20. Chopra B, et al. Cyclooxygenase-1 is a marker for a subpopulation of putative nociceptive neurons in rat dorsal root ganglia. Eur J Neurosci 2000;12:911–920.
21. Fjell J, et al. Differential role of GDNF and NGF in the maintenance of two TTX-resistant sodium channels in adult DRG neurons. Brain Res Mol Brain Res 1999;67:267–282.
22. Stucky CL, et al. Overexpression of nerve growth factor in skin selectively affects the survival and functional properties of nociceptors. J Neurosci 1999;19:8509–8516.
23. Zwick M, et al. Glial cell line-derived neurotrophic factor is a survival factor for isolectin B4-positive, but not vanilloid receptor 1-positive, neurons in the mouse. J Neurosci 2002;22:4057–4065.
24. Dirajlal S, Pauers LE, Stucky CL. Differential response properties of IB(4)-positive and -negative unmyelinated sensory neurons to protons and capsaicin. J Neurophysiol 2003;89:513–524.
25. Drew LJ, Wood JN, Cesare P. Distinct mechanosensitive properties of capsaicin-sensitive and -insensitive sensory neurons. J Neurosci 2002;22:RC228.
26. Stucky CL, Lewin GR. Isolectin B(4)-positive and -negative nociceptors are functionally distinct. J Neurosci 1999;19:6497–6505.
27. Kashiba H, Uchida Y, Senba E. Difference in binding by isolectin B4 to trkA and c-ret mRNA-expressing neurons in rat sensory ganglia. Brain Res Mol Brain Res 2001;95:18–26.
28. LaMotte CC, Kapadia SE, Shapiro CM. Central projections of the sciatic, saphenous, median, and ulnar nerves of the rat demonstrated by transganglionic transport of choleragenoid-HRP (B-HRP) and wheat germ agglutinin-HRP (WGA-HRP). J Comp Neurol 1991;311:546–562.
29. Kitchener PD, et al. Transganglionic labelling of primary sensory afferents in the rat lumbar spinal cord: comparison between wheatgerm agglutinin and the I-B4 isolectin from *Bandeiraea simplicifolia*. J Neurocytol 1994;23:745–757.
30. Kitchener PD, Wilson P, Snow PJ. Selective labelling of primary sensory afferent terminals in lamina II of the dorsal horn by injection of *Bandeiraea*

simplicifolia isolectin B4 into peripheral nerves. Neuroscience 1993;54:545–551.

31. Tong YG, et al. Increased uptake and transport of cholera toxin B-subunit in dorsal root ganglion neurons after peripheral axotomy: possible implications for sensory sprouting. J Comp Neurol 1999;404:143–158.

32. Perry MJ, Lawson SN. Differences in expression of oligosaccharides, neuropeptides, carbonic anhydrase and neurofilament in rat primary afferent neurons retrogradely labelled via skin, muscle or visceral nerves. Neuroscience 1998;85:293–310.

33. Guillery RW, Herrup K. Quantification without pontification: choosing a method for counting objects in sectioned tissues. J Comp Neurol 1997;386:2–7.

34. Coggeshall RE, Lekan HA. Methods for determining numbers of cells and synapses: a case for more uniform standards of review [published erratum appears in J Comp Neurol 1996;369:162]. J Comp Neurol 1996;364:6–15.

35. Coggeshall RE. A consideration of neural counting methods. Trends Neurosci 1992;15:9–13.

36. West MJ. New stereological methods for counting neurons. Neurobiol Aging 1993;14:275–285.

37. Stone LS, Vulchanova L, Riedl MS, et al. Effects of peripheral nerve injury on alpha-2A and alpha-2C adrenergic receptor immunoreactivity in the rat spinal cord. Neuroscience 1999;93:1399–1407.

38. Streit WJ, et al. Histochemical localization of galactose-containing glycoconjugate at peripheral nodes of Ranvier in the rat. J Histochem Cytochem 1985;33:33–39.

39. Gillen C, Jander S, Stoll G. Sequential expression of mRNA for proinflammatory cytokines and interleukin-10 in the rat peripheral nervous system: comparison between immune-mediated demyelination and Wallerian degeneration. J Neurosci Res 1998;51:489–496.

40. Hsieh ST, et al. Epidermal denervation and its effects on keratinocytes and Langerhans cells. J Neurocytol 1996;25:513–524.

41. Hargreaves K, et al. A new and sensitive method for measuring thermal nociception in cutaneous hyperalgesia. Pain 1988;32:77–88.

42. Yeomans DC, Pirec V, Proudfit HK. Nociceptive responses to high and low rates of noxious cutaneous heating are mediated by different nociceptors in the rat: behavioral evidence. Pain 1996;68:133–140.

43. Yeomans DC, Proudfit HK. Nociceptive responses to high and low rates of noxious cutaneous heating are mediated by different nociceptors in the rat: electrophysiological evidence. Pain 1996;68:141–150.

44. Caterina MJ, et al. Impaired nociception and pain sensation in mice lacking the capsaicin receptor. Science 2000;288:306–313.

45. Cao YQ, et al. Primary afferent tachykinins are required to experience moderate to intense pain. Nature 1998;392:390–394.

46. Chaplan SR, et al. Quantitative assessment of tactile allodynia in the rat paw. J Neurosci Methods 1994;53:55–63.

47. Gilchrist HD, Allard BL, Simone DA. Enhanced withdrawal responses to heat and mechanical stimuli following intraplantar injection of capsaicin in rats. Pain 1996;67:179–188.

48. Simone DA, et al. Intradermal injection of capsaicin in humans produces degeneration and subsequent reinnervation of epidermal nerve fibers: correlation with sensory function. J Neurosci 1998;18:8947–8959.

49. Bennett GJ, Xie YK. A peripheral mononeuropathy in rat that produces disorders of pain sensation like those seen in man. Pain 1988;33:87–107.

50. Wang R, Ossipov MH, Vanderah TW, Lai J, Porreca F. Nerve injury-induced down-regulation of IB4 and colocalized markers. Soc Neurosci Abstr 2001;281:1.

51. Gold MS, et al. Redistribution of Na(V)1.8 in uninjured axons enables neuropathic pain. J Neurosci 2003;23:158–166.

52. Hudson LJ, et al. VR1 protein expression increases in undamaged DRG neurons after partial nerve injury. Eur J Neurosci 2001;13:2105–2114.

53. Nam TS, et al. Adrenergic sensitivity of uninjured C-fiber nociceptors in neuropathic rats. Yonsei Med J 2000;41:252–257.

54. Obata K, et al. Contribution of injured and uninjured dorsal root ganglion neurons to pain behavior and the changes in gene expression following chronic constriction injury of the sciatic nerve in rats. Pain 2003;101:65–77.

55. Wu G, et al. Early onset of spontaneous activity in uninjured C-fiber nociceptors after injury to neighboring nerve fibers. J Neurosci 2001;21:RC140.

56. Campbell JN. Nerve lesions and the generation of pain. Muscle Nerve 2001;24:1261–1273.

57. Koltzenburg M, Scadding J. Neuropathic pain. Curr Opin Neurol 2001;14:641–647.

58. Sheth RN, et al. Mechanical hyperalgesia after an L5 ventral rhizotomy or an L5 ganglionectomy in the rat. Pain 2002;96:63–72.

59. Millan MJ. The induction of pain: an integrative review. Progr Neurobiol 1999;57:1–164.

60. Bennett DL, et al. Endogenous nerve growth factor regulates the sensitivity of nociceptors in the adult rat. Eur J Neurosci 1998;10:1282–1291.

61. Shu XQ, Llinas A, Mendell LM. Effects of trkB and trkC neurotrophin receptor agonists on thermal nociception: a behavioral and electrophysiological study. Pain 1999;80:463–470.

62. Arvidsson U, et al. Distribution and targeting of a mu-opioid receptor (MOR1) in brain and spinal cord. J Neurosci 1995;15(5 pt 1):3328–3341.

13

B Fragment of Cholera Toxin Conjugated to Saporin

Peter T. Ohara, Kanwarjit Kelley, and Luc Jasmin

INTRODUCTION

Saporin conjugates have proven extremely versatile and valuable in the selective destruction of a variety of cell types. In the nervous system, the use of saporin-conjugated toxins has generally been directed toward neurons. We were interested in whether saporin conjugates could be used to target other nervous tissue cell types, particularly the myelin-forming cells. Taking advantage of the fact that myelin is rich in G_{M1} ganglioside and that the B fragment of cholera toxin has a high affinity for G_{M1}, we used a conjugate of the B fragment of cholera toxin and saporin (CTB-sap) to target myelin-producing cells (oligodendrocytes) in the central nervous system (CNS) (Fig. 1). We found that CTB-sap is effective in removing oligodendrocytes in addition to other glial cells and largely leaves neurons intact. We successfully used CTB-sap to study demyelination and remyelination in the spinal cord *(1)*, and our preliminary results suggest that CTB-sap will be useful for inducing demyelinating lesions in other parts of the CNS.

CTB-SAP: INTERNALIZATION, TOXICITY, AND EFFECTS

The Conjugate: Structure and Toxicity

Cholera toxin is an oligomeric protein composed of an A subunit and five identical B subunits. The A subunit of the toxin massively increases cyclic adenosine 5'-monophosphate (AMP) levels; the B pentamer is the receptor-binding portion of the molecule and by itself has no toxic activity. As men-

From: *Molecular Neurosurgery With Targeted Toxins*
Edited by: R. G. Wiley and D. A. Lappi © Humana Press Inc., Totowa, NJ

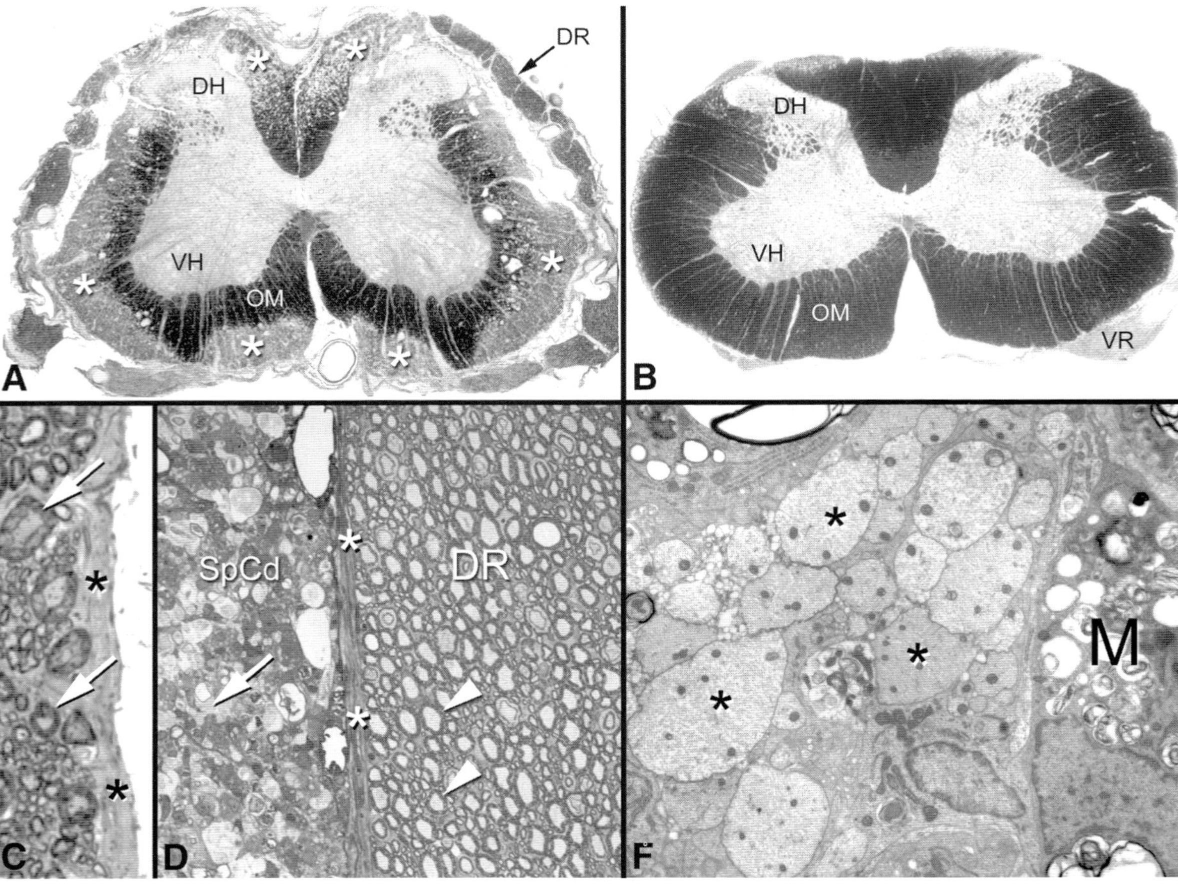

Fig. 1

tioned, the key feature of CTB is that it binds to the cell surface monosialoganglioside G_{M1} *(2–4)*. Once bound, the G_{M1}-CTB complex is internalized. By itself, CTB is innocuous and has no effect when administered into the intrathecal space or when conjugated to nontoxic marker molecules, such as horseradish peroxidase or a fluorophore, and used as a neuronal tracer *(5,6)*. It should be kept in mind, however, that CTB is a potent adjuvant to immunogens *(7,8)*, and a variety of proteins have been attached to CTB to effect an immune responses to specific antigens *(3,7–10)*. We cannot rule out the possibility that a component of the toxicity that we report below might be immune mediated.

Effects on Oligodendrocytes and Other Glial Cells

The CTB-sap conjugate binds to the surface G_{M1} receptor on oligodendrocyte myelin *(11–13)* and is then internalized where the saporin kills the cell by blocking protein synthesis. Some details of how CTB-sap gains access to the oligodendrocyte cytoplasm are not clear. We do not know whether the CTB-sap binds along the myelin sheath and is then transported to the cell bodies or if the principal site of entry is directly on the oligodendrocyte cell bodies themselves. Although the most dramatic effect of CTB-sap application is the loss of oligodendrocytes, closer study showed that

---

Fig. 1. (A) Cross-section of lumbar spinal cord stained for myelin with Luxol fast blue 3 wk after intrathecal injection of cholera toxin B subunit-saporin (CTB-sap). The inner core of oligodendrocyte myelinated axons is darkly stained; the outer rim of demyelinated axons (*) is less intensely stained. In some places more than 50% if the width of the white matter is demyelinated. The dorsal rootlets (DR) containing Schwann cell-derived myelin is also lightly stained but not demyelinated. **(B)** A section of the cervical spinal cord showing complete oligodendrocyte myelination as indicated by the uniform dark staining with Luxol fast blue. Note segments of the ventral rootlets are visible, showing that the Schwann cell myelin was only lightly stained with Luxol fast blue. **(C)** A 2-µm toluidine blue thick epon section of the periphery of a normal spinal cord. A thick pia/glia limitans layer (*) was present, and axons were myelinated (arrows). **(D)** At 3 wk following CTB-sap treatment, the oligodendrocyte myelin in the spinal cord has been destroyed, leaving bare axons throughout the white matter (arrow). In contrast, the Schwann cell myelin (arrowheads) in the DR separated from the cord by a reduced pia/glia limitans (*) appears normal. **(E)** An electron micrograph of spinal cord demyelinated axons (*) following CTB-sap application. Other than having no myelin sheath, the axons appear normal and are in the size range that should be myelinated. DH, dorsal horn; M, macrophage containing phagocytosed myelin; OM, oligodendrocyte myelinated axons; SpCd, spinal cord; VH, ventral horn; VR, ventral rootlet. Magnification: **A**, ×19; **B**, ×17; **C**, ×900; **D**, ×500; **E**, ×5400.

astrocytes and microglia are also lost. Astrocytes also express G_{M1} on their surface *(14)*, and internalization of the CTB-sap is the most probable explanation for their loss. Because unconjugated saporin or CTB alone does not cause any cell damage when injected intrathecally, we can conclude that the spinal pathology reported here is specific to the CTB-sap conjugate.

USE OF CTB-SAP FOR SPINAL DEMYELINATION

Intrathecal Application of CTB-sap

Intrathecal application of CTB-sap to demyelinate the spinal cord was used to study aspects of repair and remyelination. We used several methods for intrathecal injection of CTB-sap. Initially, we used a 33-gage polyethylene catheter inserted (ReCathCo Inc., www.recathco.com) through a puncture in the atlanto-occipital membrane of the cisterna magna and directed approx 8.5 cm caudally to place the tip of the catheter over the lumbar enlargement of the spinal cord.

We now find that a more reliable and efficient method is to use direct lumbar puncture at the L5–L6 vertebral level. This is done with a 22-gage hypodermic needle modified with a 0.4 mm wide groove aligned with the bevel *(15)*. Under sterile conditions, the needle is positioned with the bevel upward over the dorsal sacral spine, parallel to the midline and pointing rostrally, and inserted through the skin into the intrathecal space at an angle of 20–40°. A 33-gage polyethylene catheter is then laid in the groove of the needle and pushed rostrally until 4 cm of the catheter are in the lumbosacral subarachnoid space. Between 1.5 and 3 μg of CTB-sap diluted in 10 μL of sterile 0.9% saline is injected over a 1-min period. This method allows greater control over placement and subsequent diffusion of the toxin when compared to the approach via the cisterna magna.

Specific Cell Targeting and Diffusion of CTB-Sap

After intrathecal injection, CTB-sap diffuses from the cerebrospinal fluid (CSF) and penetrates the pia (the innermost meningeal layer) to gain access to the spinal cord white matter. The ability to pass through the pia is expected because other studies have shown that cholera toxin is able to traverse cell barriers, such as the epithelial layer *(16)*. The CTB-sap also has to traverse the astrocyte process that forms the glia limitans around the spinal cord.

A few days after injection there occurs extensive demyelination of the outer portion of the white matter that involves the sacral and lumbar segments and the lower thoracic segments (Fig. 1). The depth of the demyelination appears directly related to the amount of the toxin injected and the thickness of the white matter. As noted, there is an abundance of G_{M1} on the oligodendrocyte myelin, and this acts to bind a large amount of the free CTB-sap, restricting the penetration of the toxin into the cord and preventing extensive rostral diffusion. Larger doses of the toxin will lead to more extensive spinal cord demyelination, both centripetally and rostrally. For high doses, the toxin diffuses deeply in the spinal cord white matter and then reaches the gray matter, where neuronal cell death can occur. In practical terms, this is particularly a concern for caudal segments of the spinal cord, where the width of the white matter is smallest. If the end of the intrathecal catheter is placed caudal to the lumbar enlargement or high doses of CTB-sap are used, then it is common to see complete demyelination of the caudal segments and death of spinal neurons. In the latter case, bladder function is permanently compromised (e.g., the rats have urinary retention and overflow incontinence).

Biological and Physiological Effects

During the first 3 wk postinjection, rats injected intrathecally with CTB-sap showed hind-limb motor deficits that progress steadily and predictably *(1)*. The first signs occurred as early as 24 h after injection, with loss of tail tonus, and then neurological deficits progressed to a flaccid, areflexic paraplegia until approx 3 wk postinjection, when the severity of the deficits reached a maximum and stabilized. The time-course of the deficits was probably proportional to the amount of CTB-sap available. Oligodendrocytes at the periphery of the cord were exposed to a maximal concentration of the CTB-sap. As the CTB-sap diffused centripetally from the outer portions of the white matter, the amount reaching the inner white matter became progressively smaller as there was less toxin available. The oligodendrocytes in the inner white matter therefore incorporated less CTB-sap, and thus it may have taken longer to cause cell death (Fig. 2). Based on behavioral and histological data, we estimate that the maximum duration of the biological effects of CTB-sap is about 3 wk as there was no further loss of myelin after this period, suggesting that the toxin was cleared or no longer effective. Examination of the spinal gray matter up to 6 mo postinjection showed no obvious neuronal loss, indicating that the ascending paraplegia resulted principally from the loss of spinal myelin. Long term, however, a recurrent deficit occurs, the cause of which remains unclear *(17)*.

CTB-Sap Leaves Spinal Cord Axons Intact

After the oligodendrocyte and myelin debris have been removed from the spinal white matter by macrophages, denuded axons remain. These axons appeared normal when examined with the electron microscope (Fig. 1E) and are present from the pial surface throughout the oligodendrocyte-de-

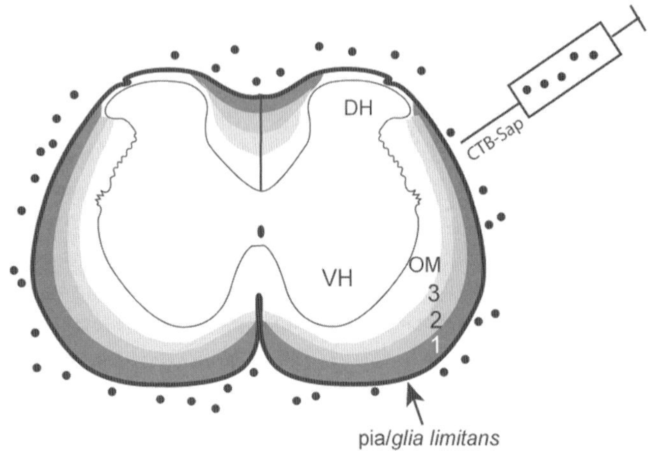

Fig. 2. Representation of the cholera toxin B subunit-saporin (CTB-sap) gradient after intrathecal injection in the cerebrospinal fluid surrounding the spinal cord. The outer rim of spinal white matter immediately under the pia/glial limitans (1) comes into contact with the full concentration of CTB-sap. The large amount of CTB-sap internalized by the superficial oligodendrocytes leads to destruction within 24 h. A significant amount of CTB-sap is bound by white matter in this region, so the concentration of CTB-sap decreases as the toxin diffuses further into the white matter (2). Less CTB-sap is available to be internalized by the oligodendrocytes, increasing the time required for the death of the cells. By the innermost region (3), there is little free CTB-sap remaining, so the amount internalized by oligodendrocytes is minimal and may take many days for the oligodendrocytes to be affected. Thus, even though the outer oligodendrocytes are destroyed within 48 h, the progression of the disease only reaches a maximum at 3 wk because of the slower degeneration of more centrally located oligodendrocytes. DH, dorsal horn; OM, oligodendrocyte myelinated axons; VH, ventral horn.

pleted area. Paradoxically, G_{M1} is also expressed on the surface of axons *(14,18–21)*, and although the axons may have come into contact with the CTB-sap, they appeared unaffected.

There are several possibilities to explain the survival of axons. First, oligodendrocytes are exposed to far more CTB-sap than the axons. A single oligodendrocyte can myelinate as many as 40 axons and thus take up CTB-sap from a very large surface area. The axon, in comparison, is completely surrounded by the myelin sheath and even at the nodes has an astrocytic covering. Thus, the axon would be exposed to less CTB-sap acutely. Only after the myelin and astrocytes have been destroyed and removed would CTB-sap have ready access to axon membranes, but by then there would be little or no free CTB-sap

1remaining. Further, there is some evidence that axonal G_{M1} is not internalized *(22)* as readily as dendritic G_{M1}, and this may be another factor protecting axons from the toxin.

CTB-Sap Is Not Toxic to Schwann Cells

In addition to sparing axons in the spinal white matter, we also saw no obvious effect of the CTB-sap on myelin in spinal rootlets adjacent to the spinal cord (Fig. 1D). When CTB-sap was injected intrathecally, we expected the conjugate to come in contact with Schwann cell myelin surrounding peripheral spinal rootlets at the dorsal and ventral root entry zones. The absence of toxicity to the rootlet myelin was unexpected because intrathecal administration of full cholera toxin or of an antiserum against G_{M1} has been shown to cause demyelination and macrophage proliferation in the spinal rootlets in a manner similar to that seen here for the spinal cord *(9)*. Occasional demyelination was observed in the spinal roots, but it was always associated with Wallerian degeneration of axons, probably from direct toxicity to motoneurons. Further study is necessary to determine whether the survival of the rootlet myelin resulted from a physical barrier (e.g., the basement membrane surrounding Schwann cells) that prevents the CTB-sap reaching the myelin or from a biochemical difference in the Schwann cell myelin.

CTB-Sap Creates Conditions for Spontaneous Entry of Schwann Cells From the Periphery

Despite the severity of the deficits seen at 3 wk postinjection, behavioral recovery occurred over the following months, and in many cases, by 6 mo postinjection only moderate deficits remained. The recovery of function was concomitant with the entry of Schwann cells into the spinal cord; they remyelinated the axons demyelinated by the CTB-sap (Fig. 3). Schwann cells are not normally present in the CNS but are capable of entering the cord under appropriate conditions. The removal of both oligodendrocytes and white matter astrocytes by the CTB-sap produced an environment conducive to the migration of Schwann cells into the spinal cord.

One notable feature of the remyelination by Schwann cells was that it did not seem to be permanent. Although the Schwann cells can remyelinate the entire demyelinated area and bring about recovery of function, after approx 3 mo the Schwann cells began to demyelinate and were replaced by newly formed oligodendrocytes *(1)*. The biology of this effect is still under investigation but may be related to the manner in which CTB-sap produces demyelination because the same phenomenon does not seem to follow demyelination by other agents, such as ethidium bromide *(23)*.

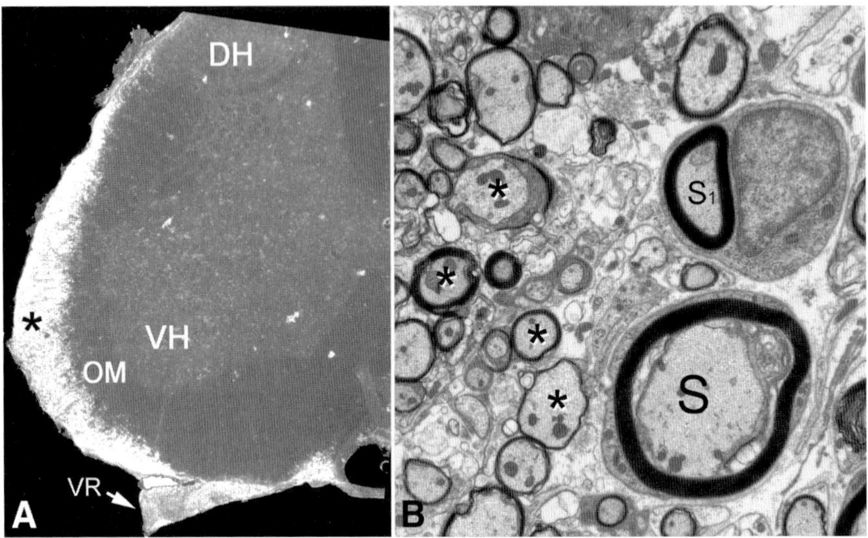

Fig. 3. By 1 mo after cholera toxin B subunit-saporin (CTB-sap) injection, Schwann cells have invaded the spinal white matter and have remyelinated the bare axons. (**A**) The invading Schwann cell myelin is immunostained with P_0, a marker for Schwann cells. Note the ventral rootlet is also P_0 immunopositive. (**B**) Electron micrograph of the interface between the oligodendrocyte myelinated fibers (*) and the Schwann cell myelinated fibers. The rim of Schwann cell cytoplasm around the myelin, basement membrane, collagen, and "signet ring" arrangement are characteristics of the Schwann cell myelinated axons. DH, dorsal horn; OM, oligodendrocyte myelinated axons; S, Schwann cell myelinated fibers; S_1, "signet ring" arrangement; VH, ventral horn; VR, ventral rootlet. Magnification: **A**, ×40; **B**, ×7200.

Intracerebroventricular Injection

In addition to intrathecal application, we have also carried out preliminary examination of the effects of intracerebroventricular application of CTB-sap. To inject the CTB-sap, a 1-cm midline incision was made in the skin over the cranial convexity to expose the skull, and a 2-mm burr hole was drilled through the bone above the lateral ventricle (AP 8.2, lat 1.6 mm) using the rat stereotaxic coordinates of Paxinos and Watson *(24)*. A glass micropipet with a 50-μm diameter tip attached to a polyethylene catheter connected to a 10-μL syringe driven by a microinjection pump was lowered 3.5 mm from the cortical surface with a stereotaxic manipulator. Then, 1 or 2 μg of CTB-sap in 5 μL of saline was injected over 1 min; the micropipet was withdrawn, and the skin sutured. The rat receiving a 1 μg dose was perfused 5 wk after injection, and the rat receiving 2 μg was perfused after 2 wk.

Path and Effects of Intracerebroventricularly Injected Toxin

Injection of either 1 or 2 µg of CTB-sap into one lateral cerebral ventricle resulted in demyelination, but in neither case was the effect as extensive as expected based on the results of the intrathecal application. The demyelination did, however, follow a path expected based on the flow of CSF. The largest region of demyelination was the corpus callosum above the lateral ventricle where the toxin was injected (Fig. 4A). The demyelination of the corpus callosum appeared restricted to the region above the middle third of the ventricle, and no demyelination was observed adjacent to the anterior or posterior horns of the ventricle. Following the flow of CSF, demyelination next occurred in a thin rim of the parenchyma surrounding the third ventricle. This demyelination of the medial hypothalamus was associated with a glial response (Fig. 4B,C) and changes in physiological behavior (*see* next section). Some astrocytic response, but minimal demyelination, was present around the aqueduct. No sign of demyelination or astrocyte response was seen in the fourth ventricle.

These results showed that CTB-sap injected intracerebroventricularly is able to cross the ependymal lining and cause demyelination. Further, the demyelination was confined to the tissue immediately adjacent to ventricle. It is noteworthy that small amounts of CTB-sap were able to produce demyelination, leading to behavioral effects and histological changes. We assume that the production and flow of CSF must constantly dilute the CTB-sap and carry it through the ventricles, limiting the time the toxin comes into contact with the tissue. Because the maximum amount of CTB-sap administered intracerebroventricularly was only 2 µg, the toxin must be very efficient in binding to or crossing the ependymal layer, making small amounts effective at causing demyelination. We presume that larger amounts of CTB-sap would result in more extensive demyelination in the lateral and third ventricles and demyelination in the aqueduct and fourth ventricle. However, in this case the effects might be too severe and compromise the survival of the animal.

Physiological Symptoms Associated With Intracerebroventricular Injection of Toxin

A number of signs of disease effects were observed after injection of CTB-sap into the lateral ventricle. Primary symptoms 1 d after injection included piloerection and a multiple sclerosis-like tremor of approx 12 cycles/s. Some loss of spontaneous movement was present in the first 2 d postinjection in the animal receiving the highest dose (2 µg) of CTB-sap despite the animal being awake and alert. Beyond these acute effects, there was a change in weight gain, presumably resulting from the demyelination of the medial hypothala-

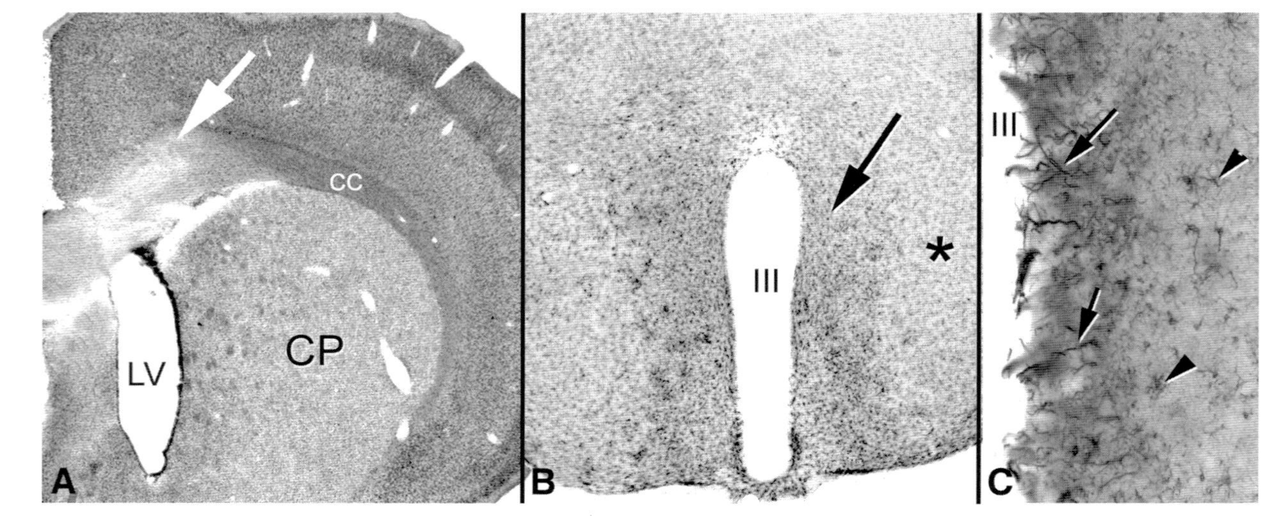

Fig. 4. Intracerebroventricular injection of cholera toxin B subunit-saporin (CTB-sap). (**A**) Following injection of 1 µg CTB-sap into the lateral ventricle, demyelination is seen in the corpus callosum immediately dorsal to the ventricle (arrow. Kluver-Barrera). (**B**) Surrounding the third ventricle (III), there is an increase in microglial activation (arrow), as shown by increased OX-42 immunostaining. Tissue further from the ventricle had normal levels of OX-42 staining (*). (**C**) High magnification of the third ventricle showing large process of activated astrocytes (arrows. GFAP). Normal astrocytes distant from the ependymal wall are indicated by arrowheads. cc, corpus callosum; CP, caudate putamen; LV, lateral ventricle. Magnification: **A**, ×14; **B**, ×25; **C**, ×320.

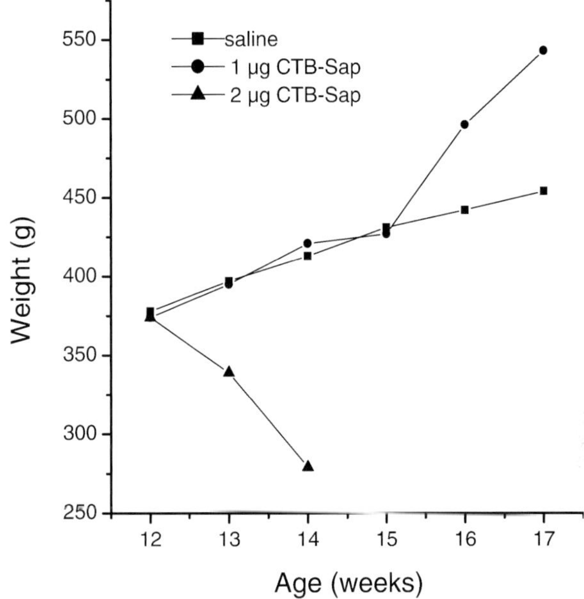

Fig. 5. Following cholera toxin B subunit-saporin injection into the lateral ventricle at 12 wk, weight changes were observed. The animal receiving the high dose showed a weight loss compared to the control population, and the rat receiving the lower dose showed a weight gain. CTB-sap, cholera toxin B subunit-saporin.

mus (Fig. 5). The animal receiving 1 µg of the toxin showed a weight gain of 39.2%; the rat that received 2 µg had a weight loss of 24.7% in 14 d, at which time the experiment was terminated. These changes fell outside of the range of normal growth rates and are most reasonably attributed to alterations of the hypothalamus; they did not occur in matched animals injected intracerebroventricularly with saline.

Intraparenchymal Injection of CTB-Sap

Injections into the white matter of the cerebellum produced focal areas of demyelination. We have no long-term data from these experiments, but they did demonstrate that CTB-sap is effective under different routes of administration and in a variety of CNS locations (Fig. 6). We note, however, that some axonal damage occurred at the core of these injections.

SUMMARY

The advantages of using CTB-sap are that it preferentially targets central myelin and spares axons, neurons, and peripheral myelin. The toxin is very

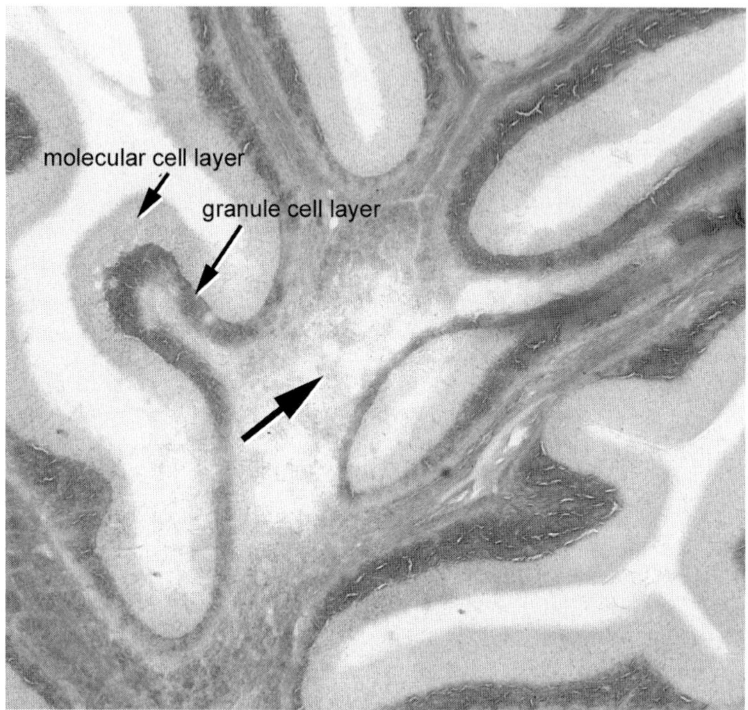

Fig. 6. Injection of cholera toxin B subunit-saporin directly into the cerebellum produced an area of demyelination (arrow) (magnification ×64).

efficient, and only small amounts are needed to produce significant effects. The amount of demyelination can be controlled by varying the amount of toxin administered and can range from small focal lesions to widespread oligodendrocyte loss. Administration of CTB-sap intrathecally or intracerebroventricularly produces a reproducible pattern of demyelination that can provide a useful model for studying basic mechanisms of myelination or for modeling a variety of neurological disorders associated with myelin loss.

REFERENCES

1. Jasmin L, Janni G, Moallem TM, Lappi DA, Ohara PT. Schwann cells are removed from the spinal cord after effecting recovery from paraplegia. J Neurosci 2000;20:9215–9223.
2. Cuatrecasas P. Gangliosides and membrane receptors for cholera toxin. Biochemistry 1973;12:3558–3566.

3. Czerkinsky C, Sun JB, Lebens M, et al. Cholera toxin B subunit as transmucosal carrier-delivery and immunomodulating system for induction of antiinfectious and antipathological immunity. Ann NY Acad Sci 1996;778:185–193.

4. Svennerholm L. Interaction of cholera toxin and ganglioside G(M1). 1976;71:191–204.

5. Dederen PJ, Gribnau AA, Curfs MH. Retrograde neuronal tracing with cholera toxin B subunit: comparison of three different visualization methods. Histochem J 1994;26:856–862.

6. Horikawa K, Powell EW. Comparison of techniques for retrograde labeling using the rat's facial nucleus. J Neurosci Methods 1986;17:287–296.

7. Gaupp S, Hartung HP, Toyka K, Jung S. Modulation of experimental autoimmune neuritis in Lewis rats by oral application of myelin antigens. J Neuroimmunol 1997;79:129–137.

8. Holmgren J, Czerkinsky C, Lycke N, Svennerholm AM. Strategies for the induction of immune responses at mucosal surfaces making use of cholera toxin B subunit as immunogen, carrier, and adjuvant. Am J Trop Med Hyg 1994;50:42–54.

9. Schwerer B, Lassmann H, Kitz K, Bernheimer H. Ganglioside GM1, a molecular target for immunological and toxic attacks: similarity of neuropathological lesions induced by ganglioside-antiserum and cholera toxin. Acta Neuropathol (Berl) 1986;72:55–61.

10. Xiao BG, Link H. Mucosal tolerance: a two-edged sword to prevent and treat autoimmune diseases. Clin Immunol Immunopathol 1997;85:119–128.

11. Cochran FB Jr, Yu RK, Ledeen RW. Myelin gangliosides in vertebrates. J Neurochem 1982;39:773–779.

12. Suzuki K, Poduslo JF, Poduslo SE. Further evidence for a specific ganglioside fraction closely associated with myelin. Biochim Biophys Acta 1968;152:576–586.

13. Yu RK, Iqbal K. Sialosylgalactosyl ceramide as a specific marker for human myelin and oligodendroglial perikarya: gangliosides of human myelin, oligodendroglia and neurons. J Neurochem 1979;32:293–300.

14. Byrne MC, Farooq M, Sbaschnig-Agler M, Norton WT, Ledeen RW. Ganglioside content of astroglia and neurons isolated from maturing rat brain: consideration of the source of astroglial gangliosides. Brain Res 1988;461:87–97.

15. Jasmin L, Ohara PT. Long-term intrathecal catheterization in the rat. J Neurosci Methods 2001;110:81–89.

16. Hansson HA, Lange S, Lonnroth I. Internalization in vivo of cholera toxin in the small intestinal epithelium of the rat. Acta Pathol Microbiol Immunol Scand A 1984;92:15–21.

17. Jasmin L, Ohara PT. Recurrent paraplegia after remyelination of the spinal cord. J Neurosci Res 2004;77:277–284.

18. Abe T, Norton WT. The characterization of sphingolipids from neurons and astroglia of immature rat brain. J Neurochem 1974;23:1025–1036.

19. Ledeen RW. Ganglioside structures and distribution: are they localized at the nerve ending? J Supramol Struct 1978;8:1–17.
20. Raff MC, Fields KL, Hakomori SI, Mirsky R, Pruss RM, Winter J. Cell-type-specific markers for distinguishing and studying neurons and the major classes of glial cells in culture. Brain Res 1979;174:283–308.
21. Robertson B, Grant G. Immunocytochemical evidence for the localization of the GM1 ganglioside in carbonic anhydrase-containing and RT 97-immunoreactive rat primary sensory neurons. J Neurocytol 1989;18:77–86.
22. Sofer A, Schwarzmann G, Futerman AH. The internalization of a short acyl chain analogue of ganglioside GM1 in polarized neurons. J Cell Sci 1996;109(pt 8):2111–2119.
23. Gilson JM, Blakemore WF. Schwann cell remyelination is not replaced by oligodendrocyte remyelination following ethidium bromide induced demyelination. Neuroreport 2002;13:1205–1208.
24. Paxinos G, Watson C. *The Rat Brain in Stereotaxic Coordinates.* 4th ed. New York: Academic Press.

Index